The Best of Health
3rd Edition:
The Best Health
Books
in the World

SHELDON ZERDEN

AUTHOR'S NOTE

This 3rd edition of "The Best of Health is the most recent step in my attempt to preserve the written record of nutrition and disease. The many outstanding reviews in this work demonstrate the purposeful devotion of scientists and researchers to discover the protocols and modalities that will enhance and extend the lives of everyone. Their goal is to discover the cause of disease as opposed to prescription medicine and its treatment of the symptoms.

The proliferation of books on disease and fitness is a reflection on the condition of health in America. Obesity is epidemic. Heart disease, cancer, diabetes, arthritis, asthma, and Alzheimer's and other degenerative diseases are rampant. Education of the public is difficult. Nutrition is almost totally lacking in our schools and inadequate in the medical schools which train our health professionals. That is why this book is so important.

The Best of Health: 3rd Edition is an excellent starting point for anyone who wishes to learn about nutrition and disease. It is a concentrated course on health through the study of the greatest literature of the last fifty years.

You, dear reader, must take control of your life. Learn the lessons in this book that the giants in the health care field left us as their legacy.

ACKNOWLEDGMENTS

I have many people to thank for their encouragement and inspiration during the preparation of this work. Nobel Laureates Linus Pauling and Albert Szent-Gyorgyi, and Richard Passwater, Robert Atkins, Ronald Hoffman, Abram Hoffer, and Gary Null were all helpful. Their recommendation of books was important. In addition, Stephen Langer, Roger Williams, John Yudkin, Hans Selye, and Carl Pfeiffer also knew the value of such a project and offered their help. In this latest work I was particularly inspired by the work of Professor Brian Scott Peskin who believes he has found the way to prevent cancer by building on the research of Nobel Laureate Otto Warburg.

I must mention my dear wife who lived in the shadow of these three works for the last thirty years. Thanks, Charlotte, for myself and all my readers.

CONTENTS

INTRODUCTION

You are about to enter the world of reality. For more than twenty years I have researched the literature of health and come up with the answers that lead to a quality of life and a longer life span.

Along the way I have come to know some of the greatest minds of the century. They are giants who have earned the Nobel Prize for their discoveries. I got to know them personally and through their books. I have selected over sixty books that encompass all the diseases that feed our $3 trillion dollar health care monster.

I have found exciting new people who will achieve great fame through their advances in the health field. Brian Scott Peskin has taken a quantum leap forward with his "The Hidden Story of Cancer." It is the last piece of the puzzle which was solved by Nobel laureate Otto Warburg.

You have in your hands the composite knowledge of the greatest minds of the last several decades. This compendium will make you a better, smarter, and healthier person.

THE TRACE ELEMENTS AND MAN
HENRY A. SCHROEDER, M.D.

Five million centuries ago, primitive, worm-like animals with spinal cords, but few brains, were swimming in vast numbers in the teeming sea. These creatures, our ancestors, whom we now call fish, eventually chose or were forced to invade the land. It took about 250 million years for fish to evolve into amphibians and amphibians to evolve into reptiles. We now come to modern man.

Synopsis

Gabriel Bertrand, the French scientist who fathered the study of trace elements, is responsible for Bertrand's Law, which states that in the absence of an essential element plants cannot live. This law applies to animals as well. Eugene D. Weinberg extended the law to say that the amount of trace elements required for growth is not necessarily adequate for an organism's optimal function. Hence, a deficiency of an essential trace element is much like a vitamin deficiency; while it is often not fatal, it can contribute to disease.

Human experiments depriving the body of essential vitamins and trace elements are seldom done, for the consequences could be hazardous, if not disastrous. Therefore, minimal human requirements of many trace elements and many vitamins are not known.

Cholesterol is a vital substance. It accounts for as much as 5 percent of the brain and pancreas, and more than one percent of the liver. Cholesterol is needed for brain function and for the hormones of the sex and adrenal glands. The skin would dry up without it. If your diet does not provide you with cholesterol (in the form of eggs, animal fats, and organ meats), your body will manufacture enough of it to supply its essential needs. And when cholesterol is consumed through diet, the liver will simply make less and excrete more. The reason that cholesterol tends to collect in the blood has nothing to do with dietary intake. It is most probably due to a problem with the body's metabolism. Studies have confirmed that when rats are given chromium, their cholesterol levels are low and they do not develop diabetes, yet without the trace metal their blood cholesterol and sugar levels rise. Due to their resemblance to man, these findings contribute greatly to our understanding of human disorders in sugar and fat metabolism.

We should change our diet and hope to build up our stores of chromium so that we can efficiently burn sugars, starches, and fats.

Avoid refined white sugar and all products containing it such as jellies, jams, candy, sweet cakes, pies, and cola drinks.

Eat whole wheat and other whole grains. Eat fish, shellfish, meats, and chicken. They contain great amounts of chromium. Meats have several times as much as vegetables, grains, and fruits.

WHY ANIMALS DON'T GET HEART ATTACKS, BUT PEOPLE DO
MATTHIAS RATH, M.D.

Synopsis

Contrary to what pharmaceutical companies selling cholesterol-lowering drugs want to make you believe, there is nothing wrong with cholesterol levels of 220 or 240. Cholesterol is a secondary risk factor because the primary risk factor is the weakness of your blood vessel walls. Elevated blood levels of cholesterol and other blood risk factors are not the cause of cardiovascular disease, but the consequences of developing disease. Drugs that block the synthesis of cholesterol and other lipid-lowering agents are now being prescribed to millions of people. These drugs are known to cause cancer and other severe side effects. You should avoid them whenever you can. Dr. Rath's prescription for optimal health and the prevention of cardiovascular and other disease is a 10 point plan:

The blood vessel system measures 60,000 miles. The heart pumps 100,000 times a day.

Vitamin C is the intercellular cement of the blood vessel walls. We need vitamin C and other vitamins. Animals don't get heart attacks because they make all the vitamin C they need.

Lysine and proline help reverse deposits. They are nature's Teflon agents.

Magnesium relaxes blood vessel walls. Arginine can be of value.

Carnitine, CoQ10, B vitamins, and other nutrients and trace elements are essential.

Important antioxidants are vitamin C, vitamin E, beta carotene, and selenium, bioflavonoids, and pycnogenol.

Stop smoking.

Moderate exercise like walking and cycling is recommended.

Eat a prudent diet. Fiber, vitamins, fruits and vegetables, and foods low in fat and sugar.

Adrenalin uses up your vitamin C. Relax, Start early to protect your cardiovascular system.

Twelve million people die of heart attacks and strokes. Animals have no heart attacks. They produce vitamin C in their bodies. In contrast, we human beings cannot produce a single molecule of vitamin C ourselves. The most important function of vitamin C is the ability to produce collagen. Collagen improves the ability for the 60,000 mile long walls of our arteries, veins, and capillaries.

Lp(a) is ten times more dangerous than cholesterol. Lp(a) is an LDL particle with an adhesive protein surrounding it. It is one of the stickiest particles in the body. Studies in Hamburg, Germany showed that atherosclerotic lesions are composed of lipoprotein (a) particles deposited in the arteries. These findings have been confirmed in further clinical studies. Lp(a) levels are determined by inheritance. The lipid-lowering prescription drugs don't lower Lp(a) blood levels. Taking vitamins are the only way to lower Lp(a).

In 1996, Newman and Hulley, in the Journal of the American Medical Association (JAMA), concluded that most of the cholesterol-lowering drugs on the market are known to cause cancer in test animals. The cardiovascular drug market is over $100 billion dollars. The multi-billion dollar drug market will collapse once millions of people learn that vitamins and other nutrients are the answer to the cardiovascular epidemic. That is why the drug industry is spending hundreds of millions of dollars advertising drugs that are known to cause cancer.

Complications occur in over 30 percent of procedures, requiring repeat angioplasty and bypass surgery. Angioplasty inevitably causes substantial damage to the artery wall. A healthy diet is the basis of any cardiovascular health program. Increased cardiovascular disease risk comes from the systematic depletion of the vitamin reserves in the body. As a consequence, the artery walls are weakened and cardiovascular disease develops. Dr. Rath recommends: eat a prudent diet, watch your body weight, and exercise regularly. Avoid too much fat and sweetened food. Above all, follow the vitamin program.

THE BROOKLYN DIET
SHELDON ZERDEN

Nutrition is the key to good health and the number one disease in America today is obesity. Since the 1980s the number of Americans who are obese has quadrupled! In fact, the epidemic is so inclusive, children are developing diabetes at 10 years of age!

59 million people in the United States have been classified as obese. That means they are more than 30 pounds overweight. The Center for Disease Control, (CDC) puts out these statistics periodically. In addition to the obese people in our country, there are untold millions who are overweight, and therefore well on their way to obesity.

There is no question in my mind that the epidemic of degenerative diseases—coronary heart disease, cancer, stroke, diabetes, arthritis, asthma, and Alzheimer's are the result of a lifelong process of malnutrition. Those who declare that we are the healthiest nation in the world are living in a dream world, a fantasy. Just look at the aforementioned list of diseases. We are truly "overfed and undernourished."

The Brooklyn Diet is my latest work. Marty Markowitz, Brooklyn borough president gave me the idea for this effort. He put the borough of Brooklyn on a diet and it stressed the need for good nutrition and the prevention of disease.

Synopsis

In detailing a way of life that will lead to a healthy, nutritious, and vital existence, it is necessary to liberally draw on the research and experience of those pioneers who absorbed the derision of the establishment. They stuck to their guns and fearlessly championed the nutritional therapies that provided their patients with the optimal quality of life.

5

The best diet should emphasize whole foods, grains, vegetables, green salads, fish, eggs, milk, nuts, seeds, fruits and berries. Vitamin and mineral supplements are required so that your intake levels are adequate. Eight to ten glasses of water are essential. Brewer's Yeast is a great source of energy, and an abundant treasure of amino acids, B-complex vitamins, and many minerals.

The Brooklyn Diet, as outlined above in general terms will take care of any nutritional problems one could have. It will also go a long way to bring your weight under control, because if you take life seriously, and eat a nutritious diet your body will respond, and thank you by avoiding disabling diseases. The foods to avoid, as much as possible, are bread, cake, pasta, rice, potatoes, and ice cream, among others.

In sum, it is not too much to ask that you agree to give your heart, brain, and other vital organs of your body the nutrition they need to operate at their maximum level of efficiency. You will know—you will feel the difference. It is the difference between lethargy and vitality. You will no longer be drifting from obesity to oblivion. Life will have meaning and purpose—and you will once again be relevant.

THE EXERCISE MYTH
HENRY A. SOLOMON, M.D.

The medical profession has played a major role in the exercise revolution, providing a legitimacy where there would otherwise be none, but not every physician who recommends exercise does it solely for profit—doctors themselves participate in vigorous workouts. They are consumers like everyone else and subject to the same ballyhoo and hype as the rest of the population.

Synopsis

The amazing exercise phenomenon, that is fueled by the profit motive and supported by a population worried about its health, has a terrible momentum. The sober truth may not stop it, but it should be stated. You may enjoy exercise, it may help you socially, you may look and feel better, but all the rest is myth. "Exercise will not make you healthy. It will not make you live longer. Fitness and health are not the same thing."

Fitness is measured physiologically by oxygen consumption. This doesn't mean a thing to your heart. Running conditions the muscles, but it does nothing for the lungs. If cardiovascular health was a product of physical training, then fit people wouldn't die of heart disease. The fact is that exercisers suffer the same ills that plague us all. The leading cause of exercise-related deaths in well-trained people is coronary heart disease.

You can be fit and healthy. You can be physically fit and ill with coronary heart disease. Finally, you can be unfit and unhealthy as well. The basic tool used by specialists to diagnose heart disease is the exercise stress test. When you are at rest it is difficult to discover the abnormalities of the heart. During activity your heart works harder, and the stress may uncover abnormal cardiac responses.

How much physical work you can do is based on how much oxygen your body can use, but oxygen consumption is hard to measure. A stress test counts heartbeats per minute, since oxygen consumption parallels the heart rate, it yields an approximate measure of how much work you do during the test. Stress tests are supposed to do two things: detect or confirm the presence or absence of heart disease, and establish a safe level of exercise.

Although physicians recommend stress tests as a matter of course, they are of very limited value and may produce misleading information with dangerous consequences.

Most people "pass" their stress test. They willingly pay their money to know they are well and can safely exercise.

But they do not know that, and neither does their doctor. The same unknowns face those who "fail" their stress test. A stress test does not necessarily detect coronary heart disease—and it normally cannot confirm its absence.

Coronary heart disease is a structural disease, caused by a narrowing of the coronary arteries, not a disease of performance . You can have nice clean arteries but a heart that does not perform well during hard work. On the other hand, you can have a heart that handles the pressure of a stress test and yet have clogged arteries. Reproducability is a great measure of liability, it is noteworthy that if a stress test is repeated the results can be completely different.

Thus, Morris's study in 1953, the confirmations in the 1960s and 1970s, and the Marathon Hypothesis combined to give credence to the notion that physical activity promotes longevity and immunity to coronary heart disease. Studies which countered this theory were ignored. For example, R.M.Oliver of Great Britain cast doubt on Morris's early findings when he studied physiques and blood fats of recruits for jobs of bus conductors and bus drivers, before the activity of the job could affect the man, and found that driver recruits were fatter to begin with, and could have higher cholesterol and blood pressure. Pre-existing characteristics rather than activity were the key beneficial factors. Runners tend to start out with lower cholesterol levels than those who choose not to run.

Some people who exercise live a long time, some do not. Doubts about the benefits of vigorous exercise are difficult to prove in the face of the ingrained idea that exercise must somehow be good.

Cardiac rehabilitation is a new buzzword. It is an idle dream. The physical condition of your heart and arteries does not improve with exercise, and neither is collateral circulation increased. Claims that it does have been contradicted by a Canadian Study: Dr. Andre Nolewajka of the University of Western Ontario studied 20 patients following a heart attack, and found no evidence that exercise increases collateral circulation in humans. Other studies have confirmed his findings.

Dr. Harold Elrick, the director of the Foundation for Optimal Health and Longevity suggests that vigorous activity does not protect people from hypertension, or guarantee low cholesterol values, both primary risk factors in coronary heart disease.

It would be nice to promise that exercise removes the fatty obstructions for artery walls, and reduces blood pressure and cholesterol, but there is no evidence to support it.

If you invest money, energy, and time in running, in the belief that it will relieve depression and improve health, you will not easily admit that you did not achieve the desired result.

"Sensible advice is overwhelmed by an overriding message: run harder, run longer, run for your life. They have the idea that to protect themselves from disease and death they must drive themselves beyond pain and exhaustion."Typical rallying cries are, "Run until it hurts," and "Push yourself to the limit and then go beyond it." Women are especially vulnerable because of their slighter bone structure and more delicate ligaments and tendons.

People do not always die in spite of exercise; they can die because of it. There is an enormous pool of undiscovered coronary heart disease in the population. Exercise deaths do occur and we cannot identify the individuals at risk

This is not an anti-exercise book. It is the other side of the exercise story. The side few people have heard and some do not want to know. Any form of exercise can be kept at a safe level if you do not overdo it. Don't do anything to the point of exhaustion or pain in the chest area. Avoid long distance running. Jogging may be all right, but drop to a walk when your body tells you to slow down. To exercise vigorously is to court disaster; listen to your body. Fitness is bit related to health. Heart attacks are not prevented by exercise, and may be caused by it.

VITAMIN C AND THE
COMMON COLD
LINUS PAULING, PH.D.

At a cancer dialogue in New York City, Linus Pauling, the double Nobel Laureate for Chemistry and Peace spoke before an overflow audience. "I am proud to be America's number one quack!" he stated. The crowd stood up and gave him a standing ovation. The reason for Pauling's remark was obvious to the people assembled. Linus Pauling had put his reputation, prestige, and very formidable standing in the world as a scientist, on the line with a book that created a storm of controversy in the medical and nutrition field. It was called, "Vitamin C and the Common Cold."

Synopsis

Professor Pauling's treatise stated unequivocally that "most colds can be prevented or largely ameliorated by control of the diet, without the use of any drugs." The answer to the common cold, he claimed, is vitamin C, also known as ascorbic acid.

The stand that Professor Pauling took pitted him against the power, the money, and the influence of the giant pharmaceutical industry with a burgeoning proprietary group of cold remedies in the hundreds of millions of dollars. There was no way that the drug industry would allow their business to be undermined by an intruder such as Pauling, who was not even a nutritionist. Pauling stuck to his guns and proceeded to amass the multitude of studies that proved his contention that colds could be prevented with the right dosage of ascorbic acid. The drug industry for its own reasons would not be interested in a substance that is available at low prices and is not patentable.

Pauling was not alone in his fight for acceptance of vitamin C as a means to battle the common cold. He was preceded by Dr. Albert Szent-Gyorgyi, the Budapest-born Nobel prize-winner who discovered vitamin C. Dr. Irwin Stone followed Szent-Gyorgyi, and spent 40 years trumpeting the advantages of ascorbic acid. Szent-Gyorgyi maintains that the medical profession misled the public because they called it a vitamin so that people would hesitate to take the dosage necessary to prevent colds.

Mammals, birds, amphibians, and reptiles have the ability to synthesize ascorbic acid in their liver and kidneys. They don't get colds. But 25 million years ago a mutational change occurred and man's ancestors lost the ability to synthesize ascorbic acid. Man must consequently make up for the lack of this substance.

The peculiar advantage of ascorbic acid is that it is not toxic. Humans have eaten 40 grams a day for a month and 100 grams for a few days with no symptoms of toxicity. The same cannot be said for medications prescribed by doctors. There is not one case of death attributed to any person ingesting too much vitamin C. Yet the Food and Nutrition Board of the National Research Council suggests 60 milligrams as the RDA, far below the amount necessary to prevent the occurrence of a cold. This regulatory group has obviously not yet learned that preventing scurvy and avoiding a cold are two separate and distinct phenomena.

Dr. Pauling states, "I am sure that an increased intake of ascorbic acid, 10 to 100 times the daily allowance recommended by the Food and Nutrition Board leads to improvement in general health and increased resistance to infectious diseases including the common cold."He also claims that in the future it will be possible to control hundreds of diseases by "Megavitamin Therapy." The best form in which to buy vitamin C is the crystals that come in 1-kilogram containers. These containers represent 2.2 pounds and are labelled "Ascorbic Acid USP fine crystals" or "Ascorbic Acid USP Powder." '

One third of all Americans are poverty stricken and poorly nourished. They suffer from a dietary deficiency. What they need is money to buy food and good sensible advice about nutrition—including information on the role of vitamins and minerals. It seems a shame that Americans spend more than one billion dollars on cold remedies that have side effects and don't prevent colds, while ascorbic acid can prevent colds if taken before symptoms develop and is non-toxic. Linus Pauling has made a major contribution to the health of the public by popularizing the facts concerning vitamin C. He is certain that millions of people can be saved from suffering the effects of future colds if they take a sufficient amount of this essential vitamin.

THE SACCHARINE DISEASE
SURGEON-CAPTAIN T.L. CLEAVE

If I were asked which book was the best one of the 100 reviewed in "The Best of Health," I would have to say, "The Saccharine Disease," by Surgeon–Captain T.L.Cleave. The book describes a single master disease—The Saccharine Disease. The author claims that there is clear evidence indicating the existence of such a disease. Saccharine (the last syllable rhymes with wine) is defined as anything related to sugar, including table sugar (sucrose) or digested white flour (white flour is transformed into glucose during digestion). It is the author's contention that these refined carbohydrates cause obesity, diabetes, and coronary thrombosis. Cleave suggests that the removal of fiber in sugar and white flour slows down the digestive process, causing stasis. This creates an unnatural pressure on the lower veins that ultimately causes hemorrhoids and varicose veins. In expanding on the dangers of saccharine, Cleave blames the enormous rise of sugar and white flour over the last 150 years for peptic ulcers, constipation, appendicitis, cholycystitis, pyelitis, diverticulitis, renal calculus, many skin conditions, and dental caries, among other problems. Of all the foods that are taken in their natural state and processed, refined carbohydrates exhibit the greatest alteration. In refined sugar, 90 percent of the sugar beet or sugar cane is removed and in white flour 30 percent of the wheat is removed. On an evolutionary scale, human consumption of such radically altered foods is a relatively recent development and people have not really been able to adapt to it. By contrast, cooking, which represents a minor alteration in constituents of food has been with us for 500,000 years. We are therefore well-adapted to it. But, to take just one example, consumption of refined sugar, in pounds per year per person, has risen from 15 in 1815 to 160 in 2003, more than a 10-fold increase.

The sharp rise in carbohydrate consumption produces harmful results in three main ways:

The removal of fiber directly affects the teeth, stomach and colon and has important repercussions in the lower venous system.

Overconsumption, (caused by the removal of fiber) leads to such diseases as diabetes, obesity, coronary thrombosis and primary E-coli infections and gallstones.

The removal of protein dangerously affects the behaviour of gastric acid causing peptic ulcers.

There are three reasons why unrefined carbohydrates are harmless. First of all, man is omnivorous; he is most typically a frugivore, or fruit eater. He lacks the carnassial teeth or rasping tongue of a carnivore (though he lacks the specialized molars of herbivore. While his gastric juice contains only a fraction of the hydrochloric acid found in the carnivore. There is no doubt that man is fully equipped to live on plant food, as almost two billion rice eaters in China and India prove today. Secondly, logic dictates that the body has evolved as a whole and that man has not had time to adapt to the current refined diet. The third and most important point is that "all the manifestations of the saccharine disease are strikingly absent in those races still subsisting on just these unrefined carbohydrates."

Individual differences in personality, race, degree of concentration of carbohydrates, and amounts consumed determine the incubation period of the saccharine disease. Moreover, the average incubation period varies among the different saccharine disease manifestations; for diabetes it may be 20 years, for coronary disease 30 years, and for diverticular disease as long as 40 years. It is now almost universally accepted that the primary cause of dental caries is the consumption of refined carbohydrates. It would be an extraordinary coincidence if damage were not also inflicted on the alimentary canal and other parts of the body by the same culprit. In fact, other diseases may well be added in the future to the list of disorders caused by refined carbohydrates. A doctor in the Transkei region of South Africa stated that, "he had not diagnosed a single case of schizophrenia in a tribal African living on an unrefined diet, while it is the most common psychosis among urban Africans."

The loss of fiber in our food is responsible for the many diseases of the colon. These include constipation, diverticulosis, diverticulitis, colitis, and cancer . Most people know that the roughage taken in foods such as fruits and vegetables improve the action of the bowel. Radiological studies made on tribal Africans who eat an unrefined diet showed that the transit time of their stools was 24 to 48 hours, as against 48 to 96 hours or longer in westernized countries. In other words, those with unrefined diets average less than half the time required by those with refined diets.

Unnatural concentration of carbohydrates (which results when fiber is removed) leads to overconsumption—and ultimately obesity. The appetite cannot be blamed for obesity since an unrefined diet does not lead to overconsumption. A wild creature in its natural environment never eats too much and is therefore never overweight. Obesity is not due to a lack of exercise. Throughout the animal kingdom no creature takes more exercise than is necessary to get its food. "Nature obviously likes to conserve the heart and certainly never inflicts on any organism the penalty of obesity for laziness." It is therefore contended that the sole cause of obesity is the consumption of refined carbohydrates.

Coronary disease has reached epidemic proportions. The enormous dimensions of the problem are suggested by the fact that heart disease accounts for 25% of all deaths in the United Kingdom and has become one of the most common causes of death in persons under 35 in Scotland. Interestingly, the medical profession suffers from coronary disease just as much as the rest of the population. The heart is a wonderful machine. In the average person its action cycle is repeated 100,000 times a day for 70 years or more without a single servicing. The environment of the heart consists essentially of the bloodstream, and since what is in the bloodstream depends on what we eat, the naturalness of the food in our diet ultimately determines the structural integrity of the heart. Our deviation from the evolutionary process through the consumption of refined foods is at the root of the coronary problem.

The most glaring departure from evolutionary principles lies in the change from saturated to unsaturated fats. Many consider cholesterol a causative factor in heart attacks because it is prominent in atheroma plaques (fatty deposits in the arteries). But cholesterol is not the only blood lipid that may be implicated in coronary disease. Triglycerides are blood lipids as well. Although there is a great deal of controversy about the effect about sucrose and triglycerides, "Any overconsumption of food and consequent energy imbalance, often leading to obesity and to pre-diabetes and diabetes , is especially prominent in increasing blood lipids, particularly the triglycerides."

We have been eating meat and drinking milk since the Neolithic era, thousands of years before the Christian era. The bible urged Jehovah's people to eat, "butter of kine, and milk of the sheep, with fat of the lambs." The new oils we are consuming now, however, are pressed from vegetable seeds (cottonseeds and sunflower seeds). Margarine, which was introduced during World War I in 1916, is usually saturated by hydrogenation to achieve a greater solidity for table use. The fact that there has been a coronary explosion since the introduction of these oils should be cause for concern and suspicion .

Fat consumption in the United States increased by only 12 percent over the 70 year period from 1900 to 1970, and the increase chiefly consisted of processed vegetable oils that were recommended for the prevention of coronary disease. While this relatively slight increase in fat consumption took place, sugar intake was increasing sevenfold. Since coronary disease rarely occurs in anyone under the age of 30 years, it has a minimum incubation period of 30 years, and perhaps much longer. This 30 year minimum incubation period dovetails with the coronary explosion when sugar consumption touched the 100 pound mark. No comparison can be made for fats since consumption of dairy products and fats increased mainly in the 1970s, after the start of the coronary epidemic.

Smoking is certainly important in the etiology of coronary disease because it constricts the terminal arteries. However, it is only an aggravating factor, not a basic cause. This is demonstrated by the fact that though there is still a considerable incidence of disease in non-smokers, there is no incidence at all in primitive societies. Furthermore, smoking cannot explain the crucial association of diabetes and coronary disease—the two occur together almost all the time.

Stress and lack of exercise must be examined because they are frequently blamed for coronary disease. If we are adapted to anything in the modern world, we are adapted to stress, and even though worry is undesirable, it is necessary in the struggle for survival.

It may cause loss of appetite, of weight, but it will not cause organic disease in a properly nourished body. As for exercise, to force exercise on someone who wants to rest is unnatural. These suggested causes of coronary disease do not merit further exploration because neither stress nor exercise can explain the link between diabetes and heart disease. We can escape the coronary danger we face today only by adhering to evolutionary principles—that is, by adopting a diet of natural foods and avoiding refined sugar and white flour.

LICK THE SUGAR HABIT
NANCY APPLETON, PH.D.

This book is a case history of a sugarholic who took control of her life, and a testimonial of the effectiveness of a diet which excludes sugar, alcohol, and coffee. Nancy Appleton describes the evils of sugar, the root cause of all the degenerative diseases.

This story has been told before, but never from the perspective of a reformed sugar addict who has taken charge of her destiny. Her exhilaration and vitality are obvious as she describes her new-found happiness.

Synopsis

Nancy Appleton was a sugarholic. She loved doughnuts, candy, and chocolate. She craved the stuff. She didn't realize it, but her body was sending her signals. She constantly had a running nose and itching in her ears. In her teen age years the addiction worsened, though her weight was under control because she was an active tennis player and burned up the excess calories. She was not fat, but she ignored the message that her body was giving her.

As an adult Appleton's life was plagued with a variety of problems— boils, varicose veins, headaches, constipation, colds, and pneumonia. With each successive pneumonia, it took longer to recover. Her immune system was being weakened by her dietary habits. Her body was out of balance and she had to learn how to listen to her body in order to restore her health.

The Department of Agriculture reports that the average American eats over 160 pounds of sugar and non-caloric sweeteners every year. More than 3 pounds a week—and when starches are added (50 pounds a year) that adds up to 4 pounds a week. Refined foods represent 25% of our daily calories. They upset our body's chemistry and have absolutely no nutritional value.

Every spoonful of sugar you eat compromises your body's health, robbing you of the nutrients needed for metabolism and digestion. "The minerals needed to digest sugar, chromium. manganese, cobalt, copper, zinc, and magnesium have been stripped away in the refining process, and the body has to deplete its own mineral reserves to use the refined sugar."

Glucose is used as a cheap filler by the food industry in foods like cereal, baked goods, sauces, and processed meats. And there is no law requiring glucose to be listed on the label of any package. Therefore, even if you do not consume large amounts of sugar directly, you can experience problems—endocrine problems, hypoglycaemia, diabetes, tooth decay, arthritis, cancer, and all degenerative diseases can be the result of a blood sugar imbalance.

A 10-ounce glass of orange juice has the equivalent of 9 teaspoons of sugar, the same as a 12-ounce can of Coke. This sugar, with your breakfast, can exhaust the enzymes needed to digest protein like eggs. If you have the orange juice when you wake up, allowing time for the juice to get through the stomach, the enzymes will later be able to digest breakfast protein without interference. It is also a good idea to dilute the juice with water.

The food industry does not support research on the effect of sugar on the body, since it relies on sugar for the manufacture of processed foods. The pharmaceutical industry also would harm itself with research. If people stopped eating sugar they wouldn't need so many drugs.

Life expectancy in the United States is over 76 years, increased from 44 years in 1900. This sounds like an amazing increase, but almost all of this gain in life expectancy is due to a reduction in deaths at birth or infant mortality. Many infectious diseases and other childhood diseases have been conquered. The sad fact is that life expectancy of a 50-year old male today is only about 2 years longer than it was almost 100 years ago.

When sugar is ingested the blood sugar level goes up, and the pancreas secretes insulin, which brings the sugar level down to normal. After a number of years of overstimulating the pancreas, the excess insulin drops sugar below the fasting level and hypoglycaemia develops, resulting in headaches, fatigue, depression, hunger, and rapid heartbeat.

Coffee can have the same effect as sugar. The best way to relieve the symptoms of low blood sugar is to remove all junk food from your diet. If sugar and refined flour are a good part of your diet you are certain also to be lacking fiber and bulk, and risk constipation, colon problems, and other diseases.

One out of two persons in the United States is afflicted with heart and blood vessel disease. Now research implicates sugar as a link in the cause of coronary heart disease. Dr. John Yudkin points out that someone taking more than 120 grams of sugar a day (8 tablespoons- a Coke has 3 tablespoons) is perhaps five or more times likely to develop myocardial infarction than one taken less than 60 grams. Dr. William Philpott finds that people who die of coronary heart disease have no detectable amounts of chromium in their arteries. Our bodies need chromium to digest sugar. Sugar leaches chromium from the body without replacing it. Philpott concludes that magnesium, calcium, and chromium must be present to resist the development of degenerative diseases.

The chocolate which covers candy bars is made with hydrogenated soy oil, also found in margarine. Hydrogenated oils have been linked to atherosclerosis, which clogs the arteries. If you don't eat hydrogenated fats or sugar, and you guard against stress, you probably will not get heart disease.

Sugar is the direct cause of a series of events that lead to obesity. "The minerals in the body become unbalanced, enzymes don't function correctly, food does not digest properly, and allergies occur. Allergies cause addiction, addiction causes cravings, and overeating is the result." Eliminate sugar and other refined foods such as white flour, spaghetti, and pizza and you will have no weight problem.

Sugar is not the only substance you must avoid to achieve the proper chemical balance in your body. "Alcohol, caffeine, rancid fats, aspirin, artificial sweeteners, food additives, and mercury, all cause problems." Dr. William Philpott finds that 95% of alcoholics are hypoglycaemic. Coffee stimulates the secretion of gastric juices that can cause ulcers, and can reduce iron absorption by 39 to 87 percent when consumed within one hour after a meal.

You now have some idea of the problems that can result from an unbalanced chemical condition. You must resolve to take control of your life and return to good health. The following list of suggestions can help you during the period of adjustment.

1) Keep sugar out of your house.
2) Avoid all forms of corn-all sugar in processed foods have a corn base.
3) Eat complex carbohydrates to avoid hypoglycaemia..
4) Snack on healthy foods such as celery, carrots, sweet potatoes, and green and red peppers.
5) Read labels. Some foods have as many as four kinds of sugar- such as dextrose, corn sweetener, invert sugar, and molasses.
6) Eat small protein snacks to raise the blood sugar level slowly.
7) Exercise to reduce your appetite.
8) Set achievable goals.
9) Avoid soft drinks, which change the calcium/phosphorous ratio.
10) Brush your teeth often.
11) Give yourself a chance to cleanse your system.

You must cut out sugar, coffee, and alcohol. The foods that will help you reach balance are vegetables, legumes, and small helpings of protein. Appleton writes that she feels better now than she has, since she was eighteen. She sleeps less, experiences less fatigue, can play tennis several hours a day, and eats as great deal of food. You can control your life and your health. It's up to you...

VICTORY OVER DIABETES
WILLIAM H. PHILPOTT, M.D. AND
DWIGHT K. KALITA, PH.D.

Synopsis

Oral diabetic drugs could be causing 10,000 to 15,000 deaths every year. They have side effects and don't lower blood glucose efficiently. The market for these drugs in the United States is $200 million – the profits are huge, and the sales promotion is intense. Drug companies spend $5,000 per doctor each year to promote oral diabetic drugs. However, nutrient therapy, (or Bio-Ecologic Medicine), as coined by Dr. Marshall Mandell) is more effective than drug treatment because it recognizes the fact that good health is based on healthy cells. It cures and prevents the causes of disease rather than treating the symptoms.

Juvenile-onset diabetes is the least common and most severe type of diabetes; one million of the nation's 10 to 20 million diabetics have this form of the disease, in which blood glucose can be as high as 1,000 mg.(1 gram per 100 ml of blood) (70 -110 mg. is considered normal). Mature-onset diabetics make up 90% of the diabetic population. This illness appears gradually, usually after the age of forty.

It is important to understand how diabetes begins. The pancreas, a gland which lies below the stomach, and weighs about half a pound, contains thousands of "Islets of Langerhans," each with about 100 beta cells which secrete insulin. These beta cells measure blood glucose levels within the body and deliver insulin, a hormone that controls the level of glucose, maintaining a healthy balance. An over-stimulated pancreas, however, eventually ceases to function normally; all addictions—food, chemical, and alcoholic—can lead to pancreatic insufficiency. Our heavy consumption of junk foods and high level of alcohol and tobacco use overtax the pancreas.

Adequate glucose levels in the body are very important. Your entire body needs the glucose to maintain the complex processes of life. Food is broken down and absorbed chiefly as glucose in the bloodstream, and stimulates a release of insulin. If high sugar levels were controlled by the use of insulin, controlling diabetes would be simple.

Pancreatic insufficiency lowers the production of lipase, an enzyme produced by the pancreas which is needed for proper lipid metabolism. Insufficient lipase causes the phospholipid/cholesterol ratio in the blood to rise, and is the foundation on which arteriosclerosis and other cardiovascular diseases are built . The pancreas also supplies proteolytic enzymes, which aid in breaking proteins down into amino acids. Insulin is composed of 51 amino acids; when amino acids are in short supply, the insulin quality and quantity are reduced. The result is high blood sugar or diabetes.

When protein digestion is faulty, undigested protein particles are absorbed into the bloodstream, where they cause inflammatory reactions throughout the body, and severe irritation to the inside lining of the arteries. These damaged areas then absorb circulating lipids in greater abundance than is healthy, and eventually form arteriosclerotic plaques, which can occlude or close down an artery. People with diabetes are 6 times more likely to have heart attacks than normal people. Insulin injections do not help this diabetic symptom; in fact, medical evidence shows that injections of insulin may be responsible for the severe cardiovascular and cerebrovascular complications of diabetes. Dr. Bernard Lowenstein reports that too much insulin stimulates the production of excessive cholesterol in the body.

The question now arises, what about cholesterol? Is cholesterol the main causative factor in heart attacks? Let's examine cholesterols function in the body and try to understand all aspects of the problem. There are many inconsistencies in the cholesterol paradigm. 80% of those who suffer heart attacks have normal cholesterol levels, and most of the cholesterol in the body is produced by the liver and therefore is unrelated to the dietary level consumed every day. "Physicians at the Mayo Clinic have shown that the severity of arteriosclerosis is not always related to the levels of serum cholesterol. People with low blood cholesterol could have just as severe arteriosclerosis."In a diet high in methionine, homocysteine could be the villain, and not cholesterol. Our contention, based on empirical and clinical evidence, is that the initial arterial damage and subsequent plaque are caused by specific nutritional deficiencies. Cholesterol and calcium are a secondary problem, following the primary vascular damage caused by homocystinuria, or a vitamin B-6 deficiency.

Even the greatest proponent of the lipid theory condemning cholesterol, the American Heart Association has modified its position; they stated in 1974 that "there is as yet no proof that a low-cholesterol, low-fat diet followed from early adult life will reduce the primary occurrence of heart attacks in Americans." We believe that plasma cholesterol levels by themselves are not the major cause of arteriosclerosis; they become a serious problem after the arterial wall deteriorates, when dangerous metabolic debris can adhere to the lesion. At that time excess cholesterol further clogs the arteries to a degree that often causes heart attacks and strokes.

Nutrients never act by themselves; they function as a team. The importance of vitamin C has been effectively demonstrated by Dr. Irwin Stone, Linus Pauling, Dr. Fred Klenner, and Dr. Robert Cathcart. It is vitamin C that builds collagen, which helps maintain the integrity of the arterial wall. The prevention of lesions in the artery by B-6 and vitamin C provide a strong defense for the diabetic in his protection against cardiovascular complication of his condition.

Dr. Evan Shute thinks that a diabetic is not being treated unless he is getting vitamin E. "Vitamin E is a powerful antioxidant; it acts as an antithrombin, preventing fatal blood clots: it prevents myocardial scarring; and it is a vasodilator, opening unused blood vessels. Vitamin Es antioxidant action can prevent polyunsaturated fatty acids from being made rancid by oxygen. Our doctors tell us to eat more polyunsaturated oils, but they don't tell us to take more Vitamin E. This could be a disaster: without enough vitamin E oxygen will turn corn oil, safflower oil, and other vegetable oils rancid by peroxidation. Peroxidation produces free radicals which cause severe irritation, and the arteriosclerotic process begins. Thus, orthodox medicine is actually "accelerating cardiovascular mortality in our population, while creating a Vitamin E deficiency."

Chromium is a micronutrient, or trace element, measured in extremely small amounts; the slightest deficiency upsets the body's proper tolerance to glucose. An increased intake of glucose or insulin calls for a release of chromium GTF (glucose tolerance factor) reserves in the body. When sugar is fed to a fasting person three things happen: blood sugar is elevated, insulin rises dramatically, and the chromium level in the blood rises, taken from the body's storage levels. The result is a net loss of chromium. Diabetic individuals excrete more chromium in their urine than normal people. The result is a significant glucose intolerance in the human body. A chromium deficiency in rats produces arteriosclerotic lesions, high cholesterol, and high blood sugar.

New theories normally evoke responses from specialists on whose areas of competence they impinge. Endocrinologists are dogmatic and don't easily alter their opinions. We don't expect an early acceptance of our observations, but the diagnosis and treatment of diabetes has been sufficiently rewarding for us to risk sharing our observations with our fellow physicians and the lay public. Hypotheses are necessary for progress. The time lag between discovery and acceptance is unfortunately too long for those who need the new therapies. We hope the reader will understand our eagerness to express our views—even if all the answers are not in.

THE HOMOCYSTEINE REVOLUTION
KILMER S. MCCULLY, M.D.

Kilmer S. McCully suffered the same fate of everyone who bucks the established order or status quo. He was fired from his position at Harvard University and his research funding grants dried up. He was up against the cholesterol goliath that has dominated the diet/heart dogma for the last half century. McCully's work has begun to unravel the overwhelming resistance of the cholesterol-fat hierarchy. He is a dedicated scientist who has devoted his life to the search for truth and the dissemination of the facts he discovered about the number one killer in the united States.—coronary heart disease. His discovery is the central theme of his book, "The Homocysteine Revolution,

Synopsis

Kilmer S. McCully, M.D. discovered that an amino acid called homocysteine is a strong, independent risk factor for arteriosclerosis.

Homocystinuria is a disease that is characterized by hardening of the arteries. McCully studied the results of ten cases in London and Belfast who had hardening of the arteries caused by cystinuria. He was curious to know why there was no cholesterol deposited in the children's arteries. Mccully hypothesized that an elevated homocysteine level caused the arteriosclerosis. This discovery was of tremendous importance because scientists in 1969 were searching for another approach to understanding coronary heart disease. There were many unanswered questions about the cholesterol paradigm. For example, why the majority of heart disease patients have a normal or low cholesterol?

McCully's ideas were denounced by the cholesterol camp. If accepted, it would undermine the conventional view of prevention and treatment of heart disease. But dietary cholesterol does not raise blood (serum) cholesterol. McCully knew that the Framingham Heart Study in 1969 showed that conclusion. He also knew that the children and animals' homocystinuria had no cholesterol in their artery walls

The vast majority of the medical community ignored the new homocysteine theory. It was not only radically different from the consensus, but it would undermine the livelihood of the alliance which had developed over the decades including the AHA, Government agencies such as the NIH, the National Heart, Lung and Blood Institute, the giant pharmaceutical industry, and the mammoth food industry. McCully was fighting a one trillion dollar colossus!

The homocysteine approach is radically different from the cholesterol theory which believes that arteriosclerosis develops from the dietary consumption of excessive amounts of fats and cholesterol. The homocysteine theory holds that arteries are damaged by the injurious effect of homocysteine on cells and tissues of the arteries, leading to loss of elasticity, hardening, calcification, narrowing of the lumen (the opening through which blood flows), and the formation of blood clots in the arteries. The homocysteine theory considers arteriosclerosis a disease of protein intoxication; the cholesterol theory considers the disease to be caused by intoxication from fats.

There is one major difference between the cholesterol paradigm and the homocysteine theory. McCully has discovered the means of preventing the buildup of plasma homocysteine, thereby preventing arteriosclerosis. Prevention can be achieved by consumption of foods that provide an abundant supply of vitamins B-6, B-12, and folic acid. Many factors contribute to the complex problem of coronary heart disease: male gender, post-menopause in women, genetics, smoking, sedentary lifestyle, high blood pressure, and thyroid disease. There are many cases of severe arteriosclerosis in which cholesterol is normal. Recent studies suggest that 50,000 American lives will be saved by adding folic acid to the food supply.

For 60 years the cholesterol-fat theory dominated the consensus. One of the shortcomings of the cholesterol-fat approach is the lack of an explanation for the rapid escalation of coronary heart disease and stroke in the mid-20th century in America and its dramatic decline in the mid 1960s and 1970s. The American diet has changed very little during the recent decades which saw a two-to-three fold decline in coronary heart disease and stroke. Cholesterol levels were the same during this period.

The time lag in the medical world is always 50 to 100 years. There has to be a"paradigm shift" about the cause of arteriosclerosis. There are too many questions about the cholesterol theory which have no answers. The success of the cholesterol-lowering statin drugs is complicated by evidence of liver and muscle toxicity and cancer in animals. (1)   evidence that these drugs inhibit the formation of ubiquinone (co-enzyme Q10), a key component of energy production in the heart and other cells.(2)

It was not until 1993 that a biochemical theory related the observations on homocysteine and vascular disease to observations in the cholesterol-fat field. Recent studies show widespread deficiencies of vitamin-6 , B-12, and folic acid in elderly and cardiac patients. Rinehart's studies with monkeys showed very little fat and cholesterol in the arteriosclerotic plaques. They were fibrous and fibrocalcific. (4)

The medical community refused to accept the homocysteine theory because it relegates cholesterol to a secondary role in the causation of coronary heart disease. The huge multi-billion dollar business that cholesterol has built is very lucrative and saturated with political intrigue. They won't give up easily. It will take an aroused public to stir representatives into action.

The Hordaland Homocysteine Study concludes that we can view arteriosclerosis as a deficiency disease. The approach is revolutionary because for the last 50 years artery disease was viewed as a disease of excess consumption of sugars, cholesterol, and fats. (3) Folic acid was added to foods in 1998 according to a decision by the United States Department of Agriculture. The dietary intake of vitamin B-12 is adequate for the population except for strict vegetarians. A future goal is to require the addition of B-6 to enrich foods which are lost in the processing. It will help to continue the decline in arteriosclerosis and improve the general health and promote increased life expectancy in the population. Kilmer McCully says that the homocysteine blood (plasma) level should be no higher than 14 micromoles.

References

1. Thomas B. Newman and Stephen B. Hulley

"Carcinogenicity of Lipid-lowering Drugs" JAMA 275: 55-60 1996 .

2. Willis, Richard et al "Co-Enzyme Q10 Levels in Rats" USA 87: 8928-30 1990 .

3. Omar Nygard et al :Total Plasma Homocysteine and Cardiovascular Risk Profile" JAMA 274: 1526-1533 1995 .

4. James F. Rinehart and Louis D. Greenberg "Vitamin B-6 Deficiency in the Rhesus Monkey, etc. AJCN 4: 318-325 1956.

SWEET AND DANGEROUS
JOHN YUDKIN, M.D.

Sugar is dangerous. It is the enemy of your health. Dr. Robert Atkins called it death! Yes- sugar is death. Dr. John Yudkin's book, "Sweet and Dangerous" states in stark terms that sugar is responsible for obesity, heart attacks, diabetes, dental decay, and a general shortening of one's lifespan. These claims are all supported with solid research .

Synopsis

Man has a natural liking for sweet things. Primitive man satisfied this desire by eating fruit and honey. In the middle of the 16th century, sugar was as expensive as caviar is today. It was only after the development of sugar plantations in the Caribbean, helped along by the slave trade, that sugar prices came down to an affordable level. As the prices fell, demand grew, and consumption rose to very high levels.

In the year 2003, the average American consumed 160 pounds of sugar and non-caloric sweeteners (corn syrup and high-fructose corn syrup). These figures are published by the Department of Agriculture. This means that we are eating more than three pounds of sugar a week. Furthermore, the consumption of starches in our diet, like pasta, bread, potatoes, and rice is adding another 50 pounds of sugar a year. The final total is four pounds of sugar a week.

This insane amount of the sweet stuff is creating havoc in a body that is not adjusted to the drastic change in man's diet. It may take 10,000 years for our digestive system to accommodate this alteration in our diet. The best known sugars are glucose, lactose, fructose, maltose, and sucrose. Fructose is fruit sugar, maltose is malt sugar, and sucrose is the ordinary table sugar you use in your coffee or tea and in making cakes, cookies, soft drinks, and ice cream. When you eat sugar or starch, glucose will be released during digestion and absorbed from the alimentary canal into the blood. As the level of blood glucose rises, the pancreas secretes insulin to lower that level to the normal state. The glucose is then converted into glycogen and stored in the muscles and liver to be called upon if the blood sugar level falls.

The body needs glucose, not the sucrose that is refined by the sugar industry. Sucrose and glucose are different in vital ways. All foods give off energy, but sugar is digested, absorbed and taken to the tissues more quickly than other foods. The speed with which sugar floods the bloodstream is probably more harmful than beneficial. Moreover, while other foods contain energy and nutrients in the form of protein and minerals, sugar contains only energy. Many people lose excess weight just by giving up sugar. If you take one spoonful of sugar in each cup of coffee and drink five cups a day, you can lose more than ten pounds of weight a year just by eliminating the sugar in your coffee. In an earlier book, "The Slimming Business," Dr. John Yudkin describes a low-carbohydrate diet as the most sensible and effective way to control body weight. This diet tells you to cut back on those foods that give you unnecessary calories and to consume more foods that give you the nutrients you require.

Although a large consumption of sugar can lead to heart disease, it is not the only cause. Other factors that contribute to heart disease are the following:

- The genetic factor — If your family has lived to a ripe old age without having disease, your chances of having a heart attack are lessened.
- Lack of exercise — If you lead a sedentary life you are inviting an attack.
- Smoking — Tobacco can affect your heart. Heavy smokers are more prone to heart disease.
- High cholesterol — It is widely accepted that one's chances of developing a heart attack are higher when the blood cholesterol is high.
- Obesity — Being excessively overweight can cause many of the ills that lead to heart attacks. Very few fat people live to an

advanced age.

Dr. Ancel Keys at the University of Minnesota was the first proponent of the ideas that diet can be a major cause of coronary thrombosis. His Seven countries Study demonstrated a strong relationship between the intake of fat and death rates due to coronary heart disease. Although considered to be a landmark contribution to the study of heart disease, this discovery has been challenged by a growing minority who believe that coronary disease is not largely due to fat in the diet.

In 1957, a study was begun of the relationship between sugar consumption and coronary disease. Soon after, a Japanese research team confirmed that relationship with a study conducted in 20 countries. Evidence began to mount, showing that a rise in sugar consumption led to higher coronary disease rates. In South Africa, the black population had almost no coronary disease. The heart attack rate now, however, is increasing with the growth in sugar consumption. In Israel, the immigrants from Yemen came in with very little coronary disease, while those Yemenites who had lived in Israel for 20 years or more were far more susceptible to the disease because of the high sugar diet of the country. The Maasai and Sumburu tribes of East Africa live largely on milk and meat, and eat virtually no sugar. They have very little heart disease. A high sugar intake can cause diabetes, though it may take up to 20 years for such a diet to produce the disease. It was formerly believed that fat consumption was responsible for diabetes, a theory wrongly based on the assumption that all carbohydrates are equal and on the fact that fat and sugar consumption were high in countries where diabetes struck a large number of people. Sir Charles Best, one of the discoverers of insulin, demonstrated in experiments that sugar produced fatty livers. He also discovered that sugar had the same effect on the liver as alcohol. Sugar will produce an enlargement of the liver, kidneys, and the adrenal glands. Knowing that sugar is bad for you is the first problem. You must have the will power to avoid it. Once you start cutting down, you will begin to savour the flavour of your foods, for sugar tends to blunt the sensitivity of your palate. You will enjoy the subtle differences of your fruit. Once in a while you can enjoy ice cream or a piece of pie.

Try to reduce your intake of sugar to 20 grams a day. The following list will help you keep track:

- 1 cube of sugar – 4 grams
- 1 level teaspoon of sugar – 5 grams
- 1 bottle of cola – 12 grams
- 1 glass of fruit drink- 20 grams
- 1 spoon of jelly, jam, or marmalade – 5 grams
- 2 ounce piece of cake- 10 grams
- 4 ounce piece of apple pie – 20 grams
- 2 ounce piece of chocolate – 30 grams 1 ounce of candy – 20 grams
- 12 ounce portion of ice cream -12 grams

If you avoid sugar you are altogether less likely to become fat, have a nutritional deficiency or a heart attack, or develop diabetes, dental decay, or a duodenal ulcer. You also reduce your chances of getting gout, dermatitis, and certain forms of cancer. In general you will increase your life span.

THE CHOLESTEROL CONSPIRACY
RUSSELL L. SMITH, PH.D WITH EDWARD. R. PINCKNEY, M.D

For the vast majority of people, diet has little practical effects on their blood cholesterol levels. 2. Blood cholesterol levels have very little relationship to coronary heart disease. 3. Overwhelming evidence indicates that diet has little or nothing to do with coronary heart disease.

These facts are contrary to everything you've heard. It is almost impossible to believe but it is true. The cholesterol paradigm is dogma—it is a religion. The big lie has sunk deeply into the subconscious of our nation.

Synopsis

We don't know what causes heart disease. Once we discover the cause, we'll be able to prevent it. We do know what doesn't cause heart disease. It is not cholesterol. It is not your diet. Physicians have learned about cholesterol the same way we do-- through the media, newspapers, magazines, and the various medical journals. They don't know all the facts. We have been overwhelmed by a tsunami or tidal wave of exaggeration, half-truths, distortions, and even outright misrepresentations of facts. There are few people left who have not been completely brainwashed.

The American Heart Association (AHA) and the National Heart, Lung, and Blood Institute (NHLBI) and their medical researchers , who are subject to the largesse (which consists of hundreds of millions of dollars in grant money) control all the coronary heart disease research and information disseminated to the public. The truth is not debatable! And it can truly set you free. The NHLBI/AHA position is the following: The great CHD epidemic during the first 60 years of the 20th

century was caused by our increased consumption of saturated fat and dietary cholesterol. No part of this position is true, and the NHLBI/AHA alliance has never published any data which even remotely supports this stand or claim. There is a very weak association between blood cholesterol and coronary heart disease, and in some people it is of questionable importance.

We are taught to fear cholesterol. What is it? What does it do in the body? How does it increase or decrease in the blood? Cholesterol is a crystal of solid alcohol known as a steroid. It is absolutely essential to our health, and is located in every cell of the body. The body contains about 5 ounces of cholesterol and only 7 percent (one-third of an ounce) circulates in the blood (NEJM 1981, Brown and Goldstein). Cholesterol is necessary in the membranes of the cells where it regulates the exchange of nutrients and waste products. It helps in the development of the brain and the nervous system and acts as a conductor of nerve impulses. It is a component in bile acids which promote digestion of foods. Without cholesterol, complex fats, vitamins A, D, E, and K, which are soluble only in fats, also could not be absorbed.

Cholesterol is a necessary substance in the manufacture of the adrenal, sex, and pituitary hormones. It is also a necessary substance in the skin which is converted to vitamin D by sunlight and creates a barrier preventing water and other fluids from entering the body through the skin.

The major producer of cholesterol is the body itself. It is mainly manufactured in the liver and the intestinal wall. But it is also synthesized in every cell in the body except nerve tissue. The body manufactures 100o mg. to 2000 mg. per day. If you don't eat dietary cholesterol your body increases its manufacture. In other words, your cholesterol level remains about constant whether you eat cholesterol or not.

The media has emphasized two specific lipoproteins: HDL (high density lipoproteins) is the good cholesterol because it picks up the excess cholesterol from the cells and removes it from the blood. The LDL (low density lipoproteins) is the bad cholesterol because it is said to deposit the cholesterol in the arteries causing atherosclerosis. Despite what you have read, it is all purely speculation.

Genetics determine the cholesterol level. Excess dietary fats tend to remain in the blood and therefore the cholesterol level may increase.

However, many people are not influenced by very much fat. Cholesterol increases with the use of nicotine, stress, pain, fear, pregnancy, lack of exercise, drugs and medicines such as male and female hormones, tranquilizers, cortisone products, vitamins A and D, diuretics, and alcohol. Various diseases affect cholesterol. These include hypothyroidism, hepatitis, kidney disease, and gall bladder obstructions. Cholesterol changes during the four seasons of the year. Therefore one measurement cannot truly represent a person's average measurement. Cholesterol measurement instruments in labs or hospitals are notoriously inaccurate. "You can't buy an accurate cholesterol measurement." In spite of that billions of dollars a year are spent on cholesterol tests. Let's see how the diet/CHD idea got started, and why it persists even when scientific evidence fails to support it.

For 40 years the AHA/CHD partnership has been chasing the diet-blood cholesterol-CHD association windmills like Don Quixote. Countless studies offered little or no support. The amazing fact is that this juggernaut has grown larger, richer, and more powerful as the mountain of negative findings accumulated. How is this possible? If you control the grant money and the media, negative findings are no problem. The public will never hear about them. This is devastating in medicine. Billions of dollars are spent needlessly and millions of lives are lost prematurely because research funding agencies have disregarded massive scientific findings and fraudulently used public monies to disseminate dogma and propaganda.

Was it money? A school of thought is an hypothesis-a theory. When scientists devote more and more of their careers, egos, and reputations to a theory, they naturally resist the notion that they could be wrong. After 10, 15, 20 or more years of publishing reports and journal articles, the die is permanently cast. There is no turning back. They began to disregard any proof that they were wrong. It is embarrassing and career-threatening to admit they have convinced others to spend millions of dollars on a faulty thesis, an incorrect idea. This causes groups of scientists to harden their position and ignore contrary ideas or conclusions. Scientific progress is totally neglected in order to preserve reputations. Money is involved for certain, but it is not the prime reason for preserving a school of thought.

In the 1980s evidence emerged which indicated a relationship between the amount of cholesterol and the CHD death rate. All of these facts strengthened the idea that diet affected the development of atherosclerosis. There was only one problem. The facts did not support the diet/CHD hypothesis. Decades passed and there was no progress in finding a cause or a cure for mans biggest killer. The AHA was anxious to show the public that their contributions were paying off. In the 1950s the AHA contracted with a team of investigators to study the concept that the fat content of the Western diet is a significant factor in the cause of atherosclerosis. In 1957, the team of researchers concluded in their report, "The proposition that the character of the American diet has so changed during the past 50 years as to increase the incidence coronary vascular disease cannot be supported! This statement, if true, would effectively destroy the entire hypothesis that diet was a major cause of CHD.

The AHA had two choices: it could acknowledge the facts and pursue other approaches, or reject the negative evidence and cling to the diet/CHD hypothesis with even greater fervor. For four years the AHA sat on the report, and in 1961 it announced that dietary fat and cholesterol was the cause of CHD and recommended that Americans "at risk for CHD" reduce their consumption of these nutrients. The AHA concluded that this recommendation was based on the best scientific information available at the present time. This institutionalized the diet/CHD paradigm and the AHA has never wavered from that position regardless of all the huge accumulation of negative evidence.

Hundreds of billions of dollars for industry has strengthened the alliance and has created an enormous financial network. Money has now become the driving force, not the elimination of CHD.

HOW AND WHY WE AGE
LEONARD HAYFLICK, PH.D.

Resolving all the causes of death would be a mixed blessing. We would certainly live longer, but we would also become weaker as the normal, inexorable aging process made our vital organs grow increasingly less efficient. The most serious objection to the argument that longevity should be extended is that doing so would exacerbate every problem faced by the world today. These problems range from mass starvation, wars, economic inequities, and health failure. The underlying problem is overpopulation.

Immortality and the complete elimination of aging are both undesirable. Many advocate a gradual slowing of the aging process. One must distinguish between life expectancy and life span. The human life span is 115 years. That is the maximum. Life expectancy has been increasing as infant mortality has decreased through the years.

Dr. Hayflick believes that only one objective is both practical and desirable, and that is to strive for maximum human life expectation by eliminating the present leading causes of death. He sees no value to society or to the individual in seeking to stop the aging process or to achieve immortality. He invokes a future in which all humans reach the maximum life span, still in possession of their mental and physical capabilities, with death occurring quickly as we approach our 115th birthday.

Synopsis

Our understanding of the basic causes of aging is nearly as primitive as it was a century ago. Aging research has been a magnet for unscrupulous persons who trade on the vanity, fears or ignorance of the elderly, making promises that cannot be kept. Science doesn't flourish when charlatans and scoundrels develop their schemes to fleece the public.

Elie Metchnikoff introduced the word "Gerontology" in 1903. It means the scientific study of the aging process. The Greek word "Geron" means old man. Geriatrics is concerned with the medical problems of the elderly. The word was coined in 1909 by Ignaz L.Nascher, an American physician. He wrote the first American medical textbook on aging in 1914, entitled, "Geriatrics: The Diseases of Old Age and Their Treatment."

Today, there is a growing belief that efforts should be made to extend life as much as possible, provided that the quality of life is maintained. I believe that extending the human life span is probably not possible, nor is it desirable. Some argue for "prolongevity," believing that aging and death can be curable, and that extending the human life span is both possible and desirable. The consequences of an ageless population would be bizarre and even terrifying.

What is Aging?

Most of the ravages of time are the result of oxidation. Aging is not merely the passage of time. It defies easy definition. We all recognize an old person when we see one, but subjective determinations on appearances are frequently wrong. More importantly, age in years does not directly correlate with biological age. We need a measurement that distinguishes biological age from chronological age. The distinction is crucial. When we remark that someone "looks young" (or old) for his or her chronological age, we are observing that we all age biologically at different rates. What we need is a few changes that can help explain why an eighty or even ninety year old is functionally only sixty years old. Longevity, aging, and death are phenomena that characterize the finality of life. Longevity is the period of time that an animal can be expected to live. In developed countries average life expectation is 75 years, and maximum life span is 115 years. The question is, why do we live as long as we do? Aging represents losses in normal function up until the time of maximum longevity. The essential question about aging is, why do we grow old? Death is the final event that ends life. Why do we die?

A vast amount of evidence supports the fact that not only physical vigour, but also the ability to resist disease decreases in humans after sexual maturation. Nature planned things so that we would die long before we became old. In that sense, efforts to extend life are really attempts to fool mother nature. There are some animals that do not seem to age. Their growth may slow as the years go by, but it does not stop. Typical examples are lobsters, many fish, amphibians (reptiles) (The Galapagos Tortoise), The Galapagos Tortoise may live for 175 years, the sturgeon for 82 years, and the carp for between 50 and 100 years. Their vital systems may not decline after sexual maturation, and they live long, but they are not immortal.

It seems peculiar that mammals, one of the latest and most sophisticated animal lines to evolve, should have a limited life span. More primitive species like sharks and tortoises do not seem to have a fixed life span or to show age changes. Some gerontologists speculate that aging and a limited life span are the "price" mammals pay for maintaining a fixed size in adulthood and the benefits of being highly evolved.

One of the most important demographic facts is the enormous increase in older people. The graying of America has been underway since the first census was taken in 1790. The fastest growing segment in our population ia the people over 85. It is 25 times larger than the corresponding population in 1900. Another important statistic concerns those people over 65. By the year 2030 there will be more than 66 million, or twice as many people over 65 in the United States as there is today.

Most Americans over the age of 65 are healthy and live normal, productive lives. Increasingly, however, health generally deteriorates and the need for care increases. Some of the people whose health makes them dependent will regain their health and become independent once again. Several social changes have occurred in recent years that have improved personal health and lifestyle decisions, such as reducing the intake of fatty foods, medical intervention with drugs that reduce blood pressure and cholesterol levels. These successes decrease the years spent in illness within our 115 year life span. For example, strokes might become more common in 80- year olds rather than in 70- year olds. Heart disease will begin to appear in 70-year olds instead of 60-year olds. We really don't know.

In recent years cytogerontologists have found evidence for the existence of a clock in cultured normal cells. The clock that determines how long a normal cell will function in culture may establish the life span of the particular species. Some interesting experiments in my laboratory suggest that the clock is located in the nucleus of the cell. The nucleus is the location of the cells genetic apparatus. It houses the chemical called DNA, which contains the fundamental genetic code and forms the genes on all forty-six human chromosomes. Recently, there have been reports that the longevity clock might be located in genes on either the first or fourth chromosome of the twenty-three pairs of human chromosomes.

In 1973, Calvin H. Harley and his colleagues at McMaster University in Hamilton, Ontario, Canada, showed that every slender chromosome terminates in a region called a telomere. Telomeres are made of DNA, the same chemical that composes all of the genes that form the chromosomes. Telomeres do not seem to contain any genetic information. Each chromosome contains tens of thousands of different genes. Immortal abnormal cells seem to have found a way to keep their telomeres from shortening at each division, thus conferring immortality upon themselves. The immortal cells produce an enzyme called telomerase, which makes more telomeres. Normal cells lack this enzyme. The interpretation in normal cells as a clock for longevity and aging is only speculative now. Biogerontologists are anxiously waiting for new developments as this fascinating story unfolds. The BLSA (Baltimore Longitudinal Study of Aging) uncovered some major surprises that have changed our understanding of how we age. The conclusions below are just some of the facts from the study.

1. There is no evidence that heart function declines with age.
2. There is a greater range of individual variation in older humans. The BLSA scientists have found extraordinary "young" 80-year olds and extraordinary "old" 40 -year olds.
3. Aging did not result in an inevitable loss of intellectual functions.
4. There is no evidence that the basic causes of aging are affected by increased exercise.
5. Sudden losses are the result of diseases, not aging. The BLSA tells us that there is no single aging process. A person's rate of aging may vary significantly from what may be predicted from the averages. There is no general pattern of aging applicable to all of our organs. Aging results from the interaction of genetic,

environmental, and lifestyle factors. Age changes are highly individualized. Chronological age is an unreliable measure of the passage of time called birthdays and receiving presents.

There is no doubt that the incidence of cardiovascular disease increases exponentially with age. It is the leading cause of death in virtually all industrialized countries. But diseases of the cardiovascular system are not the cause of aging. The proof ? People without cardiovascular disease also age. The brain is an immensely complex organ composed of an estimated one hundred billion nerve cells. There is universal agreement that the weight of the brain decreases with age. One gerontologist calculated that in one part of the brain there is an average loss of 100,000 neurons per day from the age of thirty. If this is true, you would lose about two billion cells in fifty years. The number seems large, but it accounts for less than one-seventh of an ounce of brain cells. In 1906, Alois Alzheimer, a German Neurologist, first described a form of cognitive impairment in humans that has come to be called Alzheimer's disease. The disease strikes 0.1 percent of all people aged sixty to sixty-five to as high as 4.7 percent in those over eighty-five. Today, public awareness of Alzheimer's disease is at an all-time high. It is the chief complaint of older people in respect to age-related changes in cognitive ability. Theories of aging based on random events:

Wear and tear theory— In 1882, the great German biologist August Weismann articulated the "wear and tear theory.""Death," he said, "occurs because a worn out tissue cannot forever renew itself."Weismann was correct in his hypothesis that normal cells cannot divide or function forever, but that does not explain why age changes occur. Jaime Miguel, of the University of Alicante, Spain, suggested that wear and tear occur when free radicals are formed by normal metabolic processes. He maintains that "the mitochondria," the "power plants," that provide energy for all the cells activities, are affected by molecular wear and tear.

The rate of living theory—The German physiologist, Max Rubner, developed this theory in 1908. He believes that animals are born with a limited amount of potential energy. If it is used up rapidly, aging begins early. If it is consumed slowly, then aging will be slowed. It has been referred to as the "live fat, die young' theory. In humans, life in the fast lane is also called, "burning the candle at both ends." The wear and tear theory would have you believe that a slower, laid back rate of living will let you age more slowly and you would therefore live longer. This is an appealing idea, but there is little evidence to support it.

The cross-linking theory—This theory maintains that as we age the proteins and nucleic acids in our body actually undergo a process like the tanning of leather. Fritz Verzar, the founder of the famous Institute of Experimental Gerontology in Basel, Switzerland, developed an ingenious way to measure the shrinkage of collagen. This theory is not more popular because it is based more on deductive reasoning than on experimental evidence. There is little doubt that cross-linking occurs in collagen and some other proteins, but the idea that it occurs in the DNA of living animals is only speculation. And even if it does occur, there is no good experimental evidence that it actually impedes metabolic processes or causes the formation of faulty molecules.

The Free Radical Theory – this theory is based on a chemical reaction that occurs when certain susceptible molecules in cells encounter oxygen and break apart to form reactive pieces. These molecular fragments are called free radicals. They are unstable and try to reunite with any other molecule that happens to be in the vicinity. Denham Harman, of the University of Nebraska is the chief proponent of the free radical theory of aging, although the germ of the idea was first introduced by R. Gershman in 1954.

The most convincing evidence that free radicals are involved in age changes are experiments that have been done with antioxidants. They prevent oxygen from combining with susceptible molecules to form free radicals. The most important antioxidants in our body are vitamin C and vitamin E. Enzymes called superoxide dismutase (SOD), catalase, and glutathione peroxidase also destroy free radicals.

Regardless of what the mechanism is, the administration of antioxidants does increase the average length of life. The most intriguing aspect of the studies done with free radicals is perhaps not what they might be telling us about aging, but what they are telling us about disease. Antioxidants clearly seem to postpone the appearance of cancer, cardiovascular disease, degenerative diseases of the central nervous system, and depression of the immune system. Regardless of the role antioxidants might play in the aging process, they are sending us an unambiguous message about their ability to delay the appearance of the diseases of old age, and that message should not be ignored.

With all that we know of the major theories that might explain why we age, which is the truth? The truth is that we still do not know. Gerontology as a science has been derided by mainstream biologists, mainly because there has been such a proliferation of untested theories. The most reasonable position to take at this time is to say that because gerontology is such a young science, we simply do not have a good explanation for why aging occurs. We might take comfort in the fact that there are enough dedicated scientists working in the field of aging to offer hope that the speculation might soon end.

With the exception of the discovery that age changes occur within individual cells, we do not know much more today about the fundamental cause of aging than we did a century ago. We know much more about what happens than we did before, but very little about why it happens. It is for this reason that George Sacher proposed that we have been asking the wrong question. Instead of asking "why do we age?" we should ask, "why do we live as long as we do?" Longevity has increased, and may be capable of increasing further. Let us see how we have been successful in manipulation of the aging process.

Satchel Paige, the great black baseball pitcher, has been quoted as saying, "avoid running at all times." Most people seem to exercise less as they grow older. Until recently, most older persons were expected to "act their age." Now, everyone is encouraged to exercise. The reason given for exercising is that it will increase longevity. This is only true in a limited way, because it modifies disease processes, notably that of cardiovascular disease. There is simply no evidence that exercise is capable of influencing the fundamental aging processes or to increase life span. If you exercise because it makes you feel good or because you believe that it might prevent, slow, or reverse the effects of a disease, then, by all means continue. However, if you expect to reverse aging by exercising, you should understand that there is no data to suggest you will succeed.

Scientists have discovered no more effective way to slow the rate of aging than undernutrition without malnutrition. Nor do we know of a more effective means of postponing or eliminating so many kinds of cancer and other diseases. Despite overwhelming evidence that under-nutrition will postpone disease and prolong life, few people have been motivated to opt for such a Spartan regimen. I think that for most people, the quality of their lives is more important than the quantity.

Furthermore, we do not know what the long term effects of caloric restriction might be on cognition. Many gerontologists worry that some mental processes might be impaired. My major criticism of the claim that under- nutrition increases longevity still holds. I prefer to say that over- nutrition increases disease incidence and reduces longevity. The present human life span, which developed over several million years, probably did so under conditions of under rather than over- nutrition.

"If mother nature doesn't get you, father time will."Time seems to pass more rapidly as we grow older. No one has ever shown that any medical intervention, nutritional factor, or other lifestyle change will stop or reverse the aging process. Even so, there are frequent claims that an anti-aging substance has been found. Testing the efficiency of an anti-aging compound is difficult. We simply do not know the fundamental causes of aging or what exactly determines longevity..

Because immortality and the complete elimination of aging is both undesirable, some believe that just slowing the aging process might be the best compromise. We still do not know how to slow the aging in humans, but we do know how to increase our life expectancy by eliminating or reducing the causes of death. This approach has been remarkably successful throughout most of this century. Nevertheless, the success has come at a great cost. Increased life expectancy and birth rates have resulted in an explosive increase in the world's population. Unless the number of humans populating this planet is soon reduced, there will be little purpose in considering the question of slowing the aging process or increasing the human life span. The planet will not be a place it will be worth spending more time. I've decided that there is only one objective that is both practical and desirable. That is to strive for the maximum life span, still in possession of full mental and physical abilities, with death occurring quickly as we approach our 115th birthday. If we are successful, our life expectation will not be increased, but we will eventually die from the basic aging processes that lead to failure in some vital system.

DR. ATKINS VITA-NUTRIENT SOLUTION
ROBERT C. ATKINS, M.D.

For more than thirty years Dr. Atkins forged his protocols and modalities at his center in New York. His basic tenet was to be true to the Hippocratic Oath of "first do no harm," and treat patients as individuals. Everyone is different. That is why Atkins used targeted solutions. He was trained as a cardiologist, but he gained fame as a diet doctor. He coined the term "Complimentary Medicine," which evolved into a lifetime modality that includes proper diet, nutritional supplementation, and exercise. Prescription drugs are a last resort. The result is a way of life that enhances quality, and in the process leads to a vital, happy, and longer life.

Synopsis

What is aging?-- it's what we eat. Americans eat too much sugar, refined carbohydrates, and processed fats. These foods lead to blood sugar disorders, and obesity—the first steps down the road to diabetes and heart disease. A low-carbohydrate, high-protein diet is the single most effective way to lose weight and normalize your blood sugar. Most of the information we are fed by the medical establishment is misleading. It is responsible for the physical and mental decline we call aging. You must learn to defy the authorities and educate yourself to the best techniques for reversing the aging process. The Atkins Center taught everyone the basic programs to get healthy.

Aging is simply the presence of disease. We are told to accept the fact that we are "simply getting older." Nothing could be further from the truth. Aging can be prevented or delayed through diet and vita-nutrients—vitamins, minerals, herbs, etc. Coronary disease was unheard of a century ago. If we can eradicate cardiovascular disease in the 21st century, we could extend our life expectancy by four to six or even twelve years. They would be healthy years.

We have been lied to about heart disease with such an intense barrage of misinformation that even honest researchers are repeating these whoppers. The American Medical Association, the American Dietetic Association, the U.S. Government, and the National Cholesterol Education program (NCEP) all agree to the following:

1. All dietary fats must be restricted, especially saturated fats.
2. Dietary cholesterol must be nearly eliminated.
3. Margarine is healthier than butter.
4. Carbohydrates made with white flour should be the basis of a healthy diet.
5. Eating ten teaspoons of sugar a day is perfectly good for you.

Heart attacks were so rare at the start of the 20th century that the first case was not described until 1912. In 1930, heart attacks caused only 3,000 deaths in the United States. We ate more fats than we do today. And the fats that we ate were mainly butter, lard, and tallow (beef fat) .

Don't these facts demand an explanation? Why was the American diet changed? You'll never get it from the AMA. Here's a little bit of history. After World War II, Ancel Keys, at the University of Minnesota, revealed the conclusions of the Seven Countries Study. It showed that people who ate a high saturated fat diet had higher rates of heart disease. The medical establishment embraced his conclusions. Based on Keys study and others equally flawed, the AHA started a campaign to replace butter, lard, eggs, and beef with corn oil, margarine, and cereal. Everyone fell into line except Dr. Paul Dudley White, (president Dwight D. Eisenhower's physician). He pointed out that he hadn't seen a coronary at Harvard between 1921 and 1928. He said, "Back in the myocardial infarction-free days before 1920, the fats were butter and lard, and I think we would all benefit from that kind of diet." His advice was ignored.

The diet-heart hypothesis was so firmly entrenched that it could not be uprooted. Agribusiness had too much invested in vegetable oils, corn, wheat, and highly profitable processed foods to allow any opposition—and it had the money and the government clout to bulldoze its opponents. The food industry joined the medical establishment to suppress dissenting opinions from such eminent scientists as Dr. Fred Kummerow of the University of Illinois at Urbana, nutritional scientist Dr. Mary Enig, and Dr. George V. Mann of Vanderbilt University. Their funding grants dried up when they published the truth in their studies.

Heart disease is still the leading cause of death in the United States. It killed 727,000 people in 1997. The drop in death rates from cardiovascular disease between 1950 and 2000 can be attributed to the significant decline in cigarette smoking-- 42 percent of adults in 1970 to 30 percent in 1996. Even so, the lifetime risk of developing heart disease is still one in two for men and one in three for women. T.L. Cleave in his book, "The Saccharine Disease," was ahead of his time. The one illness capable of causing premature aging is cardiovascular disease or atherosclerosis. A fatal heart attack is the culmination of a long process of heart disease that starts years earlier. The decline in blood circulation is considered a "normal" part of the process of aging. Do you believe that? Everyone ages, but not everyone gets heart disease. There is nothing normal about atherosclerosis.

The risk of heart disease is caused by oxidized cholesterol. Other risk factors are triglycerides, elevated homocysteine, lipoprotein (a), C-reactive protein, and others. Most patients are given statin drugs, the darlings of the drug industry. Taking these drugs won't help you live any longer. None of the first 80 major studies of cholesterol-lowering drugs demonstrated any significant extension of life expectancy among patients using them. In a recent study of the statin drug lovastatin (Mevacor), those who had heart attacks had three times the death rate of the control group (although there were considerably fewer heart attacks).

There's no question that antioxidant vita-nutrients such as vitamin C and vitamin E are crucial to your health and longevity. A 1995 study showed that taking antioxidant vitamins work by preventing free radical damage to the LDL cholesterol in the blood. It was published in JAMA. Yet, despite clear and convincing evidence that vitamin E life-or-death importance to your health, your conventional doctor may not suggest taking it. By keeping your levels of vita-nutrients high, you protect yourself against the free radical damage that leads to heart disease. You also protect yourself against arthritis, cataracts, and macular degeneration, and you counteract the free radical causes of aging itself.

Superoxides dismutase—(SOD) works with catalase and glutathione to disarm dangerous free radicals. Glutathione is everywhere. Without it, damage would weaken cell membranes until the cell dies. Amino acids are the building blocks of protein. You get them from your food. You need to eat meat, eggs, fish, and dairy products. Eggs are a good source of essential amino acids. Most doctors tell you to eat them sparingly because they think that eggs raise your cholesterol level. An NIH study showed that eating an egg a day doesn't increase the risk of heart disease and stroke for healthy adults.

Co-enzyme Q10—is one of the most valuable nutrients for the heart and an aid in energy dor every cell.

Melatonin—a natural sleeping pill.

Carotenoids—are a group of yellow, orange, and red- substances in the phytochemical family. There are more than 700 different carotenoids. They protect against free radical damage.

Beta-carotene—keeps LDL cholesterol from oxidizing, thereby preventing heart disease.

Lycopenes— are phytochemicals that make tomatoes red. They are found in tomato juice, watermelon, and puree.

Lutein and zeaxanthin—age-related macular degeneration can be avoided through two steps: carotenes, lutein, and zeaxanthin and stopping smoking. Egg yolks are a good source.

Bioflavonoids There are more than 1,000 bioflavonoids. They are completely natural chemicals that give foods their colours and flavours.

Green tea—contains more antioxidants and phytochemicals than any other food or beverage. It contains polyphenols that are powerful antioxidants. The flavonoids in green tea are one hundred times as powerful as vitamin C in quenching free radicals.

Quercetin—is an anti-coagulant that prevents blood clots. The best source is the onion. Other sources are apples, tomatoes, and broccoli.

Garlic—reduces the risk of heart disease. It lowers cholesterol, triglycerides, and blood pressure. A sulphur compound forms as garlic ages. Both fresh garlic and aged garlic are good.

OPCs— oligomeric proanthocyanidins found in grape seeds, berries, and pine tree bark (pycnogenol).

Ginkgo Biloba—improves the flow of blood through your circulatory system. Protects against cataracts and macular degeneration.

Vegetables—cruciferous vegetables like kale and Brusse sprouts reduce the risk of cancer.

Exercise makes you look better, feel better, and stay healthier. Regular physical activity provides heart healthy benefits. Dr. Atkins states that you must undo the damage you've suffered from the dietary mistakes of the 20th century. The so-called food pyramid is a dietary fraud foisted on the public by our own government that has caused Americans to be fatter than ever. Obesity is an epidemic. The food pyramid is heavily based on carbohydrates of the worst sort; refined grains in the form of bread, pasta, and rice. The food pyramid also tells you that protein is bad and fat is worse. You should eat complex carbohydrates such as butternut squash, potatoes, and legumes such as lentils, peas, and beans.

Simple carbohydrates are sugars. They are found in a lot of common foods such as milk (lactose), fruits (fructose), beer (maltose), table sugar (sucrose), sweets, baked goods, to say nothing of candy and soda pop. That is a big change for most people. But the very foods that you think you can't live without are usually the ones that will shorten your life. Do you love jelly doughnuts so much that you are willing to trade ten years of your life for them? I doubt it.

The great beauty of the age-defying diet is that is very easy to stick to it. You'll enjoy steaks, lobster, and an unlimited quantity of fresh vegetables. Sugary foods such as cake and cookies are permanently out the window. White rice, bread, and pasta are very limited and are replaced by whole grains such as brown rice and whole grain bread. There are three components to this diet: proteins and fats, complex carbohydrates, and simple carbohydrates. The following are the foods and proportions of your overall diet.

Proteins and fats—concentrate on meat, poultry, eggs, fish, seafood, nuts, seeds, olives, avocados, fats and oils. The range is 50 percent to 75 percent.

Complex carbohydrates — vegetables, grains, whole grain products (pasta), and legumes (beans). The range is 25 percent to 50 percent.

Simple carbohydrates — fruits, fruit juices, sweets (sugar, honey, maple syrup, etc.) milk and yogurt. The range is less than 10 percent.

The diet is designed to help you live a longer, healthier life. The basic diet is easy to understand and easier to follow. You do need a physician who can monitor your progress, take tests, and interpret the results. You can't do it alone. Dr. Atkins dedicated his life to making the world a better and healthier place. The most convincing argument that can be used for the success that can be achieved by following the recommendations in this plan is having a longer, healthier life.

THE CANCER INDUSTRY
RALPH MOSS, PH.D

The intrigue and mystery of cancer has eluded researchers who have selflessly devoted their lives to the search for a cure. The three modalities that oncologists use are surgery, radiation, and chemotherapy. Unfortunately, they have not been able to stop the inexorable rise of cancer mortality. The Center for Disease Control (CDC) announced in 2006 that cancer is the leading cause of death in the United States. The latest report showed that the total cancer deaths were 556,902 in 2003, down from a high of 557,271 in 2002.

When a researcher discovers a new approach to the cancer problem, it should be a cause for rejoicing. That has never been the case. The tragic truth, as we shall see in this comprehensive book, is that the rigid establishment structure which controls all phases of the cancer business will not yield its grip on the lucrative financial treasure that they have developed over the last 50 years. Ralph Moss has the unique advantage of being an insider. His years at Memorial Sloan-Kettering, the premier cancer facility in New York, as a public relations officer, gave him the background for writing this valuable work. It has also stirred him into shaping a career that has kept the public abreast of all the latest developments in the cancer field.

Synopsis

The emotional toll of cancer is incalculable. Most cancer victims suffer the agony of a painful, disabling, and socially stigmatized disease. They live in fear of the disease and of death. They live in fear of the orthodox treatments; surgery, radiation, and chemotherapy. Men fear castration, physical or chemical, women fear the loss of their sexuality, their breasts, and their womb. These are the bitter facts about cancer.

Equally important is the financial burden. Direct costs of $500 billion according to the Economist in 1988, and costs have increased at twice the rate of inflation. Cancer is not a charity, it is a business—a big business.

There are 50 million visits to physicians each year and American surgeons perform almost one million cancer operations each year. A major turning point came in 1985, when the U.S. government decided to cover MRI tests under Medicare insurance. Physicians buy partnership shares in these facilities. The more patients they send, the more the center earns. The arrangements are wrong because they produce a terrible conflict of interest for a doctor. CAT scans cost $300 each (more today). Dr. William B. Schwartz, a professor of medicine at Tufts University School of Medicine has said, "I find one person with a treatable lesion for every 1,000 CT scans I do." The cost of treatment is so great that cancer without insurance means second rate care and almost certain bankruptcy. 37 million Americans are currently without such coverage. One indication of the profit to be made in the field: an insurance company in Ohio paid out only 40 percent of the premiums paid out by Blue cross.

The current crisis in cancer cries out for new solutions. The personal and national cost of cancer—the suffering, plus the staggering financial waste of it all make new directions not just a dream, but a necessity. Officially all is well with the war on cancer. The cancer establishment exudes optimism about the current methods of managing the disease. Cancer is not just treatable, but curable. In fact, the ACS publication said, "one of the most curable of the major diseases in the country." "Many cancers can be cured if detected early and tested promptly."

A man who is treated for cancer and survives five years is considered cured. What happens if the cancer recurs? What happens if he dies? He will then be in the paradoxical situation of having been officially cured of cancer, and dying of it at the same time. It is obvious that the orthodox treatments have not been able to stop the rise in cancer mortality. There has been a steady increase in the cancer death rate in the 20th century and up to the present time. Cancer accounted for one in 27 deaths in 1900, one in 9 in 1940, one in 7 in 1950, one in 6 in 1960-1970, and one in 5 in 1988 (ACS, 1988).

The most central issue in the case of cancer would seem to be the death rate, which is rising. The ACS's cancer facts and figures show that in 1952 there were approximately 278,000 deaths from cancer in the United States. By 1982 there were 433,000, in 1988 the estimate was 494,000. By 1989 America for the first time had over half a million (and a million new cases). In thirty years the number of victims has nearly doubled. The ACS estimates 556,000 Americans will die from cancer in the year 2003. (The estimate was accurate as the CDC reported 556,002 deaths from all forms of cancer in 2003). The Vietnam War ended in the 1970s in spectacular defeat. In the 1980s the highly touted war on cancer disappeared into the night. The chief cancer warriors, who fought for two decades enjoyed the support of the major media, were never held accountable for the billions and billions spent on cancer research and treatment, nor for a cancer death rate half a million victims a year. A dramatic illustration of the unpredictability of the "proven" methods for diagnosis and treatment is the case of Senator Hubert H. Humphrey. Humphrey was treated for bladder cancer and died in full view of the media. He was a staunch supporter of orthodox cancer research on Capitol Hill. He was diagnosed early and doctors found tiny pinhead non-malignant growths on his bladder in 1966. By 1973 Senator Humphrey had cancer of the bladder. X-ray therapy was successful in treating the cancer. In 1976 Humphrey's doctor declared that there was no reason to prescribe further treatment. A few months later the cancer was back with a vengeance. After surgery on Oct. 1, 1976, Dr. Willard Whitmore appeared before the press and television cameras and declared, "as far as we are concerned, the senator is cured." As a preventive measure experimental drugs were used to "wipe out any microscopic colonies of cancer cells that may be hidden somewhere in the body." Within a year Senator Humphrey was dead.

In that short time he had withered from a vigorous middle-aged man to an old, balding, and feeble cancer victim. Humphrey himself blamed chemotherapy for at least contributing to his demise. He called it bottled death and refused in the end to return to Memorial Hospital for more drug treatments.

Surgery works best on cancers that are detected before they metastasize to other parts of the body and create additional tumors. Once the cancer has spread, surgery is generally useless. Surgery has come under increasing criticism in recent years for a number of other reasons. Some doctors and patients hold that much cancer surgery is unnecessary or excessive in its scope. For years, breast cancer was routinely treated with an operation called the radical mastectomy or the Halstead Procedure. Many leading experts in the field considered the operation unnecessary. The radical mastectomy was not routine in England, France, and Canada, or the Scandinavian countries. Doctors in these countries regarded it as ineffective and unnecessarily brutal. Questions were raised about the wisdom of the procedure since Dr. William Halstead (1852-1922) first widely employed and popularized it in the 1890s at Johns Hopkins University in Baltimore.

The trend is now moving toward more sparing and humane treatment. Stage I and Stage II primary operable breast carcinomas are treated by partial mastectomy (Lumpectomy) plus a standard lymph node removal. This is followed by irradiation of the remaining breast. The therapeutic results are comparable to the older operations which could be physically and psychologically devastating. It should be understood that the fee for the larger operation is also larger. George Bernard Shaw said, "the more appalling the mutilation the more the mutilator is paid." Surgeons create their own demand. In other words, the more surgeons you have the more surgery is going to be done. Surgery is the most frightening of all treatment modalities. It is therefore important to search for safer, more effective, and less traumatic methods of treating cancer.

The second method of treating cancer is radiation therapy. While many in the cancer field have called for radiotherapists, the kinds of cancer that can actually be cured by means of radiation are few. Eighty percent of patients in the early stages of Hodgkins disease (cancer of the lymphatic system) have five or more years of survival after radiation therapy. It is also very effective in cancer of the testicles, cervix, and the prostate. Dr. John Laszlo, of the ACS (American Cancer Society), acknowledges that, "it is impossible to give radiation treatment without injuring normal cells. In remarkably frank language for an ACS official, Laszlo admits that large doses of radiation can cause nausea, vomiting, loss of appetite, and reduction in bone marrow function. Some of these problems exist with chemotherapy. Nevertheless, Laszlo believes that radiation is superior to other methods in a limited number of cases.

Despite the drawbacks, chemotherapy remains a growth industry. The NCI (National Cancer Institute) estimates that 200,000 patients receive cytotoxic drugs nationwide each year. That figure has grown substantially since Moss's book was written. Yet only a few are being cured. The last decade has seen a tremendous growth in the U.S. pharmaceutical industry. The sales of chemotherapeutic agents have kept pace with this upward motion. The actual figure for cancer drug sales is close to $750 million a year, and that figure is growing higher. A large number of drugs come from a few companies. Bristol Myers Squibb controls half the U.S. market. It is hardly coincidental that the board of Memorial Sloan-Kettering has several officers of Bristol Myers Squibb. By pointing this out we don't imply that there is anything illegal or immoral going on. The drug companies predispose them to direct their research in a manner consistent with the interest of the profit-making sector. The "proven" methods of treating cancer are not working. Something radically new is needed. The country is begging for new and fresh approaches that are daring. Where will they come from? Many people believe that they will come from the well-funded orthodox research centers. Another possibility is that the most fundamental breakthrough will come from innovative clinicians of small research laboratories, which have the advantage of independence, so vital to a creative scientist. To the establishment these researchers are not innovators or scientists, they are "quacks." The ACS has a book called "unproven methods of cancer management" that can serve as a guide to orthodox thinking on quackery. While the society claims that the book is only meant to be informative, it is, in fact, a black list that resembles the list of "subversive" organizations once maintained by the house un-American activities committee. Merely including a scientists name on the list, puts the tag of quackery on him and his efforts. It is instructive to know that almost 72 percent of the methods on the unproven methods list have never been shown to be effective by any sort of rational scientific procedure. For only about a dozen methods does the ACS offer documented evidence of failure. This represents less than 20 percent of the total.

Were these methods subjected to adequate investigation before they were condemned? The answer would have to be no. Included in this "ineffective" category are such therapies as laetrile, hydrazine sulphate, krebiozen, the Gerson Method, the Hoxsey method, Glover's serum, Koch antitoxins and Revici cancer control. In no case was a double-blind study carried out on any of these procedures before it was condemned. The society appears to have made an "a priori" judgment on the worthlessness of uncommon cancer therapies, and then stretched the facts to fit its preconception. Not all of these methods are valid, and some are fraudulent, but they remain a repository of new ideas from which cancer scientists should be able to draw freely. The stigma of quackery prevents them from doing so. Pat McGrady Sr. summed it up well. "The establishment has turned the terror of this ugly disease to its own ends in seeking more and more contributions from a frightened public and appropriations from a concerned congress. Still, undismayed by the futility of funds dumped into a bottomless barrel of its "proven" methods, it remains adamant in refusing to investigate "unproven" methods."

NUTRITION IN A NUTSHELL
ROGER WILLIAMS, PH.D.

Roger Williams, the dean of American nutritionists, who discovered pantothenic acid and folic acid, repeatedly refers to this work as "this little book." This is something of a misnomer, for the significance is anything but "little." As both a biochemist and a nutritionist, the author is uniquely qualified to write about the subject of nutrition. Biochemistry has risen to the level of a separate branch of science, and those who wish to specialize in the area of nutrition must restrict their studies to that subject. Physicians, who are usually specialists in a particular area of medicine, do not really learn about nutrition. Williams states, "The future relationships between medicine, biochemistry, and nutrition are uncertain." This book is a simple, succinct, yet comprehensive outline of nutrition geared to the general public.

Synopsis

The food we eat is needed by all the cells in our body. All living cells require a multitude of nutrients. Nutrition is like a chain in which all of the essential items are like separate links. If the chain is weak or broken at any point, the whole chain fails. The absolute lack of any item, or several items, results in ill health and disease. It is not necessary that every item be furnished in required amounts at every meal or every day because our bodies always carry some reserves.

Glucose, which is necessary for brain nutrition function, can be produced in the body from proteins."Glucose puts an unnatural load on our pancreatic glands and aggravates the diabetic condition."This statement is based purely on ignorance. Glucose is the fuel on which our bodies run. We burn up nearly a pound each day. The amount in our blood at any time is small (about one-third of an ounce total), but it is replenished continually. It is essential for the nourishment of our brains, and if the level in the blood gets too low we pass into a coma.

This is the same glucose we buy in corn syrup. Natural glucose is obtained by digesting starch.

Nutrition and biochemistry are dynamic, developing sciences. Cholesterol is an important constituent of our bodies, but it is manufactured within our bodies. In some individuals, too much is produced. However, meticulous care in the avoidance of cholesterol in the diet is not warranted. A complete diet should include leaves, roots, tubers, seeds, and fruits. For the majority of Americans a diversified diet made up of plant and animal foods seems most appropriate.

Let us look at two relatively perfect foods: Milk (and dairy products) and eggs. Milk is a relatively perfect food for young animals including young children. It lacks iron—but it has many virtues. The nutrition of most people would be improved if they consumed more milk. Cheeses and other dairy products have many of the advantages possessed by milk itself. Eggs are valuable as a relatively complete food because each egg has everything required to build a complete baby chick. Cellular malnutrition, which is the basis of malnutrition, is probably at the root of 10 times as many disease conditions as rickets, scurvy, beriberi, pellagra, night blindness, and kwashiorkor. Red blood cells (5 billion per thimbleful), have oxygen-carrying bright red protein: haemoglobin. These red cells (corpuscles) are unusual, as body cells go, because by the time they mature (in mammals) they have lost their nuclei and have no powers of reproduction. They persist in the body for a few weeks until they are worn out and have to be replaced with new ones. The production of these new replacement cells involves extensive protein synthesis.

Anaemia involves a deficiency of these corpuscles or of their haemoglobin content. Without sufficient iron people and animals become anaemic. This is because haemoglobin contains iron as one of its basic ingredients. Lack of copper, vitamin B-12 (cobalt), folic acid, niacin, pyridoxine, or ascorbic acid—any one of these—produce anaemia when they are not constituents of hemoglobin.

The answer is simply this: the living cells which give rise to the red cells need these other items in order to produce hemoglobin and the red cells that contain it. Anything that can cripple these living cells is capable of producing anemia. It is revealing that so many different individual lacks have actually been proven to produce this disease.

Coronary heart disease kills more than 500,000 people annually in the

United States. The unhealthy condition of the artery wall, the deposition of cholesterol, and the tendency of the blood to clot may all be influenced by nutrition. The avoidance of cholesterol in the diet is not of prime importance because cholesterol is produced in our bodies when we consume none whatever. Hydrogenated fats, which are partially hydrogenated (margarine), are inferior in this respect to the original oil from which they are made. Good nutrition helps maintain healthy blood vessels which do not rupture easily and prevents the formation of plugs which stops blood flow.

Excessive carbohydrate consumption is contraindicated in diabetes. It is desirable that carbohydrates be produced within the body from proteins and certain other food constituents. A diabetic needs a completely adequate diet so that his pancreas, liver, adrenals, and pituitary are fully nourished. Excellent nutrition will prevent the development of diabetes. I know that there are millions of intelligent people in our country who would benefit from a better understanding of nutrition. However, if someone wants to eat heartily, grow fat, and "enjoy" life as long as it lasts, that is his right. Who needs to be educated?—everyone—everybody. It is essential that the public, including the oncoming generation of boys and girls, be educated as to nutrition and its present and future possibilities.

Who are the experts? They are trained biochemists who direct their attention to nutritional problems. They must be at home with the complex interrelationships between amino acids, mineral, vitamins, proteins, fats, carbohydrates, enzymes, hormones, nucleic acids, etc. Food manufacturers should assume the responsibility for the nutritional value of the products they sell. They should have nutritional experts who can help them produce products that are tasty, saleable, and nutritiously beneficial. Advice is easy to give, but my aim is to give good advice. I will list this advice under five main headings. Remember— every individual is distinctive and has different needs.

1. Don't be a hypochondriac—in essence, too much worry about your health can be responsible for unhinging the health you have.

2. Diversify your diet—as much as possible consider eating the following types of foodstuffs: Milk and dairy products; seed (including nut) products; meat and poultry; fish and marine products; leafy green vegetables, roots and tubers, including carrots and potatoes; fruits of all

kinds, including melons and tomatoes; fungi-yeast; mushrooms and truffles; and eggs.

3. Use and cultivate your body wisdom. Show intelligence and discrimination in your choice of food. When a hostess insists that you should eat more after you have eaten all you can stand, resist the pressure and refuse to eat more. Also, consistent, moderate exercise stimulates the circulation of blood and brings nourishment and oxygen to all the tissues. Exercise also decreases the appetite and promotes mental relaxation. In view of the known relationships between exercise, obesity, and longevity, it is hard to escape the conclusion that our sedentary way of life is harmful.

4. Avoid too much refined food. Sugar, alcohol, highly milled rice and white flour are empty calories that add no nutritional value to your diet. Substitute milk for a soft drink at mealtime.

5. Use nutritional supplements when informed opinion deems it desirable.

NUTRIENTS TO AGE WITHOUT SENILITY
ABRAM HOFFER, M.D., PH.D.

Aging is inevitable. Senility is a brain disease and a mental disease. Senility is not the same as aging. Everybody ages, but not everybody becomes senile. A healthy young adult has about 12 billion neurons, or nerve cells. Each day, the brain loses about 100,000 neurons. They get used up and die. Sixty or more years of losing these irreplaceable brain cells cause dementia and senility. On average, 25 percent of people over 75 years of age or older are senile. The number is growing. The reason is malnutrition. Senile people lose themselves in time. They fail to recognize their spouses, sons and daughters. They are helpless and require shelter, protection, and devoted nursing care.

Synopsis

Our bodies have 60 trillion cells. Our brain has its lifetime maximum at birth. By age 60 we have lost 50 percent of our taste buds, and 40 percent of our smell. Muscles lack tone, especially the face and the back of the arm. We have a clock of aging. Skin loses its elasticity. It is dry and wrinkled and it looks like parchment. Nutrition can restore elasticity. Hair turns gray, nails get brittle, and muscle mass is reduced. Skeletal changes occur as we age. Skeletons shrink, bones become thinner, weaker, and more fragile. Approximately 25 percent of women and 6 percent of men 65 or older suffer fractures of the femur and hips. Atherosclerotic plaques develop in the blood vessels. The walls of the arteries grow inelastic, heart valves become thicker, and fat and connective tissue gather around the heart. The reserve capacity of the kidneys is decreased by 50 percent, but there is enough to maintain correct fluid and mineral balance. Elderly people drink too little water. Twenty-five percent of the people in mental hospitals are dehydrated. A zinc deficiency causes a decreased taste for food and a diminished sense of thirst.   Lung function reduces with age.   Gas exchanges decrease when muscles get weaker.   The chest wall becomes less elastic and respiration is not as deep.   By the age of 90, the brain loses one-fourth of its weight.   Up to 30 percent of the neurons in a generic brain may be lost.   Many people look, feel, and behave far younger than their chronological age.   This is achieved by careful discipline involving orthomolecular nutrition, an optimal diet, and exercise.   This is the way to slow down the aging process.

Senility is a state of neuron inactivity brought on by anaerobic respiration of the cells.   If aerobic respiration is maintained at its optimum level, no one will become senile.   A number of observations have developed our hypothesis regarding senility.   Hyperbaric oxygen removed senility temporarily.   We knew that the lack of oxygen (anaerobic) had the effect of causing cancer.   This produced our hypothesis.   Otto Warburg won a Nobel Prize in (1931) because of his basic work with respiratory enzymes and cellular metabolism.   He discovered and characterized the pyridine nucleotide dehydrogenases and flavoproteins as members of the respiratory chain and worked out the mechanism whereby the energy released in the oxygenation of foodstuffs may be conserved and transferred for use in synthesis and growth.   The mechanism of cellular respiration provided the first explanation of the chemical mechanism of enzyme action.   Warburg showed that there was a relationship between aerobic respiration and cancer growth when ordinary cells in pure culture are forced to live in an atmosphere which does not have enough oxygen.   They switch the respiratory mechanism from one depending on oxygen (called aerobic), to one not dependent on oxygen (called anaerobic).   This change is apparently irreversible.   Even more important, the anaerobic cells begin to divide.   They are no longer subject to the usual growth controls and eventually become cancerous.   Warburg explained that cancer tissue was correlated with the degree of anaerobic conditions.   The less oxygen there was available to the tissue, the more rapid was its growth.   Rapidly growing tissues are generally more malignant than slow growing cancers.   Albert Szent-Gyorgyi said, "The cancerous state is a reversal to a more primitive state of the cell.   In order to remain alive, the cell reverts to an anaerobic form of respiration.   It can live in a very low oxygen tension, where non-transformed cells would soon die."   Nicotinamide-adenine-dinucleotide (NAD) made in the body from vitamin B3 enhances oxidative respiration. Warburg suggested that everyone ensure optimum levels of oxygen-carrying coenzymes B1, B2, and B3. Warburg's theory of dedifferentiation meant that evolution began with cells which lived without oxygen—in an anaerobic environment. Later on, enough oxygen developed in our atmosphere to allow cells to develop aerobic respiration. This condition is much more efficient in converting food into energy. Multi-cellular organisms didn't develop until cells became aerobic. Single-celled species has only one function—to divide (anaerobic respiration). Aerobic respiration permits growth as well as other functions. This is Warburg's theory of dedifferentiation—"Cells which switch from aerobic to anaerobic respiration." This leads to primitive cell division among those cells still retaining the ability to divide. Neurons never regenerate. There are no neuron cancers. Neurons can't divide. Dedifferentiation of neurons cannot cause cancer since neurons in the cortex are no longer able to carry on their main function and don't divide. They simply become quiescent. The result is senility. This is our hypothesis—"Senescence is neuron quiescence."

Abram Hoffer is an orthomolecular psychiatrist who has performed Nobel quality work in his home country of Canada. For more than 50 years he has proved the efficacy of niacin (B3) in the treatment of schizophrenia starting with prisoners of war who returned from Japanese prison camps in emaciated condition. Hoffer was using the orthomolecular approach years before the term was coined in 1968 by double Nobel Laureate Linus Pauling. Hoffer feels that niacin is a core nutrient along with other antioxidants for maintaining optimal health. It improves the quality of life and offers the potential for a healthier and longer life expectancy.

The closer one is to senility, the more difficult it is to prevent it. We blame the consumption of food artifacts—junk food. Good food is not enough—exercise and physical fitness is just as important. Why prolong life if we can't enjoy the added years? Stress is a limiting factor in the longevity of adult people. Hans Selye has said, "Complete freedom from stress is death." Optimal nutrition and exercise can overcome exposure to stress. Many people look, feel, and behave far younger than their chronological age. This is achieved by careful discipline involving orthomolecular nutrition, and optimal diet and exercise. This is the way to slow down the aging process. In Greece, during the Golden Age life expectancy was about 18 years—since most people died at birth or in infancy. Pericles funeral oration was delivered at the age of 69. Charlemagne (Charles the Great) ruled until 81. He handed the reins of power to his son when he was 71 when people lived an average of 22 years. Michaelangelo executed the Pieta when he was 80. Life expectancy was 32. Goethe was 84 when "Faust" was published. Disraeli became prime minister when he was 70. Life expectancy was 47. Sir Winston Churchill was 65 in 1939. He died in 1965 at the age of 89. There was no senility for these remarkable figures of history. Genes require a suitable environment for their expression. We can try to provide an optimal environment, so that even the weakest gene will serve us so much better. "My 66-year-old mother was under stress because my father was dying of prostate cancer. She was losing vision in one eye, her memory was failing and she had swollen joints. My staff and I were using niacin (nicotinic acid to lower cholesterol and triglycerides, which has an anti-atherosclerotic effect. Years ago Dr. William Kaufman in Bridgeport, Connecticut discovered that it cures common forms of arthritis. I gave my mother a 3 month's supply of niacin with the advice of taking one gram after each meal. Six weeks later I received a letter in London. She regained her vision, her memory was normal, and her arthritis was gone (Heberden bumps). Niacin therapy definitely prevents senility. This remarkable vitamin should be part of any treatment program against senility. My mother died at 87 after sustaining a stroke at 82. For 21 years she took one to four grams of niacin every day. I added vitamin C and vitamin E and other nutrients. Some people are old at 40 and others appear youthful at 80. We have the ability to approach the full span of human existence—120 years—with alert, creative, memory-filled minds. Nutritional information won't make you live longer, but it will increase the potential for a healthier life expectancy and quality of life."

DR. ATKINS' HEALTH REVOLUTION
ROBERT C. ATKINS, M.D.

The late Dr. Robert C. Atkins coined the term "complementary medicine" as his solution to the dilemma of which medicine, alternative or orthodox to select. Why not use the best of both? This book describes a whole range of treatment for diseases such as diabetes, hypoglycaemia, candida albicans, heart disease, multiple sclerosis, arthritis and cancer. Case histories of patients at the Atkins Center spotlight the benefits of nutrition-oriented treatment. Under the banner of complementary medicine, Dr. Atkins heralds the medicine of the future; a patient-oriented system that seeks the root cause of diseases. There will be a continuous search for nutritional substances that are effective and safe, with no side effects. The emphasis will be on prevention of disease through dietary means, without discarding orthodox medicines life-saving methods.

Synopsis

The history of medicine has been a constant tug-of-war between two approaches to healing: the rationalist tradition which led to medical orthodoxy we have today, and the empiricist school which evolved into alternative medicine. Hippocrates, the Greek physician whose oath doctors take at graduation, is clearly empirical. He taught physicians to work with nature, the best healer. His most significant dictum is, "primum non nocere" --- first, do no harm. Empiricism sees the human body as an integrated whole with its own healing process. Aristotle developed the rationalist, and Galen created a rationalist medicine. Rationalists treat opposites: if blood pressure is too high, lower it; if you have diarrhea, stop it; for a headache, kill the pain. Dr. Benjamin Rush best exemplified rationalist medicine. He used large doses of powerful minerals, blisters, cold baths, and bloodletting. While empirical medicine saw man in harmony with nature, rationalists viewed medicine as a struggle between man and nature.

The American Medical Association, established in 1949, serves as the voice of rationalist medicine to combat the empiricist enemy, alternative therapists. For more than one hundred and sixty years the AMA has dedicated itself to its economic self-interest, allied with the pharmaceutical industry that the Civil War gave rise to. After the war, proprietary medicines—patent medicines with identifying labels, were sold directly to the public. Advertisements indicated the specific disease which these medicines cured. Thus, physicians were relieved of the need to use their own techniques to cure patients. By 1916 there were 39,000 different patent medicines.

The pathologists of the 19th century defined diseases, creating diagnoses so that patients could be pigeonholed. As microscopes grew more powerful, and Pasteur, Koch, and others demonstrated that most illness was caused by microorganisms, the movement away from empiricism intensified. World War II ushered in the world of antibiotics, providing orthodox medicine great support in the conviction that man was a greater healer than nature. Double blind controlled experiments developed by Sir John Osler, chief physician at Johns Hopkins, became orthodoxy's religion. The Flexner report on medical education in 1910 unified the curriculum and enforced an emphasis on pharmaceuticals. Small medical schools went out of business. Those who survived adopted the uniform curriculum, with no courses in nutrition. The doctors' reliance on drugs alone to treat patients led to the total domination of orthodox medicine by a large and continually expanding pharmaceutical industry. Nevertheless, empirical medicine survived, mostly in Europe and the orient.

For almost a century orthodox medicine has been pursuing a "magic bullet" philosophy—every disease has a specific, usually pharmaceutical cure. Now, most infectious diseases—tuberculosis, syphilis, leprosy, smallpox, polio, and diphtheria have been wiped out, but we still have disease. Heart disease, arthritis, diabetes, and cancer are caused by our lifestyle. There are no magic bullets for them. Orthodox rationalist medicine uses reason and logic, what is known and what can be proved; alternative empirical medicine deals in what works, what has worked, what seems to work, and what promises to work. Alternativists identify health as balance, and disease as an absence of balance. Drugs only substitute one imbalance for another and cannot help unless there is a disease. Nutrients work in the absence of illness, and when given in optimum amounts can lead to the best of health. Both medical camps agree that it is better to prevent illness than to cure it once it is established, but the preventive medicine taught in medical schools is a science of populations and not individuals, and is woefully inadequate. Preventive medicine is the exercise of nutrition-based alternative medicine. Orthodox medicine has a formalized structure, centered around the teaching hospital, with a belief system, a ritual, and a profound faith, much like a religion. The very basis of complementary practice considers the patient as a whole and how a healing prescription must affect the whole being, in itself a humbling experience. The orthodox physician takes complete charge of the treatment, usually with prescription drugs that answer a specific complaint about one part of the body. The alternative camp asks the patient to take care of his own healing. Neither alternative nor orthodox medicine is the only answer. If a treatment works hundreds or thousands of times, why not use it? When it was shown that an aspirin resulted in 50 percent fewer heart attacks it was adopted as a therapy for heart disease. Fish oils are now becoming accepted as a cholesterol-lowering nutritional treatment, and immunology is gradually replacing toxic chemotherapy in the treatment of cancer. It can happen on a grand scale and this book can be a catalyst to that end. Heart disease is the nation's biggest killer, claiming more than 500,000 lives each year. "An orthodox cardiologist, even if he is chief of service at a medical school is probably not the best person to be treating a person for heart disease." An orthodox physician is almost certain to insist that you follow a diet that that restricts fats, salt, calories, and cholesterol. It is ironic that the medical establishment is suggesting a nutritional regimen, when they have never bothered to learn the specifics of good nutritional therapy. The 1984 Coronary Artery Surgery Study followed almost 25,000 participants under 65 years of age. Half had been treated with drugs and the other half had undergone bypass surgery. Those who were operated on showed no life-saving advantage over the drug therapy. In all cases where acute intervention was not absolutely required, a specific diet could have been prescribed to reverse the underlying causes of heart disease. A controversial treatment, chelation therapy, now offers the best chance of reversing heart disease without surgery or medication. Chelation (from the Greek word claw), a well-kept secret those who desperately need it to avoid the more dangerous bypass surgery, uses a "grabber" molecule, EDTA (ethylenediaminetetraaceticacid), commonly used in the treatment of lead poisoning, EDTA "improves circulatory function by removing toxic metals such as cadmium, lead, calcium, and iron from the body, binding with the loose, free-floating ions in the bloodstream and passing them from the body. Chelation is not a hospital procedure. It takes three hours in a doctor's office, and when you are finished you can go to work or even play your favourite sport. A typical program of chelation treatment can involve 25 to 50 visits over six to 12 months. A prescribed nutritional regimen accompanies the chelation therapy, to restore essential minerals and trace elements that have been excreted along with the toxic metals. In spite of 35 years of success with over 1,000,000 patients, orthodox medicine refuses to consider chelation therapy.

Orthodox and complementary physicians seem to agree that prevention is the best way to avoid heart disease. But to condemn cholesterol as the one villain, as medical orthodoxy does, and to ask the public to be in mortal fear of any highly nutritious food that might contain any cholesterol, is at the very least simplistic. Eggs, milk, beef, and butter are necessary for a well-rounded diet. Avoiding them in your diet may cause the very thing you are trying to prevent. Cholesterol, for all the unwarranted fear of the public, is essential for good health. Why would the body produce 1,500 milligrams of cholesterol every day for no good purpose? If you eat no cholesterol at all your liver will manufacture it. An American study showed that people with a blood cholesterol of 200 to 225 milligrams lived longer than people with levels of 150 to 200. Very low levels of cholesterol are associated with malignant and wasting diseases.

Complementary medicine is the real frontier in healing techniques. It encompasses the employment of antioxidants, gamma-linolenic acid (GLA), EPA (omega3 fish oils), mineral transporters (orotates), taurine, carnitine, bromelain, co-enzymeQ10, quercetin, pantrthine, caprylic acid, and octocosanol.

The new medicine is here.. But the medical power structure is pouring billions of dollars to maintain its own dominance. The outcome of the struggle is up to the public. There will be no help from the government, the medical profession, or the pharmaceutical industry. They are opposed to change and dedicated to the status quo. This is your revolution and it is up to you to open up your physician's mind to the things you've learned in this book. It takes an outraged public to effect change. You have the clout. Use it. Your very life is at stake.

MENTAL AND ELEMENTAL NUTRIENTS
CARL C. PFEIFFER, M.D.

Carl C. Pfeiffer firmly believes that good nutrition is the answer to the mammoth task of preventing disease in America. He is convinced that the well-nourished American is a mythical entity, and recites the work of Drs. Cheraskin and Ringsdorf, who report that 80 percent of the nation's population may be undernourished. This doesn't mean that most of us are near death; malnutrition is not the same as starvation. It simply means that any undiagnosed subclinical deficiency of trace elements or protein may cause damage to the body or brain. According to Pfeiffer, most doctors do not have the proper training in clinical nutrition and will not admit that nutrition is a problem that deserves their attention. This book clearly emphasizes a preventive approach to disease, rather than mere treatment of health problems after they develop. Pfeiffer's key to prevention is great nutrition.

Synopsis

In relation to any other material used as a food additive Proper eating habits promote productivity and longevity, while poor eating habits cause weakness and disease by depriving the cells and tissues of essential substances. More than 50 percent of Americans eat a nutrition-free diet that is high in saturated fats and refined carbohydrates. Fats account for 40 percent of the calories in the average daily diet. While a certain amount of fat (preferably unsaturated) is needed to absorb the fat-soluble vitamins A, D, E, and K and for several other functions, the body is not equipped to handle the large amount of fats in our diet. According to Denis Burkitt, refined carbohydrates lead to a high bacterial count and slow bowel movements. Dr. John Yudkin, a sugar researcher states, "If only a fraction of what is already known about the effects of sugar were to be revealed in relation to any other material used as a food additive, that material would promptly be banned."

If the current eating patterns of Americans continue, the general health of the country will deteriorate to the point where American civilization would enter a path of historical decline.

Before starting any weight control program, one should have a physical check-up to eliminate the possibility of serious physical malfunctions, such as a gland condition. Crash diets can be dangerous, for they can result in trace element depletion which will often produce "depression and even hallucinations." Any weight reducing regimen should include a nutritionally sound diet and regular exercise. A strong motivation or desire to succeed is fundamental; staying power is the requisite for a dieter. The dieter must avoid empty calories and concentrate on wholesome foods such as fish, poultry, lean meat, eggs, milk, and dairy products, green, yellow, and orange vegetables; citrus and other fruits and fruit juices; and whole grain cereals and breads. You should also supplement your diet with a mineral-free multivitamin tablet; two doses a day of 20 milligrams of zinc gluconate, 200 milligrams of B-6, and Brewer's yeast. Brewer's yeast is the best source of the B-complex vitamins. The consumption of eggs in this country has dropped precipitously in the past 40 years. In 1945, the average American ate 405 eggs a year. In 1973, the average was 292 a year. We should instead be eating two eggs a day, or 700 a year. The reduced consumption over the years is largely due to the adverse publicity that branded the egg as the cause of increased cholesterol levels. Yet studies have shown that consumption of eggs does not substantially raise blood cholesterol in the body.

A. J. Svacha et al at Auburn, Alabama, fed three eggs a day to 14 normal men. The non-smokers in that group registered only a slight rise in blood cholesterol levels. The smokers, on the other hand, had a significant 27 percent rise in cholesterol levels. A study in Japan compared 31 young men with 10 middle-aged men. N. Takeuchi and Y. Yamamura of Osaka gave nine egg yolks per day to individuals in each group. The young men had an average rise of two milligrams of cholesterol per egg. The middle-aged group had a rise of four milligrams per egg. Eggs are an excellent food. They are low in fat, rich in protein and vitamin A, low in calories, and economical. They contain choline, tryptophan, pyridoxine, biotin, folic acid, riboflavin, thiamine, pantothenic acid, selenium, zinc, phosphorus, calcium, and sulphur. (Sulphur and selenium are essential for skin, hair, fingernails, and toenails). We should not blame eggs for heart disease: "It would be wiser to concentrate on correcting an otherwise poor diet." High cholesterol levels occur when one's diet consists primarily of refined junk foods that lack essential trace elements.

In the early 1900s, Joseph Goldberger did research in the south and discovered that both pellagra and mental illness arose out of a dietary deficiency. He published nutrition studies on pellagra in 1928, but died prematurely in 1929. C. Elvehjem at the University of Minnesota was intrigued by Goldberger's work and followed it through to find the deficient substance in 1937. It was nicotinic acid, which is most often found in the liver. B-3 or niacin (other names for nicotinic acid), was therefore discovered, and since it has been added to processed flour in the United States, pellagra has almost disappeared. Niacin is also helpful in treating other diseases, especially when it is taken in large doses. Dr. Humphrey Osmond and Dr. Abram Hoffer of the University of Saskatchewan used niacin and vitamin C in daily doses of three grams to successfully treat psychotics and schizophrenics. It also aids in alleviating the pain of arthritis and keeps blood cholesterol levels down. By now, most people know that vitamin C prevents scurvy, but few realize, or are willing to admit, the wide variety of the benefits it offers. One of the body's strongest antioxidants, it keeps drugs that are easily oxidized in a stable state, it metabolizes the amino acids phenylalamine and tyrosine, folic acid coenzymes , which are vital for patients with megaloblastic anemia. Vitamin C regulates the respiratory cycle of cellular mitochondria and corpuscles; it greatly increases the absorption of iron in the intestines; collagen cannot form without ascorbate; it is an anti-stress factor; it promotes the healing of wounds, removes toxic substances from the body, and can lower blood cholesterol levels; it also prevents the formation of potentially carcinogenic nitrosamines in cured meats. The Russians have even reported success in using vitamin C to retard the aging process. The optimal dosage of vitamin C is a continuing source of controversy. The Food and Nutrition Board recommends 60 milligrams a day while Linus Pauling suggests 2,000 milligrams. The rat produces 2.4 grams per day, which is the equivalent to the amount Pauling recommends. Yet, the body's plasma level returns to normal in 12 to 13 hours no matter how much is taken. To maintain the equilibrium of the serum C level, you should take the vitamin several times a day. No harm is done with oral doses of three to four grams a day of vitamin C. The B- complex vitamins play a vital role in maintaining physical and mental health.

The study of trace elements is essential to good health is now at an exciting stage—comparable, in fact, to that of vitamins in the 1970s. The scientific community eagerly awaits new discoveries. An example is the "glucose tolerance factor" (GTF), an organic molecule containing chromium is being developed by Walter Mertz to lower cholesterol levels, make insulin more active, and generally help the hypoglycemic patient. Although aging cannot be prevented, good nutrition will help us enjoy happier and longer lives. By avoiding toxins that cause cellular degeneration, we can retard the deterioration process that begins in childhood. We must avoid processed foods whenever possible, for in the refining process they lose up to half of their vitamin and mineral value. Not only are all the known nutrients removed from the whole foods, but also all the undiscovered vitamins and trace elements. "Man cannot make an artificial orange juice, lemon juice, or egg that is as nutritious as the natural product. Processed and synthetic foods simply cannot replace nutrient-rich natural foods in promoting the good life."

BODY, MIND, AND SUGAR
E.M. ABRAHAMSON, M.D.
AND A.W. PEZET

This book arose out of Dr. Abrahamson's experience treating A.W. Pezet and his wife for hyperinsulinism (more commonly called hypoglycemia). Pezet, a professional writer specializing in medical and scientific projects for the layman, was astonished to find that so little was known about a disease that affects millions. He and Abrahamson joined forces to produce a book that explores the extraordinary relationship between body and mind, and the role that blood sugar plays in keeping the two in healthy balance.

Synopsis

The chronicling of diabetes is a fascinating record of the march of medical progress through the ages. A papyrus circa 1,500 B.C. gives a number of prescriptions for medicines to drive away the passage of too much urine (a sure sign of diabetes).. Seventeen hundred years later and 500 years after Hippocrates, Aretaeus the Cappadocian gave the first accurate account of diabetes, and in so doing also suggested the origin of the name. He wrote, "The fluid uses the patient's body as a ladder to escape downward." The Greek word for ladder is "diabeton." Webster's unabridged dictionary derives diabetes from the Latin for the Greek word meaning "to stand with the legs wide apart," as in the position of a ladder. Aretaeus had no idea of the cause or the proper treatment for diabetes. It was not until 13 centuries later that Thomas Willis described the "sweet taste of diabetic urine."The adjective "mellitus" was soon applied to the name (derived from the Latin root "mel" meaning honey), though it was still a mystery as to why sweetness had anything to do with the disease. An argument between Oskar Minkowski and his associate Von Mering over the necessity of the pancreas carried the story of diabetes into the 19th century. In 1889 they removed the pancreas of a dog to see if the animal could live without it. The dog died. They repeated the experiment with other dogs and the results were the same. Before the dogs died, the urine was recorded as containing 5 percent to 10 percent sugar. This discovery led to the determination that it is the pancreas which monitors the body's blood sugar levels. Finally, after 3,000 years, scientists could trace diabetes to the pancreas. The pancreas is a gland six to eight inches long that resembles a bunch of grapes. It lies transversely along the rear wall of the abdomen with its head touching the first part of the small intestine and its tail close to the spleen. A primary function of the pancreas is to secrete fluids that help digest proteins, fats, and carbohydrates. There are two ducts that carry these pancreatic juices into the intestine. There are other digestive juices in the intestine, some from the stomach, and other from the intestine itself. In 1869, a young medical student named Langerhans discovered a group of cells in the pancreas that were unrelated to the rest of the gland. They were given the name, "islands of Langerhans and were found to be ductless. No one knew why they were there. In 1900 a man named Opie performed an autopsy on a girl who had died in a diabetic coma. The only part of her body that was abnormal proved to be the islands of Langerhans in the pancreas. In 1916, the research team of Sharpey and Schafer suggested that diabetes was due to a lack of some secretion from the islands of Langerhans. They named the undiscovered hormone insulin.

Dr. Frederick Grant Banting and Charles H. Best , a medical student subsequently operated on a dog and tied the ducts carrying the pancreatic juice to the intestine. The dog's pancreas could not dispose of its secretion, which then backed up and produced a degeneration of the pancreatic tissue. It did not, however, injure the Islands of Langerhans tissue, and the dog did not develop diabetes. After several weeks, these degenerated pancreases were removed from the experimental dogs. Extracts were made from them and injected into diabetic dogs—who remained alive and in good health for a long period of time. Banting concluded that insulin is produced in the Islands of Langerhans, and that insulin is what kept the dogs alive. His epochal discovery saved millions of lives in the generations that followed. When insulin became commercially available, the diabetics' chances of survival took a sharp upward swing. In recognition of his work on insulin Banting was awarded the Nobel Prize. When we eat carbohydrates, they are digested and converted to glucose (animal sugar), which passes through the intestinal tract into the bowel. The glucose-enriched blood goes through the liver via a portal vein. Since there is no insulin in this blood, the sugar passes unchanged through the liver into general circulation, resulting in a higher blood sugar level. When the enriched blood reaches the pancreas, the rise in blood sugar stimulates the insulin machinery into action. Insulin is secreted by the Islands of Langerhans into the blood and is carried through a portal vein back to the liver. The sugar-rich portions of the blood are then filtered out and stored as glycogen so that the blood leaving the liver contains the proper amount of sugar. If the insulin supply is inadequate, however, the liver cannot effectively convert sugar to glycogen, and too much sugar is washed into the bloodstream. The blood sugar level rises and remains high, which characterizes diabetes. A disease discovered two years after Banting solved the diabetics' major problem when the insulin supply is too high, thereby driving the blood sugar level down too low. This condition, originally labelled hyperinsulinism, has more recently acquired the name hypoglycaemia.

In 1924, (only one year after insulin was in general use), Dr. Seale Harris, a professor of medicine at the University of Alabama, noticed that many people who were not diabetic and were not taking insulin were nonetheless showing the symptoms of insulin shock. He found their blood sugar level t o be abnormally low and called the condition hyperinsulinism. He maintained that it arises when an individual secretes an excessive amount of insulin. Dr. Harris then devised a six-hour glucose tolerance test to analyze the blood sugar level at hourly intervals. He was amazed to find that the curve plotted from the data from the first three hours were roughly the same for diabetics as they were for those suffering from hyperinsulinism.

There are now a host of facts to demonstrate that hyperinsulinism is responsible for the development of ulcers, asthma, and rheumatic fever. Medical books give the normal level of blood sugar as 80 to 180 milligrams per cubic centimetres (cc) of blood. This is the normal fasting level, though, and fasting is not a normal condition. The truly "normal" blood sugar level during the waking, working, and eating hours of the day should be an average of 140 milligrams per 100 cc. A person suffering from hyperinsulinism has a much lower level that leads to a chronic blood sugar starvation. Sugar (in the form of glucose) is required to nourish all the cells of the body. If adequate nourishment is denied, sooner or later some weak spot will break down and cause a problem.. For example, a World War II x-ray specialist diagnosed frequent cases of peptic ulcers in men saturating themselves with caffeine and sugar. Too much sugar leads to an overproduction of insulin that in turn lowers the blood sugar level too far. Thus, the staggering increase by children and teenagers in the consumption of sugar-laden, caffeine-rich carbonated drinks will undoubtedly have some effect on the incidence of diseases that result from chronic blood sugar starvation. Dr. Harris's great discovery is only vaguely known to most physicians. His findings have been challenged and ignored. Millions of Americans suffering from hyperinsulinism are being treated for heart ailments, epilepsy, brain tumors, hysteria, and neuroses. Dr. Stanley A. Portis of the University of Illinois suggests that the trouble with hyperinsulinism is that it cannot be packaged, publicized, and sold over-the-counter in a drugstore. Its treatment demands sacrifices from the patient, who must avoid candy, sugar, pies, alcohol, coffee, and sometimes smoking. Doctors prefer to write a prescription for a miracle drug than order their patients to develop habits of self-denial. Although Dr. Harris received an achievement award from the AMA (given only 12 times in the 100 years of existence), the truer reward would have been the recognition of his work and its application to millions of suffering Americans.

REVERSING ASTHMA
RICHARD N. FIRSHEIN, DO

One cannot minimize the magnitude of the problem that asthma presents to America. More than 15 million people suffer from this disease. The financial cost is great, but the toll of human misery is immeasurable. Dr. Richard N. Firshein is not merely a reporter or researcher who studies a subject and objectively reports the clinical findings. He is an asthmatic. He can describe in detail how someone with asthma feels. In fact, his story begins in the emergency room of a hospital, where many asthmatics end up when an attack leaves them gasping for breath. This book is a fascinating journey of a doctor who reorders his life and designs a program to overcome asthma. His personal experiences will be helpful to countless thousands of asthmatics as they try to deal with their problems of daily living.

Synopsis

My story starts with a visit to an emergency room. All my life as an asthmatic, I was trying to prove that I was a regular guy who could play tennis and basketball like the rest of my friends. The emergency room visit was an admission of defeat. Like most asthmatics I was living in a dream world. I had no idea how ill I really was. Now, when I look back, I can't understand how little I know about my illness. What I really needed was purified air, food sensitivity tests, a total change of diet, breathing exercises, and vitamins. I also needed a complete rest from antibiotics and asthma sprays. In essence, I needed a revolution in lifestyle. Fifteen million Americans suffer from asthma, and 4 million of them are under eighteen. The death rate from asthma has doubled since

1978. We spend about $62 billion a year on asthma. According to the National Center for Health Statistics, Americans spend $1 billion yearly on asthma medications, and adults lose $850 million a year in wages, while parents with asthmatic children lose $1 billion a year by staying home to care for their children. Yes, change is in the air. The head of the allergic disease section of the National Institutes of Health, Dr. Michael A. Kaliner, believes we have entered a whole new era of asthma therapy. The first era, from 1970 to 1990 was focused on control of symptoms. That era relied heavily on drugs that brought symptomatic relief. Kaliner publicly blasted doctors for harming patients. "No asthmatics should die, and if properly treated, very few asthmatics would die," he told the New York Times in May, 1993. Kaliner called attention to a new era which treats the underlying causes of asthma. We are at the threshold of a new paradigm of genetic medicine, and medicines fascination with asthma's underlying causes has led to many new avenues of treatment and new drugs. As I see it, asthma is the result of a disordered metabolism that occurs at the cellular level. My program looks at nutrition, herbs, the environment, and the mind-body connection. It's truly surprising how profound a difference these gentle but powerful treatments can make. Eighty percent of my asthma patients are now leading active, virtually drug-free lives. If that seems impossible—listen to my story. I became very sick before I got well.

My asthma started when I was a little kid. I missed many periods of school because of asthma attacks. However, my problems were not limited to school. At summer camp I'd wake up in the middle of the night barely able to breathe. In the 1960s, pharmaceutical drugs flourished and a new class of drugs had come upon the scene. But they still caused uncomfortable side effects and don't do enough to ameliorate this condition.

As a high school boy I lived on sprays. These drugs shaped a new generation of asthmatics who relied on their medications—and lived so-called normal lives. Those drugs allowed smokers to go on smoking, and use their sprays to continue working in moldy, toxic offices that literally bathe themselves in toxins that damaged their lungs. I was one of those asthmatics. I never left home without my spray in my pocket. What is the point of giving a person drugs if you keep exposing them to the very factors that are causing their illness.

My first crisis during my new age of drug use happened when I was sixteen. I had an attack that wouldn't go away. My doctor gave me prednisone, a powerful steroid. Long-term use can damage every organ system. I'll never forget how good I felt. I was alert. My mood was elevated. I had a general sense of well-being. This approach should be used as a last resort, not the first line of defense. Not until I entered medical school, where I worked and studied long hours, did a host of other problems begin.

I picked up allergies to chalk, foam, dust, mold, pollen, wool, and foods. My asthma worsened, and then came my first emergency room visit. I was placed on seven drugs a day, and I was taking huge doses of prednisone. As the months passed, I couldn't even get out of bed. I was desperate. I asked my physician, Dr. Stuart Young, to request an emergency admission to the most famous respiratory institute in the country, The National Jewish Center for Allergy and Immunology. It is located in Denver, at an altitude of over 500 feet, which makes it hard to breathe for normal people. For the first time I realized that if I was ever going to get better, I''d have to take complete responsibility for my health. No doctor was going to save me but myself. I had turned a private corner, I had begun my break with conventional medicine. Nutrition is the cornerstone—the most important answer to asthma. Nutritional therapy can have a powerful impact on the course of asthma. Research backs me up. I treat asthma with supplements that dampen inflammation and help the body repair itself. There is a mountain of evidence that nutrients can improve overall health, but they cannot undo the damage of an unhealthy lifestyle. As a nutritionally oriented physician, I feel that the most important medical advances of the century is our new understanding that nutrients can have profound health benefits.

The Basic Asthma Protocol

Magnesium—the one nutrient I would recommend. More than a half century ago scientists reported that magnesium sulphate worked as a natural bronchodilator, one that opened constricted bronchial tubes without side effects.

Anti-inflammatories

Omega-3 fatty acids -- are stars in the nutritional arsenal. They are found in flaxseed and fish oil. Salmon, tuna, and mackerel are high in these beneficial oils.

Bronchodilators—herbal remedies are much gentler than drugs.

Ma Huang--- reduces swelling in the mucus lining of nasal passages and sinuses.

Cayenne—capsicum, or red pepper, stimulates secretion of saliva and thins mucus plugs. It reduces edema caused by respiratory irritants.

Coleus forskholii— an Indian ayurvedic medicine that has been used for centuries to relax the bronchial muscle.

Turmeric and ginger-- used in Chinese medicines as anti-inflammatory agents.

Licorice—contains anti-allergic, anti-bronchial, and anti-inflammatory compounds.

Antihistamines

Vitamin C— I recommend 3,000 mg. a day.

Stinging Nettle— is a medicinal agent to help allergic people.

Quercetin— a potent bioflavonoid.

Histidine— an amino acid that is the building block for histamine. It reduces allergic symptoms.

Star Nutrients

Vitamin E—studies show that asthma and allergies worsen after exposure to smog. Vitamin E neutralizes the damaging effects of ozone, a major component of smog.

Vitamin C—deactivates free radicals and stimulates white blood cells to fight infection.

Beta Carotene-- is a potent free radical quencher.

B -Vitamins— they are crucial for energy production in the body.

Zinc— is an important mineral for immunity.

Vitamin A— is essential for the treatment of asthma. It ensures the health of mucus-producing epithelial tissue in the lining of the mouth, nose, and lungs.

Ginseng— is helpful in treating fatigue and low energy.

Echinacea—is an anti-infective, anti-bacterial;, and anti-viral herb.

N-acetyl-cysteine (NAC — is a free radical scavenger.

Selenium— is an antioxidant that helps maintain the integrity of the cell membranes.

Garlic—for 4,000 years the Chinese used garlic to prevent heart disease and cancer. It is not a cure- all, but garlic can reduce blood pressure.

VITAMIN B-17- FORBIDDEN WEAPON
AGAINST CANCER
MICHAEL L. CULBERT

Each year more than 500,000 Americans die of cancer. A mammoth "cancer industry" has developed over the years involving hospitals and such treatments as surgery, radiation, and chemotherapy. The business of treating cancer has become a multi-billion dollar annual operation. This pernicious "cancer industry" and the controversy that has arisen over the alternative use of Laetrile as a cure for the disease is the subject of this book.

Synopsis

Laetrile (Vitamin B-17 or Amygdalin) is an extract from the apricot pit. Proponents of its use in cancer believe that cancer results from a vitamin deficiency like scurvy, rickets, beriberi, and pernicious anaemia. The orthodox view, as expressed by the American Medical Association (AMA), the Food and Drug Association (FDA), The American Cancer Society (ACS, The National Cancer Institute, and the Pharmaceutical Industry, is that Laetrile is worthless and ineffective in the cure or prevention of cancer. Pro-Laetrile groups feel this opinion issues from the vested monetary interests of the multi-billion dollar cancer industry than from any serious evaluation of Laetrile. Dr. Dean Burk, the former chief of the National Cancer Institute, has outspokenly dissented from the official NCI view. He claims that in 1974, Southern Research Studies conducted tests that showed the validity of Laetrile in treating cancer. In a letter to a congressman he observes " once any of the FDA, NCI, AMA, ACS hierarchy so much as concedes that Laetrile antitumor efficacy was induced even once observed in NCI experimentation, a permanent crack in the bureaucratic armour has taken place, that can widen indefinitely by further appropriate experimentation." Burk's fight to have Laetrile tested on humans was aided by a leak to the press that revealed the progress of Dr. Kanematsu Sugiura's tests on mice at Sloan-Kettering. Ten months of testing has shown "significant inhibition of subcutaneous mammary tumors" as well as "significant inhibition of the formation of lung metastases." Thus, for the first time in the United States, a prestigious cancer facility had come up with positive results involving Laetrile. Though the board of Sloan- Kettering subsequently downplayed the significance of Sugiara's findings they can't reverse the facts. Although a Russian, Dr. T. Inosemtzoff, documented in 1945 successful control of two cases of cancer using Laetrile, Dr. Ernst T. Krebs, Jr. based his development of Vitamin B-17 on the obscure work of Dr. John Beard, a Scottish embryologist. Beard's work was concentrated on a cell called a trophoblast. The cell, identified in 1957 and named in 1976, plays a specific role in pregnancy by eating out a niche in the uterine wall so that the fertilized egg can gain nutrition from the mother's bloodstream. Noting strong similarities between the trophoblast and the cancer cells, Beard wondered if they might be one and the same. His studies noted that in the 56th day of gestation the trophoblast undergoes a dramatic deterioration that corresponds to the development of the secreting function of the fetal pancreas. This explains Beard's thesis that the pancreatic enzymes are responsible for the inhibition of extra-uterine metastasis of the trophoblast, which is manifested in cancer. In elaborating on Beard's views, Krebs claimed that the only real cancer-causing agent is estrogen, the female hormone present in both sexes. Krebs defined the pancreatic enzyme-immunilogical defense as the body's natural defense against cancer. He further postulated that there is an extrinsic causal factor in nutrition that constitutes the second line of defense against the disease.

The young Krebs spent nine years of university study in the area of bacteriology, physiology, anatomy, pharmacology, and medicine. He taught himself French, German, Spanish, and Italian in order to read 17,000 scientific papers, books, and research documents. In 1943 he and a pharmacist, Dr. Gurchott developed the first crystalline chymotrypsin—a pancreatic enzyme. In 1947, after years of experiments, Krebs compiled a study showing 30 characteristics that the trophoblast cell and the cancer cell have in common. He also noted the specific antithesis of chymotrypsin to cancer cells. The Krebs enzyme approach to cancer clashed with the medical world's viral theory of cancer, and his paper went unnoticed.

Krebs later realized that chymotrypsin seemed to lack the curative force that Beard has attributed to it in his theory. He then began to toy with the idea that the cyanide that caused the toxic effect in apricot pits could be the missing ingredient. Further research convinced Krebs that the key lay in refining the extract until he had what amounted to pure Amygdalin. He derived the name "Laetrile" from a compound he described as a laevo (left-moving) mandelonitrile-beta glucuronoside. Vitamin B-17 researchers are carrying on a hunt for other compounds based on cyanide beta-cyanogenetic glucosides. Dr. Krebs's theory is that these substances lumped together as Vitamin B-17 constitute the natural extrinsic prevention of cancer that is necessary when the body's intrinsic mechanism (pancreatic enzymes immunological system) is malfunctioning.

Dr. Krebs explains that cancer is a vitamin deficiency disease that has grown to epidemic proportions because of the Western diet where progress in food processing has removed Vitamin B-17 in substantial amounts from the food we eat. The Hunza people eat large amounts of apricots and apricot products, and cancer is unheard of in their region. Krebs has organized a team of 125-150 noncancerous people around the world who are regularly using Laetrile to support his contention that daily intake of vitamin B-17 will prevent cancer. So far not one of them has developed cancer.

B-17 in the pure form is a white, sugary, slightly bitter substance that is water-soluble and nontoxic. In addition to the anticancer properties, it contains thiocyanate, which reduces excessively high blood pressure. It is also alleged to prevent sickle-cell anemia. Dr. Stewart Jones further claims that B-17 helps in the prevention of pernicious anemia, and in the amelioration of hypertension and arthritis symptoms. If these claims are true, it would no doubt make B-17 one of the most potent vitamins known to man. A strong believer in the efficacy of Laetrile, Dr. Jones is convinced that a conspiracy exists among what he calls the "industrial-medical-government triumvirate." He insists that "it is far more profitable to look for a cancer cure than to find one."What is needed to oppose the cancer conspiracy is a joining of forces that would benefit from using laetrile for the prophylaxis of cancer. A partial list of such groups would include life insurance companies, tobacco companies, etc.

The American Cancer Society took in $93 million in 1972-1973 budget, yet it provided neither funds to investigate new evidence of Laetrile's effectiveness, nor any money for research on the efficacy of nutritional and vitamin therapies. The FDA and the NCI acted in the same manner, stating that there was no evidence to support the belief that Laetrile is effective in reversing tumor activity. Dr.Ernst T. Krebs, Jr. has made a lifetime commitment to the theory that cancer is a vitamin deficiency disease and that Laetrile can provide the extrinsic help that the body needs to lower the level of pain and decrease the tumor activity of cancer sufferers. He has a strong following throughout the world that includes Dr. Manuel Navarro in the Phillipines, Dr. Ernesto Contreras in Tijuana, Mexico, Dr. Hans Nieper in Hanover, Germany, Dr. John A. Richardson and Dr. Stewart Jones in California, Dr. MacDonald in Georgia and hundreds of others. The McNaughton Foundation and Dr. Dean Burk have also championed the cause of Vitamin B-17 against the pressures of the establishment. Even as the controversy rages, the fight must continue.

ORTHOMOLECULAR NUTRITION
ABRAM HOFFER, M.D. AND MORTON WALKER

Dr. Abram Hoffer is one of the outstanding pioneers in the field of orthomolecular medicine. He and Dr. Humphrey Osmond are credited with initiating megavitamin doses of niacin in the treatment of schizophrenia. The medical establishment, though, has unfortunately turned its back on the new clinical discoveries revealing the ways in which improved nutrition can help prevent disease. This close-minded attitude is a major reason why one out of four people in North America succumbs to degenerative diseases Hoffer is disturbed that the thinking of academic nutritionists has not changed since 1950. This time lag between discovery and acceptance has prevailed throughout medical history. It took 50 years for the Royal Navy to act upon Dr. James Lind's discovery that citrus fruits prevented scurvy, It is more than 50 years since Dr. Seale Harris developed his glucose tolerance test to determine the presence of hypoglycaemia, yet hypoglycaemia is still considered a non-disease. The authors of this book attempt to educate both the layman and orthodox physicians to the benefits of good nutrition. They strongly believe that orthomolecular therapy is the answer to many of today's diseases.

Synopsis

The deterioration of our food is the real villain in the dramatic increase of degenerative diseases. Even though massive sums of money are devoted to healthcare, the growing incidence of cardiovascular disease, cancer, and mental illness will continue until the "food technologists" stop stripping our foods of their essential nutrients. Close tp 75 percent of our food supply today is processed as opposed to

20 percent in 1940. We are eating ourselves to destruction with our consumption of sugar and unsaturated fats. Many of our foods suffer from a loss of fiber, vitamins, and minerals.. Orthomolecular medicine emphasizes nutrition in the prevention and cure of disease. Orthomolecular nutrition is the ingestion of the optimal level of each nutrient for each individual. Dr. Hoffer's optimum diet consists of whole foods to which man has adapted in the course of his evolution. These foods are the opposite of junk foods. They contain protein, fat, and carbohydrates in combination with vitamins and minerals. It is also important to eat whole foods because they provide the fibrous material that is so essential to the body. Without bulk digestion becomes very difficult. While certain foods must be cooked in order to aid digestion or prevent bacterial invasion, we should eat as many raw foods as possible. Vegetables such as carrots, turnips, and celery are best eaten raw to get the most vitamins and minerals, but remember to wash them thoroughly to clean away insecticides and other pesticides that may have been sprayed on.

Physicians are trained to recognize deficiency diseases. If their patients are not "dropping in the streets" they assume there is no vitamin deficiency. The average doctor still believes in the germ theory of disease that took Louis Pasteur a lifetime of heartache to teach the medical world. The discovery of vitamins is a relatively new phenomenon that those in the medical profession find difficult to believe and assimilate into their practice,. although they do administer B-12 for pernicious anemia and vitamin D foe rickets. They equate vitamins used this way with drug treatment. Doctors are generally disease-oriented and tend to treat crises instead of trying to prevent them. Certain people may require supplements to their diet. The minimum daily requirement (MDR) is useless as a guide since nutrient needs vary for each individual. The fact that people's biochemical makeup is different, requires that you experiment with vitamins, minerals, and food supplements to find the program that meets your needs. Remember, vitamins are not drugs. They are food. Consuming huge quantities of vitamins is only dangerous in the same way drinking water is--- you simply get rid of what you don't need. Orthomolecular nutrition recognizes that each person requires optimum quantities (optidoses) of each nutrient. You must start with good nutrition. Eat a sugar-free diet and only then turn to optidoses of vitamin and mineral supplements. The increasing trend toward specialization in medicine has taken the doctor further away from his patient. The physician knows the body, but in most cases does not know the patient at all. The human being is an integrated organism that functions as a whole both in sickness and good health. Holistic medicine is a counter-movement developing in the practice of medicine that takes the entire individual into account. Orthomolecular nutrition offers holistic health because the benefits of diet and nutrition are necessary in everyday life for optimal well-being. The growing success of orthomolecular therapy will help achieve the stature of acceptability from within the medical establishment. The public is increasingly aware of the need for better nutrition. People are seeking more information on how to achieve a level of good health and more doctors are willing to give them that knowledge. New ideas are essential if medicine is to advance

BYPASSING BYPASS
ELMER M. CRANTON, M.D.

Chelation therapy is the best kept secret in the medical field. It is a nonsurgical treatment that removes toxic metals such as lead and cadmium from the arteries through the intravenous administration of EDTA (ethylene-diamine-tetra-acetic acid). More than 400,000 people have taken more than 6 million chelation treatments to date (it may have reached 1 million as of this writing).

Synopsis

The most popular surgical solution of the nation's leading medical problem (atherosclerotic heart disease) is the coronary artery bypass graft (CABG). It is very costly and has grown into a 10 billion dollar a year industry (as of the publication of this book). Obviously, the figure is much higher today. The very fact that bypass surgery is so expensive has led to its position as the most popular operation in the surgical field. It costs between $25,000 dollars and $50,000 dollars. It is a medical fad, with the sternum-splitting scar as a status symbol. A well-known example of the popular status of this procedure was the life-saving quintuple bypass of David Letterman, host of television's late night show. His cholesterol was only175 by his own statement, leading one to question what was responsible for the plaque buildup that necessitated five bypasses? Would coronary bypass surgery have proliferated if it weren't so enormously profitable? Big money is involved for the cardiologist, the surgeon, the radiologist, and the hospital. "Every time a surgeon does a heart bypass, he takes home a new sports car," quipped one cynic, referring to the $15,000 dollars or more surgeon's fee that has provided some cardiovascular surgeons with incomes of $1 million dollars per year, and more. It has been estimated that by 1992 bypass surgery would become a $10 billion dollar business (obviously that figure is much higher today). That is the dilemma which Dr. Cranton had so thoroughly explored in this excellent book. A visit to a cardiologist begins with a progression of the following: an electrocardiogram, a stress test, an angiogram, and then either an angioplasty (a balloon procedure that opens the lumen of the artery to improve blood flow), and invariably the pot-of-gold bonanza called a bypass. Dr. Cranton believes there is a better way. Physicians can learn from 230 articles in the world's scientific literature that support the effectiveness of chelation therapy. It may be a vain hope, for it will take a great deal of courage and dedication for physicians to opt for the alternative of chelation, when they have to give up all that bypass surgery.

One million people die each year of coronary heart disease. It is the nation's number one killer. In addition, more than 40 million men and women suffer with heart disease symptoms. Coronary artery bypass grafting (CABG) a procedure in which occluded portions of major coronary arteries are bypassed with grafts from a patients leg veins—is currently the most popular surgical solution to the nation's leading medical problem. Bypass surgery has grown to a $10 billion dollar a year industry (that figure has grown to a much higher amount today). According to the American heart Association (AHA), 1,051,000 angioplasty procedures, 516,000 bypass procedures (CABG), 1,314,000 diagnostic cardiac catheterizations, 46,000 implantable defibrillators, and 177,000 pacemaker procedures are performed annually in the United States (based on 2001 figures). An AHA update for 2004 puts the total figure for the costs of cardiovascular disease at $368.4 billion dollars a year. Does bypass surgery prevent further health deterioration? If that were true, there would be no need to write this book. As things now stand, the operation cannot be justified by patient outcomes. A $24 million dollar study by the National Heart, Lung and Blood Institute (NHLBI), which screened 16,000 patients who underwent CABGs at 11 leading medical centers, revealed no increase in post-surgical survival rates as compared to a matched group of non-surgically treated patients. Both groups were on a par with employment and recreational status. A study in 1983 concluded that approximately 25,000 operations each year were unnecessary. That number is obviously much higher today with about 600,000 CABGs each year. Bypass surgery does not cure the underlying disease and may induce its more rapid progression. Research shows that ten years after surgery, grafted vessels have closed in 40 percent of the patients, and the remaining 60 percent had further artery narrowing. There is an inherent fallacy in bypassing one or even several portions of the body's blood vessels, when the same degenerating condition must be affecting the entire cardiovascular system. At best, the bypass operation is an expensive stop-gap measure, a risky, high-priced surgical "aspirin," providing pain relief and not much more. "What choice did I have," is a common complaint. "My doctor had nothing else to suggest." Chelation therapy is almost never mentioned. In recent years there are as many patients chelated as bypassed, with superior results. One of the main reasons for this book is to improve the quality of life for millions of people by discussing a major therapy, (chelation) that is being suppressed and discriminated against by the medical profession. Chelation is nonsurgical and requires only a series of visits to a physician's office for the FDA approved intravenous infusion of EDTA. It has little effect on cholesterol or triglycerides, but it does interrupt the disease process. Chelating physicians have been embarrassed because they could not explain why their patients showed improvement of symptoms of a whole host of diseases including arthritis, multiple sclerosis, Parkinson's disease, and psoriasis. Over time, these injections halt the progress of free-radical disease underlying the development of atherosclerosis. They give the body time to heal, and they restore adequate blood flow through the occluded arteries. Chelation is the granddaddy of all anti-free-radical treatments. It is readily available, and is a life-prolonging treatment that reverses the symptoms of atherosclerosis and almost all other age-related degenerative diseases.

Chelation therapy was pioneered by Swiss Nobel Laureate Alfred Werner in 1894. He developed the theories that became the foundation of modern chelation chemistry. Werner's concept of how metals bind to organic molecules opened the new field of chelation chemistry. EDTA proved to be effective and inexpensive as the substance used in chelation. It was patented in 1935. It was not until the end of World War II that chelation was introduced into the medical area. By the mid 1950s it was accepted as the "treatment of choice" for lead poisoning in children and adults. Clinical results are impressive. In the majority of cases, patients suffering from atherosclerosis (coronary artery disease , carotid artery occlusion that leads to stroke, high blood pressure, vascular blockage of the arteries) experience improved health. They regain physical and mental function. They begin to "live" again. As of this writing, more than 400,000 patients have received more than 6 million chelation treatments in the United States alone, without a single fatality when the treatment was properly administered and supervised. Chelation therapy does not correct defective heart valves, but after chelation valves do improve because of better heart function and increased coronary artery circulation. The question is, if this safe, tested, legal, nonsurgical treatment is so good, then why haven't we heard about it?

I completed my training at Harvard Medical School. My ambition was to have a family practice in a nice town where I could be a Dr. Marcus Welby to whole families. While in Los Angeles at a medical meeting in 1972, I heard a story that was to change my life. I was invited to a meeting in a colleague's room at the hotel to hear about the experience of an eminent and respected physician, an otolaryngologist. His name was George, he said. "I suffered a severe angina attack last year and was warned of the imminent danger of a myocardial infarct. As you can see, I am back at work full time. The way it came about is what I want to tell you about. I was playing a round of golf when all at once I felt as though an elephant had jumped on my chest." All the procedures were performed at the nation's top medical schools. I had electrocardiograms, treadmill tests, a coronary angiogram-- the works. The results were not consoling. The angiogram revealed plaque blockages of the left main coronary artery, and other arteries as well. The cardiologist recommendation was a triple coronary artery bypass. "No time to waste," the specialists agreed, pointing out the impending danger of total occlusion, and a real possibility of sudden death. During the 1970s, 10 to 15 percent of patients died as a direct result of surgery. Survivors had no assurance of long term improvement. It was a high risk surgical procedure with uncertain benefits. Today, the procedures have been improved, but the benefits are still uncertain. For George, there didn't seem to be any choice. Then fate intervened. The Christmas holidays were at hand, and the Red Cross was unable to supply the seven standby units of blood required until after New Years. The two week reprieve gave George time to talk to people and see if there was an alternative. A dear colleague who had gone to medical school with George asked, "Ever hear about chelation?""How do you spell it,?" George asked, heading for the medical library. "There are a couple of dozen or so impressive clinical reports on this chelation therapy that I'll bet most of you have never heard of." George travelled more than 2,000 miles to one of the few clinics in the country then specializing in the treatment. "After only ten of those treatments, my angina disappeared completely! Before I started treatment I couldn't walk a dozen steps without severe angina. But, I swear, I haven't had a chest pain since." "Some of the things I saw made me wonder if I could believe my own eyes. People checked in with chronic diabetic ulcerative lesions and gangrenous lesions that began healing in ten to twelve days." The usually reserved George waxed on with uncharacteristic enthusiasm, crediting chelation with astonishing cures, not the least of which was his own. "I carry a full work load. I do approximately 10 to 15 surgeries every week. I carry a full practice. I play golf. I swim 20 laps in my pool every day, and I cannot speak with any but the greatest praise for the men who are attempting to make chelation an accepted form of therapy."

In the 100 years since Pasteur made medical history, there has not been so profound a discovery as the recent development of the concept of free radical pathology as the underlying cause of degenerative diseases associated with aging. The free radical theory of aging was postulated by Denham Harman in 1962. It introduces a fresh principle: that succumbing to a degenerative disease (atherosclerosis) depends on the body's ability to defend itself against ongoing free radical attack. While the maximum life span for a species or an individual appears to be predetermined by genetics, free radicals have a decided influence on whether the limit is reached or not. When your cells are damaged, you are damaged. When enough cells die, you die. How do cells get sick and die? They succumb to free radical attack. A free radical is an oxygen molecule with an odd number of electrons in the outer ring of one of its atoms. Molecules and atoms normally contain an even number of paired electrons. If one of the electrons in a pair becomes separated an imbalance is created. This makes the molecule or atom unstable, violently restive, and very destructive. Uncontrolled, these free radicals can wreak havoc. They are deadly marauders that damage cells by breaking down delicate cell walls and damaging important protein enzymes. Chelation therapy stops excessive free radical production in its tracks, halts the development of free radical disease, and allows the body to repair the damage it has already suffered. If bypass surgery is an expensive, high-risk, limited benefit procedure, as research indicates, why then does it continue to be the winner of the "most popular operation of the year" award? Why do more than 400,000 Americans a year submit to a surgical procedure costing between $25,000 and $50,000 which will not cure their underlying disease and has a slight chance of making them worse? Good question. Almost overnight bypass surgery has become a medical fad. The sternum-splitting scar is a status symbol. "What, you haven't had your bypass yet?" one executive asks another. More recently, the question has changed to "how many arteries? Double, triple, or quadruple?" Coronary bypass surgery would not have proliferated so rapidly if it weren't so enormously profitable? Big bucks are involved. While I am clearly biased in favour of the therapies I know best, I have no quarrel with people who choose to use other therapeutic means. I have no objection to surgery where clearly indicated and appropriate, but in my view, bypass surgery should be the alternative of last resort.

THE HEART
MATTHIAS RATH, M.D.

The man that Linus Pauling chose to run his Linus Pauling Institute was not his son. He selected Dr. Matthias Rath, who conducted research with him. Rath believes in orthomolecular nutrition and therapy. It was a term which Pauling coined in 1968. Rath also believed in the importance of vitamin C to maintain the integrity of the coronary arteries. It is instructive to see what Dr. Rath considered a good program to provide for a healthy heart.

Synopsis

Dr. Rath's 10-step program for optimum cardiovascular health:

• **Be aware of the size and function of your cardiovascular system:** Your blood vessel pipeline measures 60,000 miles and is the largest organ in your body. Your body is as old as your cardiovascular system. Cardiovascular health adds years to your life.

• **Stabilize the walls of your blood vessels:** Instability and lesions in your blood vessels are the primary causes for cardiovascular disease. Vitamin C is the cement of the blood vessel walls and stabilizes them. Animals don't get heart disease because they produce enough vitamin C in their livers to protect their blood vessels. In contrast, humans develop deposits leading to heart attacks and strokes because we cannot manufacture our own vitamin C and generally get too few vitamins in our diet.

• **Reverse artery disease naturally without surgery:** Cholesterol and fat particles are deposited inside the blood vessel walls by means of biological adhesives . Teflon-like agents can prevent this sickness. The amino acids lysine and proline are nature's Teflon agents together with vitamin C They help reverse existing deposits naturally.

- Relax **your blood vessel walls:** Deposits and spasms of the blood vessel walls are the cause of high blood pressure. Dietary supplementation of magnesium, arginine, and vitamin C relax the blood vessel walls and help normalize high blood pressure.

- **Optimize the performance of your heart:** The heart is the motor of the cardiovascular system. Like the motor of your car, millions of muscle cells need cell fuel for optimum performance. Nature's cell fuels include carnitine, coenzyme Q10, B vitamins, and many other nutrients and trace elements. These essential nutrients will optimize the performance of the heart and contribute to a regular heartbeat.

- **Protect your cardiovascular pipelines from rusting:** Biological rusting, or oxidation damages your cardiovascular system and accelerates the aging process. Vitamin C. Vitamin E,, Beta carotene and selenium are the most important antioxidants. Bioflavonoids and pycnogenol are others. Above all, stop smoking.

- **Exercise regularly:** Regular physical activity is an important step for optimum cardiovascular health. Regular exercise such as walking or bicycling are ideal. They can be performed by everybody.

- **Eat a prudent diet:** The diet of our ancestors over thousands of generations is rich in plant nutrition and high in fiber and vitamins. A diet rich in fruits and vegetables and low in fat is preferred.

- **Find time to relax:** Physical and emotional stress are cardiovascular risk factors. The stress hormone adrenaline requires vitamin C.

- **Start now:** Thickening of the blood vessel walls is not only a problem of the elderly. It starts in your 20s. Early intervention equals active protection of your cardiovascular system.

STATIN DRUG SIDE EFFECTS
DUANE GRAVELINE, M.D.

Dr. Duane Graveline was a space astronaut and a flight surgeon. He was truly a space doctor. He was distressed by the total lack of honesty of the medical establishment on the side effects of the statin drugs. This book is a personal account of Graveline's experience with statin drugs and their serious side effects. It is an eye-opening account of the disruptive effect of statins, and is a warning to the millions of people who take them and to the physicians who prescribe them.

Synopsis

The most glaring deficiency of the cholesterol hypothesis is the fact that "the majority of patients with coronary heart disease and stroke have no evidence of elevated cholesterol or LDL levels."In a 1990 study, 194 male veterans, only 8 percent had total cholesterol levels greater than 250 mg./dl. The average blood cholesterol in the group was 186 mg./dl. Furthermore, autopsies in teenage soldiers in Korea and Vietnam showed lipid streaks and early atherosclerosis and their cholesterol and LDL levels were at rock-bottom level. "Natural cholesterol is innocuous. We are now learning that cholesterol manipulation is irrelevant to atherosclerosis and increased cardiovascular risk. Doctors insist that statins are not getting to everyone who needs them. They feel that the statins are the best things available for high-risk stroke and heart attack patients. They definitely reduce cholesterol in most people, but researchers in major clinical trials report that cholesterol reduction is not leading to significant reductions in cardiovascular disease mortality. In Dr. Uffe Ravnskov's "The Cholesterol Myths," he reports that the recent PROSPER trial published in Lancet demonstrated that statin therapy increased the incidence of cancer deaths, completely offsetting a slight decrease in deaths from cardiovascular disease.

Dr. George V. Mann, of the Framingham Heart Study, called the cholesterol hypothesis, "the greatest scientific deception of our time." Cholesterol is not the enemy; inflammation and statin drugs are the problem. Cholesterol is an absolutely vital substance and studies show high cholesterol is only a weak risk factor for men older than 50 years of age. Dr. Pfreiger, of the Max Planck Society for the Advancement of Science, announced on November 9, 2011, that without abundant supplies of cholesterol, normal synaptic function cannot take place. Synapses are the connections between our neurons (nerve cells). "Natural cholesterol is not the cause of our infamous atherosclerotic plaques." John Abramson, M.D., of Harvard, Jerome Hoffman of UCLA, and David Brown, M.D., of Albert Einstein and Beth Israel, in a letter dated September 23, 2004 , charged complete lack of objectivity of the originators of the National Cholesterol Education Program guidelines due to financial ties with the drug industry..There will soon be 40 million people on Lipitor and 20 million on other statin drugs. "Do we really know what we are doing?" It is well known that statin drugs have side effects. The FDA "rushed" Baycol off the market after two years of rhabdomyolysis (muscle breakdown) deaths. The number of rhabdomyolysis deaths from Lipitor, Zocor, Mevacor, Pravachol, and Crestor now far exceed those from Baycol alone.

"I was on four different statins for 10 years. I was taking 10 mg. to 80 mg.. I had muscle cramps and i put it down to aging. I was on 40 mg. of Pravachol and my cholesterol was 400 mg./dl I was placed on 80 mg. of Lipitor. Muscle pains were so bad I took early retirement in 2011. I could not get through the day. I did not suspect drug toxicity until April 2003. The only way I could walk was with a cane or walker. I am tired of defending myself from doctors who feel my disoriented thinking has nothing to do with the statins. I definitely will not take their statins! I had four amnesia episodes. The medical community fails to recognize the full spectrum of statin drug side effects—many of which are irreversible.

Inhibition of Glial cell biosynthesis of brain cholesterol is collateral damage, unforeseen by the designers of statin drugs 20 years ago. Cognitive problems are inevitable. Muldoon finds that cognitive deterioration can be found in 100 percent of statin users. Coenzyme Q10 (Ubiquinone) levels plummet when statins are initiated. This results in chronic fatigue, hepatitis, myopathy (muscle aches), rhabdomyolysis (muscle breakdown), and peripheral neuropathy. This highlights Coenzyme Q10's role in cell wall integrity and stability. Neuro-peptide formation is damaged by statin use, which is responsible for depression, irritability, hostility, aggressiveness, road rage behavior, accidents, and suicides. 30 million patients on Lipitor can lead to 150,000 cases of cognitive loss. This year alone, the medical literature is replete with reports of statin initiated amnesias and other evidence of neural dysfunction. Still, many prescribing physicians are unaware of the statin's special cognitive impairment tendency.

Canada has a warning label on Lipitor about CoQ10 depletion and L-Carnitine deficiencies. CoQ10 depletion causes liver inflammation, neuropathy, rhabdomyolysis, and kidney blockage. Seniors are unaware of a possible relationship to their statin drug. Neurodegenerative diseases such as Parkinson's, ALS (Lou Gehrig's Disease), Alzheimer's, etc. are being reported among statin users. The neurology department of California University reported a 50 percent fall in plasma CoQ10 in their group taking 80 mg. of Lipitor for 30 days. CoQ10 is arguably our most important essential nutrient. There are two grams in an adult human body. Five grams a day must be replaced, and the Western diet has only 5 mg. a day. The average physician is completely unaware of the serious side effects of statin usage. They are obsessed with lowering cholesterol. (Low cholesterol is more of a problem than high cholesterol). If a patient complains of memory gaps they call it a "senior moment," senility, or early Alzheimer's. They scoff at the possibility of Parkinson's disease or ALS. Beatrice Golomb states that "transient global amnesia" or TGA is very common with patients whose cholesterol dropped 100 points.

The extraordinary high pedestal most patients place their doctors on deserves that equally high standards are defined and maintained for the medications those doctors dispense. The annual toll of lives and serious side effects currently sustained by hundreds of thousands of patients is a heavy and unnecessary price to pay for faith misplaced.

SUGAR SHOCK
CONNIE BENNETT

It is hard to imagine that after all the great books that have been published throughout the years which have warned the public about the dangers of sugar, there are still people who aren't aware of the consequences of our high consumption of sugar. The wave of obesity and the increasing incidence of diabetes are a direct result of America's 146 pounds of sugar and caloric sweeteners per person every year. If you add the sugar that you get in white flour products, potatoes, rice, bread, and cake, etc., the total sugar consumption for the average person is about 200 pounds a year, or 4 pounds a week.

Synopsis

Connie Bennett, in her great book, "Sugar Shock" reminds us about the evils of sugar. She points out how the many severe side effects caused her untold misery and social problems Connie finally found an integrative physician, Dr. Keith De Oro, who diagnosed her condition as reactive hypoglycaemia. She cut out sugar, and a new world opened up.

Stephen Sinatra explains that as a cardiologist he treats many patients for diabetes, and his firm opinion is that heart disease is not caused by cholesterol, it is rather the consumption of sugar, and the ensuing inflammation. There have been a myriad of excellent books which deal with the problems of sugar. Among the best are, "The Saccharine Disease," by Surgeon-Captain T.L. Cleave, "Sweet and Dangerous," by Dr. John Yudkin, and many others.

The late, great, Dr. Robert C. Atkins used to say, "Sugar is death!"All of his best-selling books which featured the low -carbohydrate regimen, warned about the evils of sugar. He claimed that the heart attack epidemic started when Coca-Cola was invented. A recent study in JAMA showed that the Atkins' cohort loses more weight, and their blood pressure and cholesterol levels went down. Although it seems futile to tell Americans that they are eating wrong, it is worth the try. Someone once said that lost causes were the only ones worth fighting for. Dr. John Yudkin, in his book, "Sweet and Dangerous" showed the world that heart disease was caused by the consumption of large amounts of sugar. His studies in London hospitals confirmed his stand that it was refined sugar and white flour that led to heart disease. The world ignored his findings and he died a disillusioned man because his years of work were denied the recognition they richly deserved. Today, with decades of research and a whole new army of believers in the benefits of good nutrition, we know Yudkin was right. Connie Bennett has performed a great service with "Sugar Shock" and its overwhelming evidence of the serious diseases caused by sugar. The list of doctors who believe that sugar is dangerous is enormous. They include Dr. Mark Hyman, Dr. Robert C. Atkins, Dr. Richard Ash, Dr. Andrew Weil, Dr. Pa\tick Fratellone, Dr. Fred Pescatore, Dr. Abram Hoffer, Dr. Ronald Hoffman, and many other leading physicians and researchers. It is imperative that you educate yourself to the advantages of good nutrition and eliminate sugar and refined flour from your diet. Your health and life are at stake.

THE HIDDEN STORY OF CANCER
PROFESSOR BRIAN SCOTT PESKIN

Cancer is the number one cause of death in the United States. During the last fifty years many billions of dollars have been poured into a sinkhole, supporting the research for chemotherapeutic drugs, better and more expensive diagnostic machinery, and hospitals, etc. However, the death toll keeps rising. In 1968, 278,000 deaths ushered in President Nixon's "War on Cancer." This year there will be 570,280 people succumbing to this dread disease. A new estimate does not bode well for the future. By 2030, the total cancer mortality rate will double. Rates of cancer will grow 20 percent a year. There will be about 1.5 million new cases a year, and a total of 20 million people living with cancer. Let's face it: the war on cancer has been lost! But wait; not so fast! A fascinating new book by Professor Brian Scott Peskin called, "The Hidden Story of Cancer" has revived the brilliant work of Nobel laureate Otto Warburg, M.D., who earned his prize for physiology in 1931. He vowed to find the cure for cancer because his mother died of the disease. Professor Peskin uses Dr. Warburg's research as the core of his "Life Systems Engineering Science" solution to the problem of cancer. It is obvious that treating cancer with chemotherapy, radiation, and surgery has failed to stem the surge in mortality. It is high time to try something new, like prevention. According to Warburg, the prime cause of cancer is a low level of oxygen in the cell. Cancer cells cannot live in an oxygen environment—they are anaerobic. How does one go about keeping the cells properly oxygenated, thereby preventing cancer? It seems that Warburg didn't have the answer. However, Professor Peskin uses the scientific knowledge gained during the succeeding decades to add the missing ingredient--- essential fatty acids (EFAs). Essential fatty acids in the proper ratio deliver the oxygen needed for respiration to keep the cells normal and healthy. In the absence of oxygen the cells revert to their primordial state and the aforementioned results. It doesn't matter what kind of cancer, the primary cause is always the same—a lack of oxygen at the tissue level.

Synopsis

Cancer is now the number one cause of death in the United States. It is estimated that 570,280 people died in 2006 (data still being collected). There were 1,372, 910 cases in the U.S. in 2005. The numbers keep mounting even though we have spent $20 trillion dollars on research in the last 30 years the goal of this book is to help you live out your life cancer-free, and achieve your maximum life span. Medicine stubbornly persisted on a dead-end path during the same period that Otto Warburg was researching and presenting his brilliant work leading to the discovery of the prime cause of cancer. "If a risk factor cannot be attributed to the majority of cases of a disease, then that factor is not the primary cause of the disease." The word "theory" really means a guess. Warburg's rigorous experimentation and testing always resulted in the same outcome, making his cause of cancer a scientific law—not a theory. Warburg's work was tested a thousand times, and while that might seem like a simplistic answer to a complex problem, it worked every time.

A simple-to-correct nutritional deficiency is at the core of cancers prime cause. As we age, we become more deficient. Preventing cancer before it develops, through an understanding of the prime cause as researched by Dr. Warburg is the only way to halt this insidious disease for good. Prevention is the ultimate cure.

It took the Catholic church 300 years to admit that its condemnation of Galileo was wrong. This story is analogous with the sad story of Dr. Warburg's discovery not being put to use even though it is scientifically valid. This book will show you the solution so that you can protect yourself against cancer. The following are recommendations that are based on bad science.

1. Fruits and vegetables—they are O.K., but won't help you ward off cancer.

2. Fiber—worsens colon cancer. Fiber is cellulose-sawdust.

3 Mammograms—it is not a technique for early detection. Breast cancer is present for 8 years before it can be detected. It is a profit-driven technology posing risks compounded by reliability. It would take

1,214 mammograms to prevent 1 cancer death 14 years later. It is a very weak tool—1 percent effective—or 99 percent failure rate.

4. Heart attacks and cholesterol—75 percent of heart attack victims have normal LDL and HDL cholesterol.

5. Hormone Replacement therapy (HRT)—Therapy with estrogen and progestin results in increased risk of disease.

6. Diverticulosis—no need to avoid fruits, seeds, and nuts.

7. Blood pressure—diuretics are more effective- they are cheaper.

8. Nitrates—in hot dogs, etc. Are O.K.

9. Fish oil—worthless at best and harmful at worst.

Generic risk factors are not linked to cancers prime cause. Despite massive hype, trying to cure cancer via genetics is still far off. Any competent molecular biologist will tell you that cancer is not genetically based. Dr. Warburg warned scientists against pursuing genetic research. Many of us have been misled into believing that genetics will save us from contracting cancer. The truth of this fallacy has been publicized, but few of us know it.

Nobel Laureate Otto Warburg's discovery of the prime cause of cancer is not a theory. It is an observation he arrived at after years of experimentation and testing. Cancer does not develop rapidly. It takes decades. The body has a high resistance to developing cancer cells. That is why it takes so long to grow. The immune system protects the body against cancer. A cancerous cell can never return to normal. It's an irreversible process. Warburg's discovery demonstrates that there is an underlying cause of cancer that is the same from one person to the next. The prime cause of cancer is too little oxygen in the cell. I spent three years trying to prove it wrong. Just by decreasing a cell's oxygen content by one-third, cancer is automatically induced. Nothing more is required for cancer to develop.

Warburg found that if a cell was oxygenated early enough, cancer causation could be stopped. Once damage to a cell is too great, no amount of oxygen will return a cell's respiration back to normal. It is doomed to a cancerous life. In 1923, "The Metabolism of Carcinoma (Cancer) Cells," was published in Germany. Warburg used actual results as the basis of the scientific theory, allowing the theory to fit the facts. Today's cancer researchers have it backwards—they force the facts to fit their genetically-based theories. Glycolosis means running without oxygen. Respiration means running with oxygen. Glucose brought respiration to a standstill. Cancer tumors love sugar and sugar stopped respiration. This effect doesn't occur in normal cells. Malignant tumors produce three to four times more lactic acid per molecule of oxygen consumed than do benign tumors. Dr. Warburgs genius was unprecedented in making these seminal discoveries regarding the metabolism of cancer. The tumor cell can choose between fermentation and respiration. This makes cancer cells much harder to kill than normal cells. That is why prevention is so important. If caught early enough a tumor can be oxygenated so that cancer will not fully develop. Today we know how to achieve this result. Dr. Habib refers to EFAs (essential fatty acids) as "oxygen sponges." EFAs are the missing link that Warburg was not aware of. EFAs are "oxygen magnets." Exercise increases oxygenation to your blood but it doesn'The t guarantee the effective transfer to each organ in your body. Many people who exercise regularly still get cancer. All supposed causes of cancer in the press are secondary causes—chemical carcinogens, radiation, trans fats, food additives, cigarette smoke, viruses, and genetic mutations. Warburg warned that we are wasting our time chasing secondary causes. They all lead to the primary cause—insufficient oxygen in the cells.

Secondary causes of cancer all lead to impaired oxygen. All cancer-causing agents impair oxygen transfer to the cell and oxygen utilization inside the cell. Oxygen transfer is inhibited by (hypoxia and anoxia). The cell then turns cancerous.

The cell does not die. Instead, it loses its ability to respire and turns to fermentation. It doesn't matter what kind of cancer, the primary cause is always the same.

It's impossible to avoid all these dangerous carcinogens, but there is hope! This process can be minimized or even stopped by giving your cells the proper EFAs, vitamins, essential minerals, sufficient protein, and a detoxifier.

It is not necessary to look for further answers to a question that has already been answered. It is high time to get past the prejudices and mistakes of the past and take a look at Dr. Warbutg's revolutionary discoveries about cancer.

"Otto Warburg: A Lifetime of Important Discoveries and Advances."

Warburg was referred to as the greatest biochemist of the 20th century. His discovery ranks him with Galileo, Newton, Pauling, Feynman, and Einstein. His life's ambition was to find the cure for cancer. His mother died of cancer. Warburg did research on respiratory enzymes, certain vitamins and minerals that the body requires for the utilization of oxygen in the cell. That earned him the Nobel Prize in 1931. Today, these vitamins and minerals are termed "coenzymes."Warburg warned that no further time be spent "barking up the wrong tree." He said that by concentrating in the wrong areas (genetic and viral causes) huge numbers of people would die unnecessarily.

Warburg was eccentric. He was the first to admit it. He avoided food with chemical additives. Dr.Warburg was Jewish, and Hitler's obsession with contracting cancer caused him to insist that Warburg stay and continue his research. You can imagine how all the other scientists and medical researchers must have felt about this. They hated Warburg because of his blunt truthfulness and lack of tact.

The answer to cancer is EFAs, oxygen magnets. These unsaturated fats attract the oxygen in your blood stream and transfer it into the cell just like little "oxygen sponges." This happens in all of your 100 trillion cells. EFAs need to be replaced every day in our food. They are integral to the structure and function of cellular respiration. Without a high respiration efficiency, cancer is sure to follow. Decreased oxygen utilization is precisely the circumstance that Dr. Warburg demonstrated that leads directly to cancer. This is the process we know how to stop cold with EFAs. Before cancer can start a deficiency of EFAs in human cell membranes, making them less able to absorb oxygen- was only possible by taking into account Dr. Warburg's discovery of the prime cause of cancer—insufficient oxygen in the cells. An EFA deficiency is the missing link that holds the key to the health of your cells and body.

Parent EFAs comprise the basic raw material for your body. Parent omega-3 (alpha-linolenic acid, or ALA and omega-6 (linoleic acid or LA).

Your body can't make either ALA or LA. That is why they are called essential. We must obtain them from foods or supplements. We need both ALA and LA. They have complementary functions. There are also substances called EFA "derivatives."Your body makes them out of your parent omega- 3 and omega- 6 EFAs that you eat.

The most common omega-3 EFA derivative you'll see in stores are EPA and DHA, and the most common omega-6 derivatives are CLA and GLA. The most critical factor is the correct proportion of parent omega-6 to parent omega-3. The correct ratio of EFAs is a range of one part to two parts omega-6 to one part omega-3.

Just for the record, GLA is gamma-linolenic acid and CLA is conjugated linoleic acid. EPA is eicosapentaenoic acid and DHA is docohexaenoic acid.

The body uses a much greater quantity of parent EFAs than derivatives—up to twenty times more. EFAs have been proven in numerous studies to prevent cancers from developing. Some of these studies also show that EFAs can inhibit the growth of cancer already present in the body.

Mitochondria are "cellular power plants." A cell typically contains hundreds or even thousands of mitochondria which occupy up to 25 percent of the cells cytoplasm. Each mitochondrion is supposed to be loaded with EFAs.

What you should eat:

Each red blood cell contains about 280 million hemoglobin molecules. For maximum anti-cancer protection, we require highly oxygenated haemoglobin in our red blood cells. Your body needs lots of iron. Eat plenty of animal-based protein like eggs, poultry, meat, cheese, yogurt, and fish. People can't deny themselves ice cream, pie, and soda. The cravings overpower them, and they never go away. Excessive carbohydrates are the worst foods to consume if you want anti-cancer protection.

The following list shows the content of EFAs in oils

Omega-6 (linoleic acid)		Omega-3 (alpha-linolenic acid)
50%	Corn oil	0%
65%	Sunflower oil	0%
75%	Safflower oil	0%
20%	Flaxseed oil	55%

45%	Sesame oil	0%
Omega-6 (linoleic acid)		**Omega-3 (alpha-linolenic acid)**
43%	Pumpkin oil	15%
74%	Evening Primrose oil	0%
38%	Borage oil	0%
8%	Olive oil	0%
	Nut oils	
28%	Walnut oil	5%
4%	Hazel nut oil	0%
8%	Cashew oil	0%
10%	Almond oil	0%
23%	Brazil nut oil	0%
29%	Peanut oil	0%

Warburg's 19 Principles

• The prime cause of cancer is cellular oxygen pressure that is too low.

• The prime cause of cancer is the replacement of respiration of oxygen in normal body cells by a fermentation of sugar. Carbohydrates are utilized as cancer's prime fuel instead of proteins or fats.

• Minerals (coenzymes) are critical to the cellular respiration function (oxygen transfer).

• Cancer has no genetic and no viral basis. It's proteins, not genes that count. Genes cannot explain cancers prolific (enormous) increase in less than 80 years. Our genes haven't changed in the last 100 years.

• Iron is important. Anemia increases the risk of death by cancer by 65 percent. Bio-available iron is found in animal-based protein sources such as meat, chicken, eggs, steak, etc.

• Cancer could be prevented if the respiration of the body's cells is kept intact.

• Cancer prevention is the key. Once oxygen deficiency damage is done to a cell, it can't be repaired. Fermentation causes proliferation and the spreading of cancer.

• To prevent cancer, you must keep the speed of the bloodstream so high that the venous blood still contains sufficient oxygen.

• Keep high concentrations of haemoglobin in the blood.

Haemoglobin is a protein. Fish, eggs, yogurt, and cheese give you iron and protein.

Add respiratory enzymes (minerals) to food in your diet.

- Avoid additives, preservatives, artificial sweeteners, hormones (steroids), and other carcinogens.

- There are many secondary causes of cancer. They bring about the "prime cause of cancer"—insufficient oxygen.

- Normal cells meet their energy needs by the respiration of oxygen. Cancer cells' energy needs are supplied by fermentation of glucose (sugar). Cancer cells love sugar—the fuel of fermentation.

- Cancer cells grow in the body with almost only the energy of fermentation.

- Cancer metabolism is an irreversible process. It must be prevented.

- Thirty-five percent inhibition of oxygen respiration brings about the transformation of cell growth.

- When oxygen respiration fails, fermentation appears and cancer develops.

- The first harm to the cell that occurs is likely to be the harm to its respiration.

- Warburg warns that the pursuit of secondary causes of cancers such as viral agents and carcinogens is obscuring the true cause of cancer--- the lack of oxygen

Peskin's Grand Premise

"Long term EFA deficiency in the modern diet resulting from food processing has created the exact cellular malfunction in the population that was discovered by Otto Warburg to be the prime cause of cancer.--- an insufficiency of oxygen in the cells. In addition, an EFA deficiency perpetuates cardiovascular disease, which in a vicious circle that becomes the body's resistance to cancer by lowering blood speed and spreading cancer throughout the body via blood and metastasis.".

"Warburg's views on the significance of the metabolic characteristics of cancer cells were not shared by the majority of experts—though none of the facts on which they were based have been refuted." (Hans Krebs)

Warburg's facts were verified over one thousand times in experiments all over the world.

There is no doubt that the prevention of cancer will come, because man wishes to survive. How long prevention will be avoided depends on how long the prophets of agnosticism will succeed in inhibiting the application of scientific knowledge in the cancer field. In the meantime, millions of men must die of cancer unnecessarily.

FOOD FOR NOUGHT
ROSS HUME HALL

This book condemns what the author feels is a technologic manipulation of food inimical to the interests of the consumer. Hall claims that the mass production of food is geared to what the public wants, but the public has been manipulated to "want" items profitable for the producer. Moreover, he attacks the food regulatory agencies for not truly protecting and defending the best interests of the consumer. Diet and nutrition can have a direct effect on disease, and the public must be as well-educated as possible to develop and maintain good health.

Synopsis

Since Roman times, white has been associated with goodness, purity, and higher standards of living. But white refined food in the roman era was also accompanied by a large rise in dental decay. In modern attempts at "refinement" the new technology has excluded the bran and germ and left the starchy endosperm in the form of a highly refined white flour. The public loves food that is sweet, smooth and visually appealing, and food producers are only too glad to provide it. It seems ridiculous, though, to refine the vitamins out of the flour and then add them back in at a greater expense. The addition of B vitamins and iron to our white breads has successfully eliminated B vitamin deficiency diseases from America. The USDA says, "it is useless to try to persuade the American people to eat foods that are nutritionally good for them. Instead it should be put into the foods that the public likes. Frankfurters and candy should be beefed up with vitamins, minerals, and proteins.

The food industry treats crops not as foods, but as a raw material to be manipulated and manufactured into numerous products. One example is the production of baby food. Chemically modified starches have been a boon to the commercial baby food industry for about 20 years. The baby food can be stored at room temperature or at refrigerator temperature for long periods of time. Although questions have been raised over the safety of this material and its nutritional benefits for young children, 25 billion jars of baby food have been sold. Professor of food protection and toxicology at the University of California at Davis, G.F.Stewart, claims, "most practicing food technologists have very little nutritional background and also little appreciate the impact of their efforts not only on the nutritional value of the food, but also on the nutritional well-being of consumers." Arthur Odell of General Mills is quoted as saying, "you can't sell nutrition... Hell, all people want is Coke and potato chips."

Food is a new growth area for chemists and chemical engineers. E.M. Fallen, a former executive of Agway, Inc. In Syracuse, stated that 7,500 new products are introduced every year. Most of them fail quickly, for consumers waste no time informing the food industry of what is acceptable. Rapid changes and enormous product variety is the order of the day.

Nutrition science has failed to develop any new knowledge about the effects of modern food technology on human health and well-being. It clings to the ancient 19th century studies that classify food stuffs as proteins, fats, and carbohydrates and accessory factors.

Nutritionists provide no insight into what constitutes nutrition in the latter part of the 20th century. One aspect of nutrition that they can measure is the amount of vitamins and minerals in food. Many vitamins are destroyed by heating and many minerals are lost in the cooking water. When food is prepared in institutional quantities and chefs must thaw out 50-pound cartons of meat and cook vegetables in 300 gallon kettles, the preparation time increases considerably. You can imagine what happens to the vitamins and minerals during this process. Can the "food value"required by the FDA on the label of manufactured food be a screen behind which the methodology of food fabrication escapes public scrutiny? Even more frightening, is the possibility of a world food shortage in the near future and a diet consisting of totally synthetic food.

The FDAs labelling regulations for percentage of daily values of proteins, vitamins, etc., will not insure good nutrition. The food industry can easily add synthetic products to balance the numbers. Unfortunately, nutrition science has failed to exercise its responsibility in watching over such actions; it simply lacks the necessary intellectual resources to do so. The medical profession with some obvious exceptions, can't seem to bring itself to admit that inadequate nutrition leads to health problems.

The regulatory agencies entrusted with monitoring the food we eat maintain the outward appearance monitoring food safety, but their interests don't parallel that of the public.. Food additives are ostensibly supposed to be of "an advantage to the consumer" with antioxidants used to prevent rancidity, antimicrobial agents employed to discourage mold growth, and solvents used in preparation of protein. About 1,800 chemicals are routinely added to manufactured food with no more than an FDA-created list known as the GRAS list (generally regarded as safe."

It is interesting to note that the FDA, which is charged with the responsibility of regulating the foods we eat, is often deficient in its duties. Dr. Herbert Ley, when he was forced to retire as commissioner of the FDA in 1969, said, "the thing that bugs me is that people think the FDA is protecting them... it isn't." Dr. Ley claims that he was forced to retire as commissioner of the FDA because he was consumer oriented.

There is a continuing controversy regarding coronary heart disease. The official hypothesis accepted by medical science is that a diet heavy in saturated fats and cholesterol promotes the onset of coronary thrombosis. Dr. Ancel Keys, of the University of Minnesota, is in the forefront of those who assert that high serum cholesterol levels increase the risk of heart attacks. Other researchers have come to different conclusions. Dr. John Gofman, at the University of California at Berkeley, notes that cholesterol and other lipids are transported in the blood in the form of lipoprotein complexes Gofman and his associates claim that analysis of particular lipoprotein classes can be of great help in predicting the likelihood of a heart attack.

The results of independent research further undermine the established belief that saturated fats and cholesterol in the diet promote heart disease. At the Yale Nutrition Laboratory, it was found that the effects of high cholesterol in the diet were nullified by a superior diet of proteins, minerals, and vitamins. These findings were corroborated at the Tufts University School of Medicine. Roger J. Williams, at the University of Texas, has been examining the emphasis on polyunsaturated fats. He said that Americans are eating more than they did in 1900, but are getting fewer antioxidants such as vitamin E.

Dr. Hugh Trowell pointed out that heart disease is practically unknown among Bantu tribesmen. Their whole diet is high in fiber. Drs. Cleave and Campbell state that "coronary disease should be related solely to the consumption of carbohydrates."

Dr. John Yudkin is another maverick who does not subscribe to the central belief that dietary fat causes heart disease. His work has convinced him that refined sugar and other refined carbohydrates are at the root of the problem. Cleave and Campbell concur in this belief. They see no correlation between fat intake and heart disease. They note that the common factor to all tribal diets is the absence of sugar and refined carbohydrates. A survey of 400 Maasai men in Tanganyika in 1962 showed little or no evidence of atherosclerosis, although they ate meat and milk exclusively and their serum cholesterol levels were low.

The official view of heart disease calls for Americans to follow a diet of fewer calories, cholesterol, and saturated fats. Millions of dollars have been spent on research in an attempt to prove that eggs, which contain large amounts of cholesterol, increase the risk of heart attacks. There is no scientific evidence to corroborate this theory. The AHA recommends that Americans limit their egg consumption to three a week.

The "benefits" of polyunsaturated fats are questionable due to the refining process they undergo. Some scientists have even wondered whether refining results in a product that is unrefined. Vegetable fat in the refining process is subjected to many chemicals and a high degree of heating that reduces the nutritional value to a great extent. Margarine may sell more cheaply than butter, but is the economic gain worth what may well be a nutritional loss?

The scope of this book is vast, and its conclusions are not unanimous. However, they help you develop a rational approach to good health through a complete understanding of nutrition.

YOU CAN DO IT!
SENATOR WILLIAM PROXMIRE

A nutritious diet program must be followed in concert with the exercise plan to achieve the greatest benefit. Fresh fruits, juices, melons, lean meats, chicken, fish, veal, cottage cheese, and skim milk--all in moderation – are the basic foods you should have in your diet.

Synopsis

Most bread in America is a disaster. Sprouted wheat bread is excellent, but any whole grain bread is good. Such a diet makes eating more pleasurable than ever, for moderation increases enjoyment. If you are hungry, a sliced tomato can be a tasty treat. Avoid refined sugar, ice cream, cakes, and pies. The American breakfast is designed to foster and encourage heart attacks.

Beware of bacon and eggs, hot or cold cereal and cream, and commercial bread and butter. The cardboard box of dry cereal is more nutritious than the cereals they contain! The coffee break at homes, offices, and factories creates another nutritional disaster. Coffee with cream and sugar, a sweet roll, Danish pastry or a piece of coffee cake, are all just empty calories. They make you fat and provide no nutrients or vitamins.

The cocktail hour is the most destructive habit in the world. It leads to 35,000 out of the 50,000 auto deaths each year. It also destroys the health of millions and adds empty calories that convert to sugar. TV snacks, crackers, potato chips, candy, cookies, and soft drinks are dead—they're nothing foods. Eat a balanced diet that has nutrients, vitamins, and minerals, but don't overeat even those foods that are good for you

This book is for those who are drifting aimlessly toward a middle-age that is destined to make them a burden to self, spouse, and family. Remember, no one can feel your pain, your shame, or your inner insecurity. Your life can be exciting, full of fun, good health, vitality, and happiness.

You   can   alter   your   course—you   can   do   it!

Author's Note : This book was the catalyst that inspired me to develop "The Best of Health: The 100 Best Health Books."

LIFE BEYOND 100
NORMAN SHEALY, M.D., PH.D.

A life expectancy of more than 100 years is no longer the stuff of science fiction. Dr. Norman Shealy's recommendations for optimal health and longevity are grounded in a long and successful career using both conventional and complementary medical practice.

Years of clinical practice have convinced Dr. Shealy that the medical establishment and the pharmaceutical industry have increased longevity by the use of prescription drugs. The treatment of symptoms rather than the prevention of disease has condemned hundreds of thousands of people to an old age that is worse than the alternative.

This book is a guide to youthful aging, and there is no reason why healthy aging to 100 is not only possible, but the potential for an extended quality of life is assured, using the approach of this eminent physician.

Synopsis

Living well past 100 is a radical concept. "Energy does not age." It is the nature of the human energy system. We must examine the importance of nutrition, diet, exercise, sleep patterns, depression, and vitamin intake. Don't underestimate the critical role of self esteem. "Self-esteem is the "make or break" power of the individual. It connects the psyche to the spirit.

Do we want to live to be 100 and beyond? Is there a fountain of youth? The human spirit is a key factor in the paradigm of health. Many energetic, enthusiastic individuals are ready to redefine old age. A new concept of longevity is 100—some to 120. They may live healthily to 120-160 just by adding a few simple activities to their daily lives.

Three Rules for Increasing Longevity:

- Keep DHEA level healthy—add 13 years.
- Keep Calcitonin level optimal--- add 13 years.
- Keep free radicals low—add 13 years.
- Average life expectancy--- 140 years.

Genetics may add or subtract 20 years. All health-conscious people should live at least 120 years. Those with the best genetic potential could live to be 160.

Steve Austad, a gerontologist at the University of Idaho, believes that a 150-year life span is quite feasible. Future discoveries will extend the potential even further. I will present evidence that supports a 140-year average potential.

Since 1985, I have continued to seek safe alternatives to drugs and surgery for 85 percent of the individuals who do not need these approaches. Every cell in the body is replaced within seven years. At 101 my grandmother was busy canning in her kitchen. After World War II, children were responsible for aging parents. Today, elderly parents are often rejected or sent to nursing homes.

People who are active remain happy. "Longevity is a greater spiritual challenge than a physical one." "Western culture worships youth. The elderly are often abandoned and warehoused. Medical science emphasizes advances that may enhance life, while the media extols youth. Retirement is forced on many vibrant leaders at 65 while AARP recruits people at 50, speeding up the concept of aging.

The use of antibiotics over the last 60 years has become widespread. Good health does not depend on drugs. "Drugs rarely return an individual to robust health. The firmest foundation for health is attitude."

Many diagnostic tests are administered primarily for the medical and legal protection of the physician. Often these tests are not helpful to the patient. I maintain that no more than 15 percent of all illnesses require drugs. If you want to age healthily, it is your responsibility to get there.

After 50 years of the war on cancer, life expectancy has increased by only 4 months quality of life, even less Deaths from prescription drug use in the United States is 113,000 per year. Other medical therapy deaths total 137,000. "There are more deaths from drugs than lives saved by drugs."

Dr. Robin says that "one should avoid hospitalization except for serious illnesses." At least 50 percent of hospital admissions are unnecessary. One of the requirements of life beyond 100 ia to "avoid medical care that is not essential to life or function." In 2002, Tommy Thompson, secretary of HHS said, "The American medical system is on the verge of collapse."

An essential component of the "fountain of youth" regimen is the following:

- Fruits, vegetables, nuts, fresh foods—fish, beef, chicken, pork, etc.
- Whole grains, (potatoes, starches in moderation), 100 percent whole grain bread (two to three slices a day).
- One or two eggs daily (unless your family has high cholesterol).
- Old-fashioned peanut butter (never hydrogenated or with sugar).
- Supplements-exercise-relaxation-meditation-avoid stress.
- Sex—enjoy sex with your partner.
- Water—2 quarts a day.
- Cholesterol—under no circumstances should you take any cholesterol-lowering drugs. They are dangerous.
- Avoid fast foods and carbonated drinks.
- Go on a low-carbohydrate diet.
- Avoid homogenized milk.
- Brown rice-oatmeal (no boxed cereals).
- Dried legumes cooked—up to one cup daily

DHEA (dehydroepiandrosterone), is a major feedback modulator of all the hormones in the body. It is made from cholesterol. It may be converted into estrogen and testosterone. Low levels of DHEA are found in every major disease. Dr. Hans Selye, (the father of stress) demonstrated the progression of alarm to adaptation to maladaptation to degeneration and exhaustion or burnout. I feel that this progression is highly correlated with DHEA levels.

A magnesium deficiency is more common than any other chemical or nutritional deficiency. It is the third most prevalent mineral in the human body. It is a natural calcium channel blocker. Magnesium is inside cells—calcium is outside cells. Magnesium regulates the electrical potential in nerve cells. Every single disease is a symptom of a magnesium deficiency. Magnesium is helpful in fibromyalgia, depression, diabetes, hypertension, and most other illnesses. The soil in every country except Egypt is depleted of magnesium. Magnesium taurate is the best absorbed oral supplement.

You must be willing to make the healthy choices discussed in this book. You have the opportunity to enjoy life beyond 100. The fountain of youth is now in your hands.

LIVE LONGER NOW
NATHAN PRITIKIN, JON N. LEONARD
AND JACK L HOFER

The American profession in America can be justifiably proud of its record in the past few generations. Infectious diseases that plagued our people early in the 20th century have virtually been defeated. TB, smallpox, malaria, and typhoid fever have practically disappeared as causes of death. Does this mean that we should be satisfied with the state of health in our country? The answer is definitely NO! The authors claim that we have not made a dent in another class of diseases—the degenerative diseases. It is the goal of this book to draw attention to the threat of such diseases, and to offer advice and how to prevent and possibly reverse them.

Synopsis

Heart disease, stroke (cerebrovascular disease), diabetes, atherosclerosis, hypertension, and gout involve the degenerative breakdown of the individual cells that leads to a breakdown of the whole person. The World Health Organization (WHO) claims that we are faced with the greatest epidemic in history. More than a million people die of degenerative diseases each year. The total is more than half of all deaths from all causes in the country. There has been some progress in decreasing the fatalities from high blood pressure, gout, and diabetes through drug treatment, but these diseases are only a minor segment of the degenerative diseases. We can only measure progress by our success in dealing with those disorders resulting in a greater number of deaths – i.e. heart disease, stroke, and atherosclerosis. The introduction of anti-hypertensive drugs in 1956 has helped decrease the incidence of cerebral haemorrhages, but the average American is still as likely to die of heart disease and stroke today as he or she was in 1910.

Atherosclerosis is a disease of the arteries that causes most heart attacks and strokes. If we can prevent this disease it would help to eliminate the degenerative diseases. It is neither necessary nor desirable to take drugs or wait for medical breakthroughs—the prevention and reversal of the degenerative diseases is at hand. It is simply a matter of what you eat and how you exercise your body. The billions of dollars spent each year by Americans to pay for the cost of heart attacks can be saved if the atherosclerosis causing the attacks were prevented. Yet we do not think to ourselves "that person died of atherosclerosis."

The American diet consists of 42 percent fat, almost half of our calorie intake. Primitive societies have a diet that contains 10 percent fat or less. In 25 primitive societies that were examined, none displayed a high incidence of heart disease. During a five-year period in the 1950s, the Nkama Nune hospital in southern Africa did not report a single Bantu death from heart disease. Furthermore, there is proof that genetic immunity is not the reason for resistance to heart attacks. When indigenous people moved to a large city and ate the high-fat, Westernized diet, the incidence of heart disease started to climb.

In the early 1950s, when the link between high blood cholesterol levels and heart disease was still uncertain, a great misunderstanding occurred. It was found that unsaturated fats (corn and safflower oil) reduced the cholesterol level in the blood. Soon, the dairy industry, which made billions on margarine, and the American Heart Association championed the use of unsaturated fats. They claimed that the substitution of unsaturated fat s for saturated fats would produce less heart disease. The sad fact is that they were wrong. Heart disease is still the number one killer in America. All fats are bad and should be drastically reduced in the diet.

Lester Morrison, a doctor in California, placed a group on a low-fat (15 percent) low-cholesterol diet. After 12 years, every single person in the control group had died, but 38 percent of the experimental group had survived. Morrison did not use a drop of unsaturated fat in his diet, yet the blood cholesterol levels of the experimental group showed the largest decrease (28%0 of the 12 studies shown in his book In spite of these facts, the unsaturated fat concept persists.

Diabetes is similar to atherosclerosis in that it can be prevented and treated by diet. Dietary fat is the culprit in both diseases. The evidence of a lack of diabetes in primitive societies has brought forth the low-fat, low-carbohydrate diet as the best means of preventing and treating diabetes. Diabetes can be caused in normal individuals by feeding them enough fats and simple carbohydrates to raise the fat level in the blood. High levels of fat reduced the effectiveness of the insulin in these people. With less effective insulin, sugar levels build up. The miracle of insulin, which was discovered 80 years ago has had its image tarnished by complications such blindness and heart disease. It has also become known recently that insulin injections can seriously damage the pancreas and the body's capacity to produce its own insulin.

Hypertension, or high blood pressure, is caused by atherosclerosis, excessive salt intake, and specific diseases of the kidneys, the adrenal glands, and the arteries. Millions of Americans are afflicted with this disease; one out of eight people examined in a recent study in Chicago (Schoenberger and Associates)were found to suffer from hypertension. There is a convincing association of atherosclerosis and hypertension. Studies reveal that the New Zealand Aborigines, who are free of heart disease and atherosclerosis have no hint of hypertension.   Blood pressure can be brought under control very quickly with anti-hypertensive drugs, but prolonged use of these drugs can cause various undesirable side effects. To get away from drug use for the control of hypertension, one should switch to a diet that is salt-free, low in fat, cholesterol, and sugar.

The role of exercise in the prevention and reversal of degenerative diseases is well-known. The Framingham Study (conducted since 1948) showed that the death rate from heart disease was five times greater for inactive men than for those who exercised. Exercise over a long period of time builds additional routes of blood supply. The growth of new capillary articles, and other new routes of blood flow results in a freer less encumbered flow of blood, which keeps the heart thoroughly oxygenated.   Hypertension is dramatically reduced by exercise alone. When a diabetic exercises, he uses blood fats for energy rather than using blood sugar as a non-diabetic does. With continued exercise, the fat level decreases and his insulin becomes sensitized and more effective. F.I. Buys and his associates in Johannesburg reported that in seven out of eight diabetic patients, the symptoms of diabetes disappeared after eight months of daily exercises.

The exercise program consists of what is called "roving." It is a combination of walking and jogging. You decide when to jog and when to slow down to a walk. Set your limit and travel that distance four or five times a week. Time does not matter. Roving will increase the efficiency of your heart in delivering oxygen to the body's various tissues. Collateral circulation will result in a significantly greater amount of oxygen in each quart of blood. The elasticity of your arteries will be increased, blood pressure lowered, and fatigue and stress, both mental and physical, will decrease.

Program 2100 is a personal program and a goal toward which you must strive. It will change your way of life. Your nutrition and exercise habits are clearly defined. If you follow the program, your life will be extended and will take on new dimensions of health, happiness, and quality.

THE 24-HOUR-DIET
PROFESSOR BRIAN SCOTT PESKIN

Professor Brian Scott Peskin takes a heroic stand for the truth against the establishment's status quo. Our health care costs have mushroomed to more than $2 trillion dollars, and we are now faced with an epidemic of obesity and diabetes.. It is imperative that we change the trend toward "Armageddon." It's sad that he has to apologize for being "insensitive" and "politically incorrect."

Peskin hurls the harpoon of truth into the whale of lies (the fairy tale) that the American public has been brainwashed to believe. He presents a diet regimen that is based on science. A decade of research in the world's most prestigious medical journals and textbooks validate his proposal for a diet regimen that will make you lean-for-life.

He takes up the "lost cause" of the nutrition imperative. Someone once said, they are the only ones worth fighting for." Peskin exposes the myths about saturated fats, cholesterol, fiber, soy, exercise, fish oils, and others. The scientific truths that are revealed in "The 24-Hour Diet" can be a shock to the public. Billions of advertising dollars have lulled the average person into believing the lies of the food industry, the pharmaceutical industry, the Food and Drug Administration (FDA), and other government agencies. (I refer to the Department of Agriculture, the National Institutes of Health, the National Heart, Lung and Blood Institute (NHLBI), and thousands of researchers in academia..

Every generation, someone emerges to challenge the domination of the powerful forces of the medical establishment. We now have a new voice that has been heard around the world. Peskin has aroused the public with his "The Hidden Story of Cancer," "The 24-Hour-Diet" is a logical extension of that monumental work, and will be a boon to the thousands of readers who will benefit from his scientifically developed protocols.

Synopsis

I had a problem. My abdomen was too big. I ate low carbohydrates and avoided sweets for more than a decade, but my stomach fat never diminished. I went to the gym and trained with weights. It didn't help. Something was wrong. Then the science hit me over the head!

This book is the story of my discovery. I wrote this book to save your life. You only need 24 hours of one day of will power at a time. My goal is to give you the scientific facts that will help you discover a unique system for becoming lean-for-life with boundless energy. I have spent many years of research to bring you the science from the world's leading medical textbooks.

My mission is to reverse America's and Europe's epidemic trends. Most of us have tried many diets and failed. This book is intended to bring you the truth about obesity—its prime cause and prevention.

I have no interest in being "politically correct" because the truth should be blind to outside influence. My conclusions will be different from everything you've heard on the subject. If people find fault with these conclusions, then they should be able to offer a better solution. These conclusions are drawn directly from science.

Why don't doctors know this information. The best reason is that they are overwhelmed treating patients' symptoms. Years ago, there was no type 2 diabetes. Men in their 30s didn't get heart attacks. Today, it is common. More than 50 percent of us contact cancer. More than 60 percent of us are overweight. Almost everyone we know is sick. Physicians are overloaded with patients. They don't have time to understand this information./ You have to learn the correct information on your own.

You can rest assured that everything in this book is validated by personal experience. "The 24-Hour Diet" doesn't use "weasel words" like "may," "possible," "suggests," "likely," and "could." You will learn about fat, protein, and carbohydrates.

PEOs (parent essential oils) are unprocessed, natural, parent essential oils commonly called EFAs (essential fatty acids) including fish oils, which are not the vital parent forms. Your body can't make these oils on its own. That's why they are called essential. Every one of our 100 trillion cells need essential oils for oxygen to reach the cells. Most supplement manufacturers don't distinguish the "parent" EFAs from the "derivative" EFAs. It is vital for you to know the difference.

We must get the PEOs, not the mistakenly termed EFAs, because stores sell oils they call "EFAs," including fish oils, which are not the vital parent forms. Your body doesn't need to consume many of the derivatives because it makes its own out of the parent essential oils you consume. Taking fish oils and other health food store "EFAs" can overdose you with derivatives and harm your health.

It is imperative to make sure you are taking more unprocessed parent Omega-6 than parent Oega-3. The ratio should be more than one part Omega-6 to one part Omega-3 and less than 2.5 parts parent Omega-6 to one part Omega-3—and no fish oils.

Everyone is overdosing on Omega-3. I've found that at least 3,000 mg. of PEOs in the above ratio reduces carbohydrate craving and increases your energy level. I also recommend a supplement that includes at least eight essential minerals – magnesium, manganese, iron, chromium, boron, copper, selenium, and zinc. The minerals must be chelated. True chelation binds the minerals to amino acids in the correct form for full utilization by your body. Minerals are coenzymes. They work with vitamins to assist in all of your biological processes. Vitamins are found in our food, so taking a mineral supplement is even more important than taking a vitamin supplement.

I highly recommend a gentle herbal detoxifier based on the long standing Essiac concept formula. These three vital supplements work well together along with my dietary recommendations.

I used to crave two large pizzas a week. I would bring them home and eat them myself at 10 p.m. before going to sleep. I would also crave hot fudge sundaes and vanilla cake with chocolate frosting. Banana splits were my favourite. Things are different now. My program has solved the carbohydrate addiction for me and people around the world. All you need to do is trust the science behind the program for 24 hours at a time.

Questions about the program

Q. Are fruits and vegetables the gateway to good health?

A. Excessive sugar from fruits, vegetables, grains, and starchy carbs are not all good for you. I don't think so. An apple a day is fine, but a quart of apple juice will not help you lose weight.

Q. What do you think of fish oils?

A. They are worthless at best and harmful at worst. They overdose you with Omega-3 derivatives. Parent omega oils in the proper ration are the answer. Top medical journals have recently reported the hazards of fish oil.

Q. Why don't you recommend 8 to 10 glasses of water a day?

A. "Force feeding" yourself on water when you are not thirsty is one of the worst things you can do if you want to stay lean-for-life.

Q. Doesn't exercise (running and aerobics) help you lose weight?

A. Exercise hasn't kept Americans thin as a nation. We have never been more exhausted or fatter in spite of the increase in exercise.

Q. Isn't too much protein bad for the kidneys? How much protein should we eat daily?

A. Protein can't even enter the kidney—and it doesn't leach calcium from bones. You need at least eight ounces of animal-based protein such as cottage cheese, eggs, poultry and meat to stay lean-for-life.

Q. I love carbs. How could they be bad?

A. The more you eat, the more you want. This makes you overweight for life because it short-circuits nature's natural fat-burning mechanism.

Q. Aren't carbs the source of energy?

A. If weight loss is your primary goal, this is the worst thing you can do.

Q. Should I count calories. Why do you say calories don't count?

A. "The calorie theory" was disproved in 1893 by Adolph Fick, M.D.

Q. How do I get rid of my flabby stomach?

A. Follow the 24-Hour-Diet.

Q. If I cut carbs I feel weak and tired. How can i avoid this?

A. Don't remove carbs too quickly. Gradually cut down from two to four weeks.

Q Do I need a lot of fiber in my diet?

A. No. You want less fiber in your diet. Fiber irritates your colon and recent studies show it actually increases the risk of colon cancer.

Diet and nutrition advice is contradictory. Books in most cases are based on opinion, not reality. There is only one correct answer. Believe no one. Believe the science, period.

This book will give you all of the science needed to become lean-for-life. My idol, Nobel Laureate Richard Feynman, said it best.

"It does not make any difference how smart you are, who made the guess or what his name is. If it disagrees with real-life results, it is wrong. That is all there is to it."

For 50 years Americans have become bigger and sicker by the decade. I founded "Life systems Engineering Science" to help solve the problems in human health. I was shocked to find that the so-called "solution" to our weight and health problem was actually the cause of the problem. We are causing our own demise but don't know it. Scientists know how to keep us lean-for-life. The popular press misinterprets most of what they say.

Carbohydrates are the number one reason for acid reflux. If it isn't protein like meat, fish, chicken, or eggs and it isn't fat, like butter, cheese, cream, or oils, then it is carbohydrate. Carbohydrates are composed largely of sugars and starches. They include bread, cereal, fruit, cream, milk, popcorn, rice, pasta, and potatoes. Carbohydrates are everywhere, and they are not your body's preferred energy source. We have been misled to believe that carbs are necessary for energy and this is the primary reason Americans are overweight.

The Basic Medical dictionary clearly states, "The body oxidizes (burns as fuel) more fatty acids each day than any other fuel."

The medical textbook, "Scientific Foundations of Biochemistry in Clinical Practice" makes it clear. Just 1 percent of your pancreas is capable of treating all that sugar. The remaining 99 percent is supposed to treat fats and proteins so you can digest them, but a high carbohydrate diet overloads this 1 percent, making it do the majority of the work.

If you stop insulin generation by decreasing carbohydrate consumption, then fat storage will be blocked. In other words, all you need to do in order to stop fat from being stored is to stop your body from constantly producing insulin. The only way to do this is to stop your carbohydrate consumption. Less insulin equals less fat storage. My standing joke is that on a carbohydrate-based diet, by eating a complex carbohydrate like brown organic rice, instead of candy or soda, you get just as fat—only 15 minutes later!

A high carbohydrate diet is a dieter's worst nightmare. It causes you to stay hungry. The more candy, cakes, and ice cream you eat. The more you want. The insulin response makes you crave an ever increasing amount. For decades the average American has consumed 60 to 70 teaspoons of disguised sugar in the form of juice, oatmeal, fruit, cereals, rice, bagels, spaghetti, food bars, etc. "Contrary to popular opinion, protein and natural fats are wonderful and extremely healthful for you."

If you want to start a low-carb regimen, be sure to gradually reduce your carbohydrate intake. A sudden change can shock your system. Reduce your carb portions to about half for a month, then each week, reduce them a little more.

Cholesterol—we are being misled about the dangers of saturated fat and cholesterol. You'll soon be on the path to enjoying delicious foods like whipped cream, chocolate, eggs, and butter because you will learn the truth about cholesterol. Television and print ads bombard us with comments about "bad cholesterol" coming from genetics and the food you eat, but LDL cholesterol is not bad. If it was, we'd all be dead, and humans would have ceased to exist eons ago.

LDL cholesterol isn't bad and HDL cholesterol isn't good. LDL brings those important PEOs into each of our 100 trillion cells. Any problem with cholesterol lies elsewhere. The Journal of the American Medical Association (JAMA) published the truth

- The study reports that "cholesterol levels in and of themselves are meaningless.

- 1,700 patients analysed with heart disease show more heart-related disease with cholesterol below 250 than between 300 and 400 or higher.

- Food processors have ruined our food. They create trans-fats in the hydrogenation process and ruin healthy oils—all in a n attempt to prevent spoilage. LDL cholesterol acts like a "poison delivery system" bringing trans-fats into the cells. It's these oxidized parent Omega-6 fats that clog the arteries, not the saturated fat.

A protein rich diet has greater reductions in blood pressure. LDL cholesterol, and triglycerides than a carbohydrate –rich diet. Medical journals and textbooks report conclusively that a high-protein diet is superior to the politically correct diet that follows popular opinion and "conventional" dietary wisdom. Instead of following science, "you will end up fat, dumb, and dead." I realize that this commentary is shocking and you might find it insensitive. I listen to the science, not "popular opinion."Protein can't make you fat! There is no mechanism for storing excess dietary proteins. India is one of the most diabetic countries because of improperly practiced vegetarianism. The Association of

Official Analytical Chemists International concludes that traditional diets have serious deficiencies. The point is clear. Vegetable-based protein is inferior to animal-based protein. The utilization of the protein in rice and beans is approximately half that of an egg! Since rice and beans have only half the protein of eggs, that means they have only one-quarter the protein of eggs.

At least 8 ounces of animal-based protein needs to be consumed each day. Eggs, cottage cheese, and full-fat yogurt, as well as meat, poultry, and fish are part of the diet. Hemoglobin, the oxygen transporter in blood, requires lots of protein for its manufactures. 2-3 ounces of protein is not enough! The more animal-based protein consumed, the less osteoporosis. Bone loss results from vegetable-based proteins. /the bone matrix is composed of protein-based collagen, and it needs PEOs too.

Protein adds calcium to bone. Protein from meat stops bone fracture. A study of 32,000 women showed that women eating the most meat were 68 percent less likely to break a hip. Vitamin B-12 can only come from animal sources. We have always heard, "protein harms your kidneys." Wrong! Uncontrolled blood sugar levels harm your kidneys. That's why diabetics have the highest rate of kidney failure. Meat doesn't cause cancer. It is rather the hormones, pesticides, and other additives that are at fault. That is why I recommend organic meat, cheese, and eggs.

Americans have unknowingly damaged their health by eating lots of soy. Soy is touted by nutritionists, physicians, and health and beauty publications extolling its virtues. This advice is not based on science. Soy is the second largest cash crop in America, generating $14 billion dollars a year. Evidence against the use of soy has been available since the 1960s. Soy is not a health food. Don't eat too much soy because it is harmful to humans and can actually increase the risk of developing cancer.

Soy milk is not milk. It does not require refrigeration. The Chinese eat only 10 grams a day, only one-sixth of the amount Americans are encouraged to eat. The Japanese consume more soy than Americans and their cancer rates are higher than Americans. The Asian diet uses soy as a condiment (soy sauce). In America, tofu is sold as a meat replacement. Women have been told that soy prevents cancer. I wish that were true. In 1996, researchers found that soy protein isolate increased hyperplasia—a condition often leading to malignancy—(cancer of the uterus). A year later another study showed that genistein (found in soy) was found to affect womens' breast cells negatively.

Common Questions About Soy

Q. Is soy a good source of protein? Can it replace meat?
A. No!
Q. Is soy good for the blood? A. No! It contributes to arterial blockage and heart attacks.
Soy has never attained GRAS (generally regarded as safe) status by the FDA.
Infants on soy formula have experience thyroid problems.

Key Points of the 24-Hour-Diet

* Eat when you are hungry.
* PEOs will help satisfy you.
* Eat primarily proteins and natural fats.
* Meats, poultry, eggs, and cheese.
* More parent Omega-6 than parent Omega-3.
* The 24-YHour-Diet gives your overworked pancreas a much needed rest.

Great Protein Foods
* Full-fat cottage cheese and full-fat yogurt.
* Fish is wonderful.
* Ground sirloin burgers are my favourite food.

I cook two half-pound burgers in a fry pan and top them with ketchup at least three times a week. I then have sauteed green beans, and a glass of water.

I am so fulfilled with real food that sweets have lost their grip on me. A great snack is celery stuffed with cream cheese, or a handful of organic nuts like pecans or almonds, and freshly made whipped cream.

Buy an accurate scale. Weigh yourself in the morning, before breakfast. Friday night and Sunday there is no dieting. Holidays—enjoy them—indulge.

FEEL BETTER, LIVE LONGER WITH VITAMIN B-3
ABRAM HOFFER, M.D. AND H. D. FOSTER

In this book we present evidence that over half the population would benefit by taking extra doses of vitamin B-3 (niacin) ranging from milligram to gram doses, depending upon basic physiology of the body. For the average healthy person I suggest 60 to 100 milligrams daily would be beneficial." (from E-mail by Dr. Abram Hoffer to Sheldon Zerden).

For people too low in high density lipoprotein cholesterol (HDL) the recommended dose is 3 to 9 grams. Some schizophrenic patients have gotten better on up to 30 grams daily. I have found it also helped in cases of brain damage depending on the severity of the damage and for how long it has been present. It is part of Dr. Klenner's treatment of multiple sclerosis.

The following is a list of the properties of vitamin b-3. The literature evidence is given in Hoffer and Foster's book.

- Anti-pellagra.
- Antidote to adrenochrome and LSD.
- Therapeutic for the schizophrenias.
- Therapeutic with vitamin E for Huntington's Disease.
- Therapeutic against Parkinson's induced psychosis.
- Excellent anti-stress.
- Decreased tendency to get Alzheimer's disease.
- Anti-anxiety including alcoholism.
- Anti-aging—my patient, the oldest in Canada, aged 112, died in 2006. She was on niacin for 42 years. Sge did cross-country skiing at age 110.
- Therapeutic for arthritis.

- Elevates HDL- the world's gold standard for this.
- Lowers LDL.
- Lowers triglycerides.
- Lowers lipoprotein (a).
- Decreases arteriosclerosis and decreases the ravages of the cardiovascular system.
- Protects against diabetes.
- Heals Bright's disease (glomerulonephritis)
- Mild ant-convulsive properties.
- Anti-cancer and protects against radiation and chemotherapy induced cancers.
- Prevents degeneration of brain cells.
- Therapy for delirium tremens.

Brain cell damage and Vitamin B-3

Humphrey Osmond and I began to study the therapeutic properties of niacin and niacinamide in 1962, the precursors to the Nicotinamide Adenine Nucleotide (NAD) cycle. We confirmed the observations that had been reported in the literature by 1952 and found some new ones which were very surprising. The term vitamin B-3 refers to the two basic terms of this anti-pellagra vitamin.

I have always wondered why it is so versatile. I know that giving this vitamin increased NAD levels in cells, and that NAD is a very important component of enzymes in the body which control many reactions. When it is not present in adequate amounts the person develops pellagra, a deadly disease, which at one time killed 30,000 Americans in the Southeastern United States. Over 100 years ago it was one of the major pandemics, not only in the United States, but around the Mediterranean, where corn became a staple food. Central Americans were much more intelligent. They also ate a lot of corn, legumes, and other vegetables. However, they treated their corn overnight with alkali, which released the vitamin so it can be absorbed. They did not get pellagra.

I concluded that it was as important as the NAD cycle. It is so important in almost every reaction in the body and when it is not present in adequate amounts the cells are not able to convert food into energy as well. NAD is the key molecule for cellular metabolism. But there was no evidence for this hypothesis until recently.

Sasaki et al found that substances which are used in building the NAD cycle will prevent damage to the axons of nerve cells in rats. The nerve axon is the long nerve originating in the nerve cell (neuron). It is damaged in many neuropathological conditions such as diabetic neuropathy, demyelination disease (multiple sclerosis) and neurodegenerative diseases such as Alzheimer's, Amyotrophic Lateral Scerosis (Lou Gehrig's Disease) (ALS). In these diseases the axon degeneration may precede the damage of the nerve cell and according to these authors may contribute significantly to the clinical symptoms. Anything which increases NAD formation (niacinamide, niacin, tryptophan, and pyridoxine), but niacinamide itself was not protective. It has to be converted into NAD. Practically, this means that NAD levels should always be kept at normal levels and will be protective against these diseases rather than curative. The author concluded, "in summary, we found that multiple manipulations that increased activity of the NAD pathway can promote axon protection, supporting the hypothesis that increased NSDF availability is a likely mechanism responsible for the delayed axon degeneration" 1

Kaneko et al from Harvard medical School studied rats with the equivalent of multiple sclerosis. They found that niacinamide reduces the inflammation and demyelination. Niacinamide, they suggest may be a promising candidate for a neuroprotective treatment of MS patients and other axon degenerative relevant diseases. They did not test niacin, but i expect the results will be similar or even better. 2

- Sasaki et al Journal of Neuroscience
2006: 16: 8484-8491
- Kaneko et al Journal of Neuroscience
2006: 26: 9794-9804

THE SECRET HISTORY OF THE WAR ON CANCER
DEVRA LEE DAVIS, PH.D., MPH

The Greek playwright Euripides said it more than 2,500 years ago, "Nothing so evil as money ever grew to be current among men." That statement is as true today as it was then. Devra Davis, an epidemiologist and director of the Center for Environmental Oncology at the University of Pittsburgh in Pennsylvania. USA has undertaken one of those lost causes that are truly the only ones worth fighting for. She has courageously taken on the whole cancer establishment and dared to tell the truth about the incestuous relationship between researchers and industry. The government has also dragged its fight against this deadly disease. Richard Nixon's war on cancer in the early1970s was doomed to failure because it was mainly targeted to the symptoms of cancer and not the causes. The ultimate answer to cancer is prevention.

The tobacco companies, the chemical industry, the petrochemical industry, etc. Are a multibillion dollar reason why researchers are compromised into accepting fees as consultants while they are at the same time passing judgment on the safety of asbestos, vinyl chloride, pesticides, benzene and other toxic substances. It is hard to believe that environmental causes of cancer were known by researchers in the 1930s. The scientists in Nazi Germany were the pioneers of modern industrial chemistry. They were also pioneers in epidemiology. German researchers knew about the link between smoking and cancer.

Dr. Davis lost both of her parents to cancer. She weaves the personal story of her life into a very thorough and comprehensive look at the effects of pesticides, toxic wastes, CT scans, MRIs, cell phones, aspartame, x-rays, lead, mercury, PCBs, and polyvinyl chloride (PVC). This monumental work is something to be praised. Nothing can be said by the forces of greed and inaction that can alter the truth that is contained in the pages of this great book.

Synopsis

Cancer has become the price of modern life. In America and England one out of every two men and one out of every three women will develop cancer in their lifetime. In America there are 10 million cancer survivors. Cancer is the leading killer of middle-aged persons and the second leading killer of children. As we age, the body loses the ability to defend itself against the damaging effects of being alive.

We inherit genes from our Parents. Genes tell cells when to die and when to get food. Attacks on our genetic base are repaired in the blink of an eye. It's amazing. Without these repairs none of us would survive. An aging population does not explain why five times more men and women get brain cancer in America than Japan, or why rates of testicular cancer in men under age 40 have risen 50% in one decade in industrial nations. It also doesn't explain why women of generation are getting twice as much breast cancer as their grandmothers did, and why black women die from breast cancer in greater numbers than their white counterparts do? Aging does not explain why so many more children have developed cancer. What can we do to reverse the trend?

Despite progress, more than half of all those diagnosed with cancer will not last a decade. People who lead clean, exemplary lives—still get cancer. Nine out of ten women who develop breast cancer are born with perfectly healthy genes. What causes cancer is a complicated matter of intense debate. More than 80,000 chemicals are in widespread use. There have been toxicity tests on fewer than 1,000.

Cancer is the only disease that merits its own war. 40 years--$69 billion dollars of taxpayer money—the war goes on. Talk of imminent victory has grown muted.

In the 1930s German scientists showed that tobacco use increased cancers and other diseases in humans. In 1936, Alton Ochsner reported nine cases of lung cancer in six months. He suggested that cigarette smoking lay behind the sudden surge in the disease. In 1940, Argentine researcher Angell Roffo identified tobacco tars, rather than nicotine, as the principal cancer-causing part of cigarette smoke. He founded the world's first cancer institute in Buenos Aires. Even when nicotine was taken out of tobacco in his experiments on animals, tumors occurred. This made it clear that tars in tobacco were the chief culprits.

In the 1930s, Dr. Franz H. Muller, at the Jena Tobacco Institute, created the first irrefutable modern proof that smoking causes lung cancer in humans. In three decades the disease had gone from a rare occurrence to the second leading cause of death in Germany.

Two major figures, Wilhelm Hueper and Robert Kehoe, were in the forefront of the research and public understanding of the environmental causes of cancer. Hueper warned the DuPont Company that they could expect to see many cases of bladder cancer at its plant in Delaware. At the Beta Napthylamine manufacturing plant, an industrial dye caused bladder tumors in dogs that looked like those found in men in Europe. In November 1937, Hueper was warned not to publish any of his findings. In 1038, Hueper was fired. He ended up at the National Cancer Institute from 1948 to 1968, when he retired. He is the person Rachel Carson credited in her ground breaking book, "Silent Spring," for exposing the connection between the environment and cancer.

Robert Kehoe was a central figure in public health circles. His experience led him to as lucrative corporate job after serving as a professor at Cincinnati and director of the Kettering Laboratory. Kehoe had signed contracts with major corporations, but before issuing public reports, the manuscripts had to be submitted to the donors for "criticism and suggestion." Kehoe, like many doctors who worked for industry, believed that the details of workplace hazards were best kept confidential. Kehoe was a captain in the U.S. Army. After the war in Germany ended, he interviewed German scientists and brought back critical studies ranging from chemical warfare, pesticides, pharmaceuticals and industrial materials

Ethyl Corporation, which was jointly owned by Standard Oil of New Jersey (Exxon) and General Motors, was truly a global firm. Germany was one of its most important clients. Harry Truman termed the alliance with I.G. Farben "treason." I.G. Farben was Hitler's biggest donor. Its members included BASF, Bayer, Hoechst, and others.

Kehoe visited some of the concentration camps. Surely he saw the ovens. He kept photos of the corpses. Yet, he makes no mention of the genocide that was carried out. Lt. Colonel Richard Seibel entered the camp at Mauthausen and stated, "We've come across this big camp, we don't know what it is. People are dying everywhere—people don't do this to people."

Kehoe's depictions of the camps were clinically detached. The Germans came up with diethylstilbestrol (DES). It was the first synthetic estrogen created. It was added to animal feed to fatten cows. Pigs, and chickens for the German nation. Boys that worked in the factory that made DES developed painful, swollen breasts. DES was made from coal tar. It could make a scrawny cow put on several hundred pounds in a few months. This was valuable to a wartime economy. It is now banned in industrial countries. Just as Hueper had warned Irenee DuPont in 1932, bladder cancer was rampant in dye workers.

Kehoe found that the amount of time spent working at the Bensisine Plant in Leverkausen, Germany (1946) exponentially increased the workers' likelihood of contracting bladder tumors.

0-5 years- 10%
5-10 years- 20%
10-15 years- 20%
15-20 years- 50%
20-25 years- 90%

After 20 years or more—everyone had bladder cancer. Kehoe reported to OSS (CIA) with the warning that the subject matter was a "trade secret" and was not to be compromised or released to the public. Many years later lawsuits were filed alleging earlier knowledge of some of these hazards. Thus, the lives of Hueper and Kehoe became connected. Kehoe resumed his highly profitable career with the same firms that employed him in the 1930s.

Archives at the University of Cincinnati show that Hueper's work continued under Kehoe's secret direction. Benzidine was studied at Kettering laboratories by Hueper in the 1940s. He knew that rats with bladder tumors were caused by benzidine dyes at DuPont. For 20 years after Hueper left DuPont, no new cases of cancer were reported. In 1980 it was revealed that 364 cases of bladder cancer has occurred in one factory alone (The Chambers works). Hueper and Kehoe shared a confidence that the assembly of facts would lead to a better world. They had fundamentally different views. Hueper ended his career as an alienated outsider. Kehoe remained at the top of his profession—and was hailed as the founder of modern industrial toxicology.

In 1928, a Greek American researcher named George Papanicolaou found a way to inspect the opening of a womb. A few cells can be swabbed that would reveal the health of the cervix. This is now called a "Pap test" or a "Pap smear." In the 1930s, the medical world was not moved by Papanicolaou's work, and women continued to die at an alarming rate. The American Cancer Society began promoting the Pap smear in 1957, 15 years after it had been shown to save lives, and 30 years after it was first developed.

Democracies rest on an informed public. In 1933, Evarts Graham, a top surgeon of the day, achieved fame for the first removal of a cancerous lung. Graham was a chain smoker and could not accept that cigarettes were a hazard, but Ernst Wynder would soon change his mind. Born Ernst Weinberg in Germany in 1922, Wynder fled the Nazis and arrived in America in 1938. He served as a U.S. Army intelligence officer from 1943 to 1945. He learned about the Nazis' stunning research on smoking and health. Wynder's studies of Graham's patients would change his mind. More than 600 men with lung cancer were all heavy smokers. The first study linking smoking and lung cancer was published in JAMA on May 27, 1950. Graham managed to quit smoking in 1953. It was too late. He died four years later from lung cancer.

S. Cuyler Hammond, ACS chief of Epidemiology trained an army of women to gather information on their lifetime smoking habits of their neighbours. Hammond accumulated detailed information about the smoking habits of 187,766 men in nine states and confirmed that those who smoked were most likely to die of cancer and heart disease. Hammond presented his findings to the board.

According to one of his family members, Hammond was threatened with financial ruin if he released any of his work. The previous director of the ACS, Clarence Cook Little was summarily canned, so Hammond knew this was no idle threat.

The tobacco czars were in a panic. A new strategy was adopted. Create doubt. If new studies emerged on the hazards of smoking, flood the media with assertions that nothing had been proven. The Tobacco Industry Research Council (TIRC) tapped Clarence Cook Little, the former director of the American Society for Cancer Control (ASCC). With millions of dollars at his disposal, he funded research on the hazards of tobacco, and could therefore claim that the issue was not settled. Little stated, "There have been many experiments here and abroad, and none have been able to produce carcinoma of the lung in animals." What he neglected to say was that when exposed to the levels of tars and smoke that humans took in regularly, most mice died. Dead mice don't get cancer. Little pointed out that not all smokers get cancer.

The AMA and the ACS refused to take a firm position on the dangers of smoking. The tobacco industry had circled its wagons brilliantly.

Three big bombs fell on the tobacco industry in the 1960s. In 1962, The Royal College of Physicians issued a report which concluded that smoking was a health hazard. "Cigarette smoking is a cause of lung cancer and bronchitis, and continues to the development of heart disease." The same year the ACS finally weighed in on the issue. "Clinical, epidemiological, chemical, and pathological evidence demonstrate beyond a reasonable doubt that cigarette smoking is a major cause of lung cancer." Two years later (1964), the U.S. surgeon general echoed the evaluation of the Royal College of Physicians, that cigarette smoking causes cancer.

For more than a decade after the surgeon general's report, the AMA continued to accept funding from the tobacco industry. The ACS, however, joined the fight against tobacco. In 1994, a team of investigators led by Stan Glantz at U.C. at San Francisco received a box containing thousands of pages of documents from the Brown and Williamson Tobacco Corporation. Those documents, known as the "cigarette papers" made it clear that the tobacco companies, with the help of the ACS and the AMA, prolonged the uncertainty about their products throughout the 1950s.

The ACS is not alone in its historical reticence. The AMA hardly mentions its work with the tobacco industry. When Clarence Cook Little died in 1971, at the age of 83, his obituary in the New York Times made no mention of his earlier work at the TIRC, or his earlier work at the American Cancer Society. His family left unreported his last 25 years, which he spent magnifying uncertainties about tobacco products.

Mammograms

Today, new computerized systems digitize and magnify what can be seen within the breast. Some radiologists have never seen a microcalcification they can leave alone—and surgical biopsy—is booming. New machines take higher resolution and find microscopic changes that could not be seen a decade ago. (MRIs) Magnetic Resonance Imaging of the breast costs between $2,000 and $3,000 a procedure. There is no way to know whether increased testing is truly better for women's health.

The marketing of mammography, ultrasound, and breast MRI has a life of its own. The National Breast Cancer Coalition (NBCC) believes that there is insufficient evidence to recommend for or against mammography. The fact is oncology is a business, as well as the grounds for trying to keep people from dying of cancer. Sometimes, its business side stands in the way of its larger, more noble goals. Those on the front line today do not have the capacity or the incentive to be disinterested observers.

Asbestos

The dangers of asbestos are no longer disputed. It is one of the best studied workplace hazards in the world, partly because it was so widely employed as an insulator in buildings, ships, power plants, and factories.

Unfortunately, asbestos degrades into invisible, floating particles that slip into the fragile sacs of the lung, leaving permanent scars. Chronic exposure leaves a person with less and less working lung tissue. Eventually he or she suffocates.

Asbestos fibers inflame the lung, sending white blood cells called microphages to try to get rid of the unwelcome foreign bodies. When this fails, other cells grow around the attacked area, leaving distinct scars. Sometimes the heart gives out from all the extra work that has to be done just to get sufficient blood through the lungs.

Germans officially compensated the surviving families of dead asbestos workers in 1936. Italy followed suit in 1943. How did the industry respond? They set up secret studies in private laboratories to see if animals responded in the same way reported in workers. Much of this work was done in the 1950s and did not surface until 1978. Lawyers representing men and women who had died of asbestos pried these records from the previously secret files of the asbestos industry.

Sarma, Ontario is an industrial center that is known for the highest asbestos exposure ever recorded anywhere. The town has five times the level of mesothelioma as the rest of the region. Almost 1,500 cases of the disease were diagnosed between 1981 and 2001, about one new victim a week. That is impressive for a town with a population of 70,000.

Sarma doesn't have a single asbestos mine in the region. Sarma is home to 20 percent of Canada's petroleum refineries. An editorial in the Toronto Star reads, " The men went to work every morning, proud to earn a livelihood for their families, and they came back each evening carrying death in their clothes. Asbestos dust blew so thickly into the street that the traffic would come to a halt.

Despite a century of evidence on its dangers, the market for asbestos is booming in India, China, Iran, Kazakhstan, Thailand, and other developing countries. Regarding future deaths that this will bring, those making the decisions know, but they don't care, much like the factories around China leaking benzene into the rivers.

The terrific profitability of the industry, the role of asbestos in wartime, And the shifting grounds of public health research kept this hazard from being fully indicted for more than three decades

The chances that asbestos workers who smoked would die of lung cancer did not just add up, they multiplied. Those who worked with asbestos and did not smoke cigarettes had a fivefold risk of the disease than the general population. Those who smoked cigarettes alone had a tenfold greater risk. But the poor fellow who worked with asbestos for twenty years and smoked a pack a day had a more than fifty times greater chance of dying of lung cancer than one without such exposure.

"In a world where information on the health and safety of workers remains locked up in company files, wrapped in the protections of confidentiality, independent information and independent experts to make sense of it are an endangered species."

100,000 chemicals are used in commerce. Most have not been studied as to their ability to affect our health. For three out of four of the top 3,000 chemicals in use today, we have no public record of their toxicity, "We have come full circle. In the 1930s, the world's leading cancer experts identified many important causes of cancer in industry, nutrition, and behaviour. The evidence has been stretched, reviewed, revised, etc. And put back together again." It is a huge dilemma.

THE WHOLE SOY STORY
KAALA T. DANIEL PH.D. CCN

Soy is a phenomemom. It is a healthy alternative to meat, non-allergenic dairy, low-cost protein, a "wonder food." Soybean production and processing is one of the world's largest growth industries. It is already a $14 billion dollar business. Soy promotion is aimed at vegetarians and the poor.

The industry has a waste problem-- the leftover sludge from soy-oil manufacture. This developed into a campaign to sell soy products to upscale consumers as a miracle substance that would prevent heart disease and cancer, build strong bones, and keep us young forever. University professors demonized meat, milk, cheese, butter, and eggs. The funds behind this push for soy are enormous. Farmers pay a fee for every bushel of soybeans they sell. Ultimately, it goes towards the promotion of the most highly processed foods of all—imitation meat, milk, cream, cheese, yogurt, ice cream, candy bars, and smoothies made of soy.

The late Dr. Robert C. Atkins, defender of beef and butter has been seconded to the cause. Low-carb bread, pastry, and pasta, the foods Atkins warned against are made with high protein soy. Soy is found in most supermarket breads. Soy milk plants are found in Kenya. Hindus in India are eating lentils made of extruded soy protein. China, where people want more meat, not tofu, is building soy factories. The USDA's menu program shows unlimited use of soy in student meals.

Pages and pages of full-color ads for soy-based candy bars are featured in Men's Fitness magazine. If their readers were warned that soy lowers testosterone levels in men, advertising revenues would dry up and the magazine would fold. Soy producers pay $80 million dollars annually to support domestic and foreign markets for uses of soybeans and its products. Archer Daniels Midland spent $4.7 million dollars on

Meet the press and $4.3 million dollars on Face \the Nation.

The science behind soy- the whole soy story- needs to be told. The public need to hear. It will burst the soy bubble. Soy represents a threat to our health and our future.

Synopsis

The Chinese valued the soybean, but they did not eat it. Five sacred grains- rice, millet, barley, and wheat. The soybean is a legume, not a grain. Soy was a nitrogen fixing root. About 2,500 years ago it became a fermented food. Until then the Chinese considered the soybean inedible. They knew that soybeans remain toxic after ordinary cooking. Soy promoters claims that soybeans have been a major part of the Asian diet for more than 3,000 years, or from "time immemorial" are not true. Miso arrived in Japan 540 and 552 A.D. Chinese missionaries developed miso in 896 and 938 A.D.

Tofu- a precipitated product- monks noted that randy behaviour declined when consumption of tofu went up. Soy lowers testosterone levels. Tofu was a staple in Buddhist monasteries. It spread through China, Korea, and Southeast Asia. By 700 A.D. It was a meat or fish substitute. Is soy a staple? Proponents of soy foods state that soy is a staple food in Asian countries. The fact is that soy foods accounted for only 1.5 percent of calories in the Chinese diet(1977 publication).China, Korea, Vietnam, Thailand, Indonesia, Mongolia, and Japan don't eat very much soy. In Indonesia tempeh is the soybean food of choice. They have 41,000 tempeh shops.

It wasn't until 1995 that soybeans were grown for food. Europeans and Americans were slow to welcome soy into Western cuisine. John Harvey Kellogg, M.D. (1852-1943) championed the health benefits of the soybean. He harangued against the evils of meat. ArtemyAlexis Horvath Ph.D. , in his manifesto, "Soya Flour as a National Food." Henry Ford had great plans for soy. Ford's secretary described a soybean biscuit as "the most vile thing ever put into human mouths." Adolph Hitler promoted soybeans, vegetarianism, and natural foods. Benito Mussolini ordered the formation of a committee to require soy flour as an ingredient in the Italian staple polenta. In the Soviet Union the Communist party pushed soy protein and margarines as the solution to low-cost feeding of the masses. Soybeans were not seriously considered for food in the U.S. until World War II. Shortages created a demand for a cheap source of protein. The myth that soy is eaten in great quantity in Asia is an invention of the soy industry.

DuPont is the largest producer of soy protein. It owns 20 joint ventures in China with a total investment of $700 million dollars. In America, soy is aggressively marketed as an "upscale health food" that can prevent heart disease and cancer despite a lack of any real proof of these claims. Soy foods are one of the fastest growing sectors in the food industry. Retail sales grew 21 percent in 2000, with the strongest increases in sales of soy milk, energy bars, meat analogues, and cold cereals.

Soy foods are now nearly as expensive as meat and pricier than dairy. The largest food companies now manufacture soy foods. They include Kraft, Kellogg, Conagra, General Mills, Heinz, Unilever, Best Foods, and Dean Foods.

Soy is listed on the FDA's "poisonous plant database." It reveals 256 references that include studies that warn about goiter, growth problems, amino acid deficiencies, mineral malabsorption, endocrine disruption, and carcinogenesis. Because scientists have been unable to prove the health benefits of soy, industry efforts have led to a mastery of the art of ambiguous health claims. The campaign has been brilliant and soy hype has led to higher profits.

All soybeans contain anti-nutritional factors (anti-nutrients) and toxins. They can harm us unless soybeans are properly processed to neutralize them.

Allergens- can cause allergies. Goitrogens-can damage the thyroid. Lectins-can cause red blood cells to clump together and may cause immune system reactions. Oligosaccharides-are the pesky sugars that cause bloating and flatulence. Oxalates-can prevent proper absorption of minerals such as zinc, iron, and calcium. Isoflavones-are the phytoestrogens (plant estrogens) that act like hormones that affect the reproductive and the nervous systems. The best known are Genistein and Daidzein. Protease inhibitors interfere with the digestive enzymes protease and trypsin .notably trypsin inhibitors which interfere with the digestive enzymes protease and trypsin. Saponins are substances that bind with bile and may lower cholesterol and damage the intestinal lining/

Most people agree that mature dried soybeans must never be eaten raw. 2 hours of pressure cooking or 7 to 9 hours of boiling on a stove top are necessary. Soybeans must be soaked, cooked, and fermented in order to be edible. Fermented soybean products enjoy high honor throughout Asia as digestive aids, patent medicines, powerful energizers, stamina builders, and longevity elizirs. Miso, Shoyu, Natto, Tempeh, and other products are examples. Similar culturing turned milk into clabbered milk, grapes into wine, cabbage into sauerkraut, cucumbers into pickles, and fruits and spices into chutney.

Westerners should regard reports about "the good old soys" with a grain or or two of salt. Popular news stories tend to treat all soy foods alike, but the traditional products bear little or no resemblance to the modern soybean products promoted by the soy industry and sold in the American grocery stores. Asians simply do not eat any soybean products in great quantity. They are used in small amounts as condiments or seasonings, mot as main courses, and rarely more than once a day.

Modern spy sauces contain dangerous chemicals known as chloropropanols which are produced when soy sauce production is speeded up using acid hydrolyation methods. In Great Britain 25% of soy sauces were found to contain dangerous levels of these chemicals, and products were recalled in 2001. There have been no recalls in America, but the same process is used, so safety of commercial soy sauces cannot be assured.

Soy milk is a lactose-free dairy substitute that is made from soybeans that have been soaked, ground, crushed, and steamed. Sales were $600 million dollars in 2001. They are projected to reach $1 billion dollars by 2005. The Chinese did not value soy milk. The Japanese found the flavour and color of soy milk undesirable. In the late 1970s the industry began advertising soy milk as a "beautiful pick-me-up energy drink." Sales then picked up. Taste is what most concerns the soy industry.

The soy industry is in a quandary. The only way it can make its soy milk please its consumers is to remove the very toxins that it has promoted as beneficial for preventing cancer and lowering cholesterol. In 2003, Time magazine wrote, "the soy-based yogurts we tried were chalky, gritty, and sour, with a chemical aftertaste. A typical reaction from our tester was "awful." Most soy milk-derived products contain a thickener derived from a red seaweed known as carrageenan. This water-soluble polymer or gum often serves as a fat substitute. Recent studies show that carrageenan can cause ulcerations and malignancies in the gastrointestinal tract of animals.

Soy cheeses are increasingly used by fast food operators such as Pizza Hut, Casein, a cow's milk protein is added to make the ersatz product taste more like "real cheese." Without it, soy cheeses that are heated will soften but not melt and stretch. Professional reviewers have described these imitation cheeses as "barely edible," "yukky," "disgusting," "plastic," "rubbery," and "smelling like old stinking socks." Although promoted as healthful with the phrase "no cholesterol," many brands of soy cheeses contain dangerous partially hydrogenated fats-with the highest levels in the brands that taste the best.

Soy milk is so dangerous to infants that commercial manufacturers carry strong warnings on their cartons. On June 13, 1990, Stuart Nightingale, M.D., assistant commissioner for health affairs at the FDA issued a warning about the use of soy milks saying they were "grossly lacking in the nutrients needed for infants," and asking all manufacturers to put warning labels on soy milks so they would not be used as formula substitutes.

American ingenuity has created a whole new era in soy foods. Names like Soysage, Not Dogs, Fakin' Bacon, Sham Ham, etc. Are made to look like the meat and dairy products they are meant to replace. These products cost so much they no longer carry the stigma of "poverty food." The higher prices have given soy the image of an upscale health food. More and more Americans are unknowingly eating soy protein hidden in fast-food burgers, spaghetti sauces, breads, cookies, and other processed foods in restaurants, supermarkets, and other outlets. Soy protein isolate (SPI) is mixed with nearly every food product sold in today's stores-energy bars, muscleman powders, breakfast shakes burgers, and hot dogs. SPI is a major ingredient in most of today's soy infant formulas.

Soy protein isolate is a highly refined product that is deficient in many vitamins and minerals. During the production of SPI the level of toxins and carcinogens are increased. The manufacture of SPI is a complicated procedure. Defatted soybean meal is mixed with a caustic alkaline solution to remove the fiber. It is then washed in an acid solution to precipitate out the protein. The protein curds are then dipped into alkaline solution and spray dried at extremely high temperatures. Is there any nutritional value left in SPI.

The only economical way to obtain soybean oil is a high-tech process that includes grinding, crushing, and extracting, using high temperature, intense pressure, and chemical solvents such as hexane. During these processes, the oil is exposed to light, heat, and oxygen, all of which damage the oil by creating free radicals. The resulting rancidity affects the taste and smell.

Most of the world's soy oil never gets poured into a vegetable oil bottle. It undergoes a process known as hydrogenation, which turns polyunsaturated oils that are liquid at room temperature into fats that are solid at room temperature. The soy oil is thus made into a bland, odor-free solid fat that is dyed pale yellow if it is to be sold as margarine, or bleached white if it is intended as shortening. Neither refined soy oil nor hydrogenated soy oil products were ever eaten in China, Japan, or other countries in Asia. They are modern, Western, industrial era food produce.

Many people don't realize that they are consuming spy oil. In 1978, 84% of all vegetable oil was soy. The term vegetable oil gives the manufacturer the freedom to throw whatever vegetable oil happens to be cheap and available. Soy oils go incognito because most are processed by hydrogenation into margarine or shortening.

Today's "regular" stick margarines are usually 80% hydrogenated soy, corn, or cottonseed oil. Unlike margarine, shortenings are all fat. The best known is Crisco. It took creative advertising by the American soybean Association and magazine manufacturers to convince the public that margarine was a tasty and healthy alternative to butter. The vegetable oil industry has kept people in the dark about the sordid secrets of margarine manufacture, particularly the crucial process of hydrogenation.

Hydrogenation begins with a cheap oil from corn or soybeans, one that is rancid from the process of extraction. It is mixed with a catalyst, usually nickel oxide- then blasted with hydrogen gas with temperatures as high as 400 degrees. Soap-like emulsifiers and starch are mixed in, followed by a high temperature steam cleaning, bleaching, dyeing, and flavouring. The product is then compressed into sticks, bars, or tubs that will be sold in the supermarket.

Soy margarines and shortenings are used in all readymade foods from baked goods to frozen dinners, ti fast –food fries and non-dairy whipped toppings. Commercially they work very well, healthwise they wreak havoc throughout the body. The culprit is trans-fat, an artificial form of fat formed during the hydrogenation process that has been implicated in heart disease, cancer, learning disabilities, autism, obesity, and other ills. Dr. Joseph Mercola, D.O. warns, "don't let these companies fool you with their expensive alternatives to the real thing: butter. This new non-trans-fat margarine is still liquid plastic."

Formula for Disaster

Soy formula was never used traditionally in Asia. Babies who were not breastfed received dairy formulas. Yet the myth persists that soy formula has been around for centuries, so it must be safe. From the 1940s to 1960s reports surfaced of deficiencies of vitamins A, K, B-12, and the minerals zinc, iron, and calcium from soy formula. The specter of thyroid damage emerged in 1939. By 1961, formula manufacturers added iodine, but risks to the thyroid remain. Soy formulas also lack cholesterol, a vital substance needed by the growing baby's brain. Soy is allergenic, and worst of all, soy formulas contain high levels of phytoestrogens (plant estrogens) known as isoflavones which put the infant's developing endocrine, nervous, and immune systems at risk. Despite such clear and present dangers, soy infant formula now represents a 25 percent market share in the United States.

Soy Protein - The Inside Scoop

Methionine is a sulphur-based amino acid that is a precursor of SAM (S-Adenosyl methionine) made by our liver. Kilmer Mccully M.D. author of "The Heart Revolution: The Extraordinary Discovery That Finally Laid the Cholesterol Myth to Rest," and "The Homocysteine Revolution," and winner of the Linus Pauling Award, notes that diets high in soy protein can lead to reduced SAM synthesis because of methionine deficiencies, which in turn lead to increased levels of homocysteine, an atherogenic amino acid, which, if elevated in the blood indicates a greater risk if heart disease and stroke.

In November 1999, the FDA approved a health claim that permits food processors to label many soy products with the phrase "diets low in saturated fat and cholesterol that include 25 grams of soy protein a day may reduce the risk of heart disease ." that health claim fails to earn the hapless consumer that the benefits are spurious, that the risks are grave, and that the public's "number one consumer protector is not only asleep on the job, but in bed with big business."

Trans-fats

Trans-fats stiffen the membranes, inhibit enzyme activity, block transport of nutrients, and inhibit the elimination of wastes. Mounting evidence suggests that trans fatty acids contribute to and even cause heart disease and cancer. Hundreds of medical and scientific journal articles link hydrogenated oils to heart disease, cancer, obesity, diabetes, immune disorders, birth defects, infertility, vision problems, allergies, attention deficit, hyperactivity, and senility. Trans-fats pose such a danger that the National Academy of Sciences Institute of medicine concluded recently that the only safe level of trans-fat is zero.

How much trans-fats do Americans eat? Mary G. Enig, Ph.D. estimates we eat an average of 13.3 grams per person per day. Junk food eaters, who subsist on deep-fried nuggets, fast-food fries, doughnuts, chips, and cookies , eat far more. Enig's estimate is considerably higher than the ADA's estimate of 5.3 grams of trans-fatty acids per day. Over the years the ADA has been a cheerleader for the processed food industry, and earns money for its journal by running ads for processed foods.

Tests by Mary G. Enig revealed that most margarines contain at least 31 percent trans-fats and many shortenings contain more than 35 percent. Parkay margarine leads the pack with 45 percent trans-fats. The last word goes to Enig who asks, "if the trade association truly believes that trans-fatty acids do not pose any harm to humans and animals, why are they concerned about any levels of consumption?

Soy Estrogens

One thing is clear: soy estrogens are not weak. Yes, popular health writers repeat the misinformation that soy phytoestrogens are safe, useful, and effective because they are "weak" estrogens. They claim that phytoestrogens are 10,000 to 1,000,000 times less potent than human estrogen, Estradiol . According to studies by Markewicz et al in 1993, the correct figure is 1,200 times less potent than human estrogen.

Soy and Cancer

Soy protein and soy isoflavones supplements are heavily promoted as "miracle cures" for cancer. The idea that a simple food could save lives sounds like very good news indeed. Unfortunately, the truth is another soy story. A few studies suggest that soy isoflavones might help prevent cancer, but far more studies show it to be ineffective or inconsistent. Some studies even show that soy can promote or even cause cancer.

The idea that scientists could even consider soy for a cancer health claim is ludicrous. Soy isoflavones-the plant estrogens in soy are listed as "carcinogens" in many toxicology textbooks. Women eating soy to prevent breast cancer risk developing the very disease they are trying to prevent. Studies in the 1970s show that soy causes proliferation of breast cancer cells.

The story of soy sheds light on the dirty little secrets of the food processing industry, the power of public relations, the corruption of scientific inquiry, and the collusion of the FDA, which is mandated to protect us. Sadly, big business and big government have usurped the dream of John Harvey Kellogg, Henry ford, and others- using soy as the solution to world hunger. Whole soy foods that are healthy if eaten in moderation have given way to ersatz products that lead to malnutrition and disease. Gigantic corporate farms and billion dollar soybean-crushing and food processing plants have driven out the small farmers. The result worldwide is an epidemic of disease- a kind of cancer on the body of mother earth.

What will the coming years bring? Unfortunately, it will bring more false claims for soy protein and soy oil while the grassroots movement demands honesty, integrity, commonsense and "real food?" The challenge and choice is yours.

GENOME
MITT RIDLEY

The most exciting advances in the history of medicine are now at hand. We are on the threshold of discoveries that will transform the practice of medicine and change the way we live. The Human Genome Project is a $3 billion dollar a year effort to map and sequence 80,000 genes. The knowledge that we gain will enable scientists to prevent and cure all the diseases of man. It will generate both medical and ethical controversy within the scientific community

Genome is a book that captures this exciting concept. It is mind-boggling to think that man can be disease-free and extend his life span to 150 to 200 years. It is early in the game. Many companies in the genetic research area are years away from developing commercial applications for their gene-mapping successes. This book examines the future potential of the genetic discoveries that lie ahead.

Synopsis

Human beings are an ecological success. There are nearly six billion of them. They thrive in every continent except Antartica. No doubt, this ecological success of the human comes at a high price and we are doomed to catastrophe soon enough. For a successful species we are remarkably pessimistic about the future. But for now we are a success. We come from a long line of failures. We are Apes, a group that went extinct fifteen million years ago. We are Primates, a group of mammals that almost went extinct forty-five million years ago. We are Synapsid Tetrapods a group of reptiles that almost went extinct 200 million years ago in competition with the better designed Dinosaurs. We are descended from limbed fishes which almost went extinct 360 million years ago. We are Chordates that survived the Cambrian Era 500 million years ago. Our ecological success came against humbling odds.

LUCA, the last universal common ancestor, looked like a bacterium and she lived in a warm pond. LUCA lived about four billion years ago. Three billion years passed during which trillions and trillions of single-celled creatures lived, each one reproducing and dying every few days or so. About a billion years ago, a new world order developed, with bigger, multicellular bodies- a sudden explosion of large creatures. Within a blink of a geological eye (the so-called Cambrian explosion may have lasted only ten or twenty million years), creatures of immense complexity (nearly a foot long), carved out a niche for themselves. Single-celled creatures still dominated each successive age. The Paleozoic, Mesozoic, and the Cenozoic, the brains of animals grew larger. The genes had found a way to build bodies capable of survival. They had the intelligence to migrate to friendly environments that did not threaten their existence with winter storms. They also could build a shelter.

From four billion years ago to just ten million years ago, we pass insects, fishes, dinosaurs, and birds to the biggest-brained creature on earth (probably our ancestor), the ape. The gorilla is the ancestor of the chimpanzee and the human being. The chimp-human split occurred possibly less than five million years ago. We are 98% chimpanzees and they are 98% human beings. Chimpanzees are 97% gorillas and humans are 97% gorillas. In other words, we are more chimpanzee-like than gorillas are. There is no known part of the immune system, the digestive system, the vascular system, the lymph system, or the nervous system that we have and chimpanzees do not, or vice-versa. There is not even a brain lobe in the chimpanzees that we do not share.

It is less than 300,000 human generations since the common ancestor of both species lived in Central Africa. The difference between human beings and chimpanzees are genetic differences and virtually nothing else. Some two percent of the genome tells the story of our ecological and social evolution from that of chimpanzees and theirs from us.

On February 28, 1953, in the Eagle Pub, Francis Crick announced, "we've discovered the secret of life." Watson was mortified. He still feared that he might have made a mistake. They had not. DNA contained a code written along the length of an elegant, intertwined staircase of a double helix, of potentially infinite length. This discovery is considered the most momentous discovery of the century, if not the millennium. The code itself, the language by which the gene expressed itself, retained its mystery. Cracking the code required true brilliance. It was a four-letter code –A, C, G, and T. And it was translated into the twenty-letter code of amino acids that make up proteins. But how? Where? And by what means? By 1965 the whole code was known and the age of modern genetics had begun. It would have dazzled Gregor Mendel and Charles Darwin whose genius formed the foundation of the genomic revolution.

To define genes by the diseases they cause is as absurd as defining organs of the body the diseases they get. Livers are there to cause cirrhosis, hearts to cause heart attacks, and brains to cause strokes. The only thing we know about some genes is that their malfunction causes a particular disease. In the late 1980s, various groups of scientists began the search for the "asthma gene." The one thing you cannot argue is that asthma is on the increase because "asthma genes" are on the increase.

The genes have not changed that quickly. There are many candidate genes on several chromosomes which are possible in varying orders of importance in any combination of them. Each gene has its companion and feelings run high. To the outside world the sheer nastiness of scientific funds comes as a surprise.

Politics, by contrast, is a relatively polite affair. This is the reality of gene hunting. There is a tendency for ivory-towered moral philosophers to disparage such scientific research as gold-diggers seeking fame and fortune. The simplistic headiness of the press can be very misleading. Yet anybody who gets evidence of a link between a disease and a gene has a duty to publish it. If it proves an illusion, little harm is done. The genome is as complicated and indeterminate as ordinary life, because it is ordinary life.

Genes are not there to cause disease. It is time to penetrate the genetic forest that harbors the inheritance of intelligence. Toward the end of 1977, a brave scientist announced to the world that he had found a gene for "intelligence." It was on chromosome 6. Skeptics could not accept the idea that mother nature could entrust the determination of our intellectual capacities to the blind fate of a gene or genes. Yet this is what Robert Plomin and his colleagues discovered. There is no accepted definition of intelligence. Is it thinking speed, reasoning ability, memory, vocabulary, mental arithmetic, or the appetite for intellectual pursuits that marks them as intelligent? Let us accept the plainly foolish definition of intelligence as the thing that is measured by the average intelligence tests. As you grow up, you gradually express your own innate intelligence and leave behind the influences stamped on you by others. You select the environments that suit your innate tendencies to the environments you find yourself in. This proves two vital things: that you genetic influences are not frozen at conception and environmental influences are not inexorably cumulative. Heritability does not mean immutability.

Plomin's gene (IGF2R) is enormous, with 7,473 letters in all, but the sense-containing message is spread out over a 98,000 letter stretch of the genome, interrupted forty-eight times by nonsense sequences called introns. Plomin's gene, if it proves real at all, will be one of the many that can influence intelligence in many different ways. One form of the gene is about twice as common in a group of super-intelligent Iowan children as the rest of the population, a result extremely unlikely to be accidental. But this version of the gene only adds four points to your IQ. It is certainly not a "genius gene." The Frenchman Alfred Binet, the most famous pioneer of intelligence testing, argued that the putpose of IQ tests wass not to reward gifted children, but to give special attention to the less gifted ones. Genes may create an appetite, not an aptitude. The heritability of intelligence may therefore be about the genetics of nurture, just as much as the genetics of nature.

DNA fingerprinting has arrived. It has revolutionized not just forensic science but all sorts of other fields as well. It was used to confirm the exhumed corpse of Josef Mengele in 1990. It confirmed the presidential parenthood of the semen on Monica Lewinsky's dress. It was used to identify the illegitimate descendants of Thomas Jefferson in 1998. A company called Identigene placed billboards on freeways all over America reading, "Who's the father? Call 1-800-dna-type." They received 300 calls a day asking for their $600 dollar test.

Cholesterol is a word that is pregnant with danger. It is the cause of heart disease, bad stuff, red meat. You eat it you die. Nothing could be more wrong than this equation of cholesterol with poison. Cholesterol is an essential ingredient of the body. It lies at the center of an intricate system of biochemistry and genetics that integrates the whole body. Cholesterol is a small organic compound that is soluble in fat but not water. The body manufactures most of its cholesterol from sugars in the diet, and could not survive without it. Five crucial hormones are made from cholesterol, each with a different task.

A startling discovery showed that British civil servants working in Whitehall get heart disease in proportion to their lowliness in the bureaucratic pecking order.

A massive long-term study of 17,000 civil servants yielded an unbelievable conclusion. The status of a person's job was more able to predict the likelihood of a heart attack than obesity, smoking, or high blood pressure. The same result emerged from a similar study of a million employees of the Bell Telephone Company in the 1960s.

The conclusion undermines almost everything you have ever been told about heart disease. It relegates cholesterol to the margins. It relegates diet, smoking, and blood pressure to secondary causes. It also relegates to a footnote the old and largely disqualified notion that stress and heart failure come with busy, senior jobs or fast-living personalities. Instead your heart is at the mercy of your pay grade, or the status of your job. What on earth is going on?

Dopamine and norepinephrine are so-called monoamines. Their cousin, another monoamine found in the brain, is serotonin, which is also a chemical which determines personality.

If you have high levels of serotonin in your brain you will be a compulsive person, given to tidiness and caution, even to the point of being neurotic about it. Obsessive-compulsive disorder can be alleviated by lowering serotonin levels.

At the other end of the spectrum, those who commit impulsive violent crimes or suicides, are often those with less serotonin. Dean Hamer concludes that serotonin is the chemical that abets, rather than alleviates anxiety and depression. He calls it the brain's punishment chemical.

Yet all sorts of evidence shows that you feel better with more serotonin, not less for some people, a genetic minority (though no gene version has yet been found that correlates with susceptibility to this condition) The dark evenings of winter lead to a craving for carbohydrate snacks in the late afternoon. Such people often need more sleep in the winter, though they find the sleep less refreshing.

The explanation seems to be that the brain starts making melatonin, the hormone that induces sleep. Melatonin is made from serotonin, so serotonin levels drop as it gets used up in melatonin manufacture.

The quickest way to raise serotonin levels again is to send more tryptophan into the brain, because serotonin is made from tryptophan. The quickest way to send more tryptophan into the brain is to secrete insulin from the pancreas, because insulin causes the body to absorb other chemicals similar to tryptophan, thus removing competitors for the channels that take tryptophan into the brain, and the quickest way to secrete insulin is to eat a carbohydrate snack.

Even drugs and diets designed to lower blood cholesterol can influence serotonin. It is a curious fact that nearly all studies of cholesterol-lowering drugs and diets in ordinary people show an increase in violent deaths compared with control samples that usually matches the decrease in deaths from heart disease.

In all studies put together, cholesterol treatment cut heart attacks by 14 percent, but raised violent deaths by 78 percent. So treating high cholesterol levels has its dangers. It has been known for twenty years that impulsive, antisocial, and depressed people, including prisoners, violent offenders, and failed suicides—have lower cholesterol levels than the population at large.

In the MRFIT trial, in which 351,000 people from seven countries were followed for seven years, people with very low cholesterol and very high cholesterol were twice as likely to die at a given age as people with moderate cholesterol.

The extra deaths among low-cholesterol people are mainly due to accidents, suicide, or murder. The 25 percent of men with the lowest cholesterol count are four times as likely to commit suicide as the 25 percent of men with the highest count. The link between low cholesterol and violence almost certainly involves serotonin. Monkeys fed on low-cholesterol diets become more aggressive and bad-tempered, and the cause seems to be a drop in serotonin levels.

The telomerase genes are as close as we may get to finding "genes for youth." Telomerase seems to behave like the elixir of eternal youth for cells. The Geron Corporation hit the headlines in August 1997 for cloning part of telomerase. Its share price promptly doubled, not so much on the hope of eternal youth, but rather the prospect of making anti-cancer drugs.

Tumors require telomerase to keep them growing. Geron scientists immortalized cells with telomerase. In one experiment they took two cell types grown in the laboratory, both of which lacked   natural telomerase, and equipped them with a gene for telomerase. The cell continued dividing, vigorous and youthful, far beyond the point where they would grow old and die. At the time the result was published, the cells had exceeded their expected life span by more than twenty doublings, and they showed no sign of slowing down.

The lack of telomerase seems to be the principal reason that cells grow old and die, but is it the principal reason that bodies grow old and die? There is some good evidence that cells in the walls of arteries generally have shorter telomeres than cells in the veins.

Arteries are subject to more stress because arterial blood is under higher pressure. They have to expand and contract with every pulse beat, so they suffer more damage and need more repair. Repair involves cell copying, which uses up the ends of telomeres. The cells start to age, which is why we die from hardened arteries, not from hardened veins. There is great variety in telomere length between different people, from about 7,000 DNA "letters" to about 16,000 per chromosome end, and telomere length is strongly inherited, as is longevity. Jeanne Calment, the French woman who lived to age 122 may have had many repeats of the message TTAGGG. He brother lived to 97.

Aging is turning out to be under the control of many genes. One expert estimates that there are 7,000 age-influencing genes in the human genome, or 10 percent of the total. This makes it absurd to speak of any gene as "the aging gene."

Cancer requires active telomerase. The prime risk factor for cancer is age. So we have a paradox. Shortened telomeres mean higher cancer risk, but telomerase, which keeps telomeres long, is necessary for a tumor. The resolution lies in the fact that the switching on of telomerase is one of the essential mutations that must occur if cancer is to turn malignant. It is now fairly obvious why Geron's cloning of the telomerase gene caused its share price to rocket on the hopes of a general cure for cancer. Defeating telomerase would condemn tumors to suffer from the rapid advance of old age themselves.

One of the first calls for the sequencing of the human genome came from the Italian Nobel Prize winner Renato Dulbecco in 1986. He argued that it was the only way to win the war on cancer.

For the first time in human history, there is a real prospect of a cure for cancer, and it has come from reductionist, genetic research. Those who damn the whole science as dangerous should remember that these are early days in gene therapy. Some think it will be as routine as heart transplants are today. But it is too early to tell if gene therapy will be the strategy that defeats cancer or whether some other treatment based on angiogenesis, telomerase, or P53 wins the particular race. Whichever, never in history has cancer treatment looked so hopeful.—thanks almost entirely to the new genetics.

The media, as usual, rapidly polarized the debate with shouting matches between extremists on late-night television, and interviews that forced people into simplistic answers: are you for or against genetic engineering? The truth is that genetic engineering is as safe and as dangerous as the genes that are engineered. Some are safe, some are dangerous. Some are green, some are bad for the environment.

Transgenic animals such as sheep, cattle, pigs, and chickens have commercial applications. Sheep have already been given the gene for a human cloning factor in the hope that it can be harvested from their milk and used to treat haemophiliacs. (The scientists who performed this procedure cloned the sheep Dolly, and displayed her to an amazed world in 1997). It sounds rather easy. The technical obstacles to breeding a transgenic or a knockout human being are becoming trivial for a good team at a well-equipped laboratory. In a few years from now you could take a complete cell from your own body, insert a gene into a particular location, on a particular chromosome, transfer the nucleus to an egg cell from which the nucleus had been removed, and grow a new human being from the embryo. The person would be a transgenic clone of you.

None of this is as yet possible—but is very unlikely to remain impossible for much longer. When human cloning is possible, will it be ethical? For the moment, society is willing to place a moratorium on cloning or germline gene therapy and strict limits on embryonic research to forego the medical possibilities in exchange for not risking the horrors of the unknown.

THE DOCTOR WHO LOOKED AT HANDS
JOHN M. ELLIS, M.D.

Some men are born with a mission. The country doctor who authored this book is such a man. Many of Dr. Ellis's patients in his Texas clinic were big, fat, eaters who were susceptible to all the ills related to fat consumption, including coronary thrombosis. He decided to treat them by changing their diets, and in the process of doing so he made some startling discoveries.

Synopsis

Dr. Ellis read about Dr. Lester Morrison of Los Angeles who was treating victims of coronary thrombosis with a low-fat diet. The diet itself was not unusual; it merely substituted lean meat in place of fat meat, increased the amount of vegetables and fruits, and required vegetable oils for cooking. It was planned for an adequate balance of vitamin and mineral nutrition. Dr. Ellis used the Morrison Diet for patients who ate large quantities of fat, and showed symptoms that predisposed them to arteriosclerosis. The diet worked wonders for his patients. Many of them lost weight and the pain in their elbows and shoulders disappeared.

Dr. Ellis was especially impressed with one patient who was so thrilled with her recovery that she said, "If I knew how to play the piano, I could play it!" Before the diet the woman could hardly flex her fingers. Afterward her hands and fingers were so relieved that all movement was easier. This remarkable improvement started the doctor's concentration on his patients' hands and fingers. Another thing happened to his patients after they had been on the diet for a little while. They lost inches off their waistlines. By deduction, Dr. Ellis concluded that it was the content of the diet that brought such marked changes in his patients.

Fat consumption is certainly a bane to the American population, but it was the discovery of vitamin B-6 that was soon to obsess Ellis. As he developed his own theories of the vitamin's value in relieving edema of the hands, tingling and numbness in the fingers, pain in the shoulders and elbows, and possibly bursitis.

Back at the clinic Ellis turned his attention to one of his patients suffering from parasthesia of the fingers, and a tingling sensation that was relieved by the Morrison Diet. He administered the B complex to the patient every other day for two weeks. The doctor's artist wife documented the improvement by drawing sketches of the fingers before the injections and two weeks afterward. Ellis was amazed to see how the patient came to be able to flex his fingers and press the palms with the tips of his fingers. She then tried an experiment with another patient. She was a cook in the school cafeteria where Dr. Ellis's children ate lunch every day. He had tingling and numb fingers, chest pain, and her arms and shoulders ached. She also had cramps at night. Her hands and fingers were puffy and swollen in the morning. After two weeks of B complex injections all the pain was gone, as were the edema and swelling. It shocked Ellis that American school children were being subjected to a diet grossly deficient in B vitamins. This woman ate the same food that the school children did in the cafeteria.

Ellis decided to try to narrow down the field of B vitamins to see if one in particular was effective. He determined that nobody had ever described a syndrome for B-6 deficiency in adults. The doctor then prepared the first B-6 experiment and lined up two different patients.

One was a black woman, eight months pregnant, weighing 195 pounds. After giving he the second injection of 50 milligrams of pyridoxine hydrochloride (B-6), Dr. Ellis received what he said was the greatest thrill in medicine. The woman's feet were wrinkled, pliable, and loose. He shoe almost dropped from her foot to the floor. What he had seen was the relief of edema of pregnancy. An identical procedure was used on another pregnant woman with the same result—elimination of edema of the feet, hands, and fingers. There was no doubt that a vitamin B-6 deficiency was causing the edema.

A number of subjects were placed on a high-fat diet with no instructions to limit their salt intake. Could it be that vitamin B-6 regulates the body's use of salt? From his experiments, Ellis conjectured that B-6 must allow potassium and sodium to travel back and forth through the cell membrane. If B-6 is not present, a nerve can throw a muscle into spasm or else become momentarily paralysed itself. In other words, B-6 allows potassium and sodium to stay in proper balance inside and outside nerve cells.

Dr. Ellis theorizes that many Americans have five to seven pounds of excess fluid in their bodies that can be eliminated with vitamin B-6. He believes that B-6 can protect and preserve cartilage of the joints by altering the secretion of aldosterone and cortisone produced in the adrenal gland. He speculates further, "B-6 was assisting the pituitary gland in the control of all the endocrine glands. This would mean that vitamin B-6 might aid in the prevention of other diseases of the endocrine glands such as diabetes and hypothyroidism. These are all, however, just ideas floating through Ellis's mind. He has no proof of anything except his patients with a B-6 deficiency were loaded with fluid that could be relieved by the daily administration of 50 milligrams of B-6.

The vitamin B-6 deficiency that existed in so many people in Dr. Ellis's community raises the whole question of diet. Optimum health depends on 20-odd essential proteins, 13 vitamins, and 10 to 14 minerals. A diet should be divided into two parts: calories for energy and vitamins, minerals, and protein for nutrition. Protein should come from lean beef, skimmed milk, fish and chicken, Fresh or frozen fruits should be eaten every day. Vegetables should be eaten raw. "Quantitative adequacy is the secret of good nutrition, and one has to be forcing useless calories out of his diet constantly. Fat calories and sugar calories do not contain vitamins and minerals." A vitamin B-6 deficiency is prevalent in the United States. Americans overcook green vegetables, and thereby boil out all the vitamins. In addition, multivitamins on the market today have so little B-6 that they can't prevent parasthesia of the hands. Most preparations have only 1 or 2 milligrams of B-6—not enough to remove edema or swelling of the hands.

Ellis sums up his four years of deliberation about the American diet with this statement, "There is no doubt that coronary thrombosis is of dietary origin, stemming from a vitamin B-6 deficiency."

THE HEALING FACTOR
IRWIN STONE, M.D.

Dr. Stone presents in this book a detailed explanation of the evolutionary role of ascorbic acid, and particularly its critical role in human history. He is convinced that Vitamin C is "The Healing Factor" and has numerous therapeutic applications.

Synopsis

Unlike fishes, amphibians, and reptiles, which produce ascorbic acid in their kidneys, higher vertebrates and mammals produce this life-essential substance from glucose in the liver. However, through a genetic mutation in the biochemical makeup of an ancestral primate, man lost the enzyme that enables all other creatures (except the guinea pig and the fruit-eating bat) to manufacture their own ascorbic acid internally. Fortunately, man needs a relatively low amount of ascorbic acid to survive, and as long as he inhabited tropical or semitropical regions where the food supply was abundant and contained ample external sources of ascorbic acid, he was able to overcome his enzyme deficiency. But when human civilization spread throughout the world, man was more susceptible to diseases and epidemics, notably the violent outbreaks of scurvy that contributed to the Black Death in the Middle Ages and decimated much of Europe's navies in succeeding centuries. Not until the mid-eighteenth century was it discovered that citrus fruit is valuable in the prevention and cure of scurvy, and not until 1933 was the specific "healing factor" or vitamin C isolated and identified.

An outstanding attribute of ascorbic acid is its lack of toxicity, even in large doses. In some hypersensitive individuals such side effects as diarrhea or rashes may occur, but they will clear up when the dosage is lowered. One can avoid these reactions altogether by building up gradually to the desired dosage. It is best to take ascorbic acid with food or before meals. There are no large storage depots for ascorbic acid in the body, and any excess is rapidly excreted when saturated. The whole body may contain up to 5 grams, which dictate the necessity for a continuous fresh supply to replenish the losses.

One of the most important functions of ascorbic acid is the formation and maintenance of a protein-like substance called collagen. As the body's most important structural substance, collagen acts as a cement to hold the organs and tissues together. Collagen cannot be formed without ascorbic acid. It is the substance that strengthens the arteries and veins, strengthens the muscles, toughens the ligaments and bones, supplies the scar tissue for healing wounds, and keeps skin tissues soft, firm, supple, and wrinkle-free. But it cannot be formed without Vitamin C; when collagen was missing, scurvy results, brittle bones fracture on the slightest impact, weakened arteries rupture and hemorrhage, muscles become weak to the point of incapacitation, joints are too painful to move, teeth fall out, and wounds and sores never heal. Collagen is intimately connected to the entire aging process.

Ascorbic acid is also a potent detoxicant that counteracts and neutralizes the harmful effect of many poisons in the body. It detoxifies carbon dioxide, sulphur dioxide, and carcinogens. It is the only immediate protection we have against the bad effects of air pollution and smoking. Vitamin c is a potent virocide. At relatively high doses it destroys the infectivity of a wide variety of disease-producing viruses such as poliomyelitis, herpes, vaccinia, foot-and-mouth disease, and rabies. Moreover, the National Cancer Institute reported that ascorbic acid was lethal to certain cancer cells while harmless to normal tissue—a potentially important breakthrough in cancer therapy and research.

Since 1933, when ascorbic acid was discovered as the anti-scorbutic substance identified as vitamin C, thousands of research projects have undertaken to pit the vitamin against almost every known disease. Unfortunately, though, most investigators use the small dosage levels that had been fund to be satisfactory for scurvy. This bias toward low dosage has led to failures and confusion and has cast doubt on vitamin C's effectiveness as a therapeutic substance. It was not until the late 1940s and early 1950s that Dr. Fred R. Klenner of North Carolina provided the foundation of megascorbic therapy by successfully treating viral diseases with large doses of vitamin C.

Taking 3 to 5 grams daily of ascorbic acid will give you a high resistance to respiratory diseases. At the first symptom of a cold, take up to 2 grams of ascorbic acid and repeat at half-hour intervals. Usually, by the third dose the virus will be effectively inactivated. Clinical evidence has shown that large doses of vitamin C can also be effective on bacterial infection, cancer, heart disease, arthritis, rheumatism, ulcers, stress, and many other diseases. The lack of a convenient dosage form, however, has been a major impediment to the development of megascorbic prophylaxis. What is needed now is a pleasantly flavoured chewable wafer supplying 2 to 3 grams of ascorbic acid. The situation is even worse for doctors who want to use megascorbic therapy by injection. Ampoules contain at most one gram. There should instead be ampoules with sterile solutions containing 20 to 40 grams of sodium ascorbate suitable for injection. Unfortunately, the wheels of progress grind slowly, especially in the field of medicine. The odds are that it will take many years for the therapeutic and preventive claims made for vitamin C to be accepted by the medical establishment and the public.

SOLVED: THE RIDDLE OF ILLNESS
STEPHEN E. LANGER, M.D.
WITH JAMES E. SCHEER

It was discovered more than 100 years ago that an inoperative thyroid gland caused myxedema (a swelling of body tissues) and arteriosclerosis, but the significance of clogged arteries meant nothing to the medical world in 1877, because heart attacks were not a major problem at that time. The importance of the thyroid was again demonstrated in Austria, where Empress Maria Theresa made autopsies mandatory, creating a veritable research laboratory for the medical world. Hundreds of pages of records showed the clogged arteries of people whose thyroid glands were removed. The medical world remained unmoved. Indeed, it created a cholesterol hysteria which scared American people away from all the best and most nutritious foods.

Synopsis

Dr. Stephen E. Langer graduated from the New York College of Medicine at Buffalo, where he studied medical psychology. He holds that belief systems are not sacred; ideas should change if something better comes along. His practice was revolutionized by the work of Dr. Broda Barnes, one of the world's foremost authorities on the thyroid gland. After 50 years of clinical experimentation, Dr. Barnes stated that 40% of the adult population of the United States suffers from hypothyroidism. Dr. Langer was sceptical, until he used Dr. Barnes's method—and found a slightly higher percentage. Millions of people suffer needlessly: the Barnes Basal Temperature Test of thyroid function is simple and accurate, and thyroid hormone is one of the cheapest substances on the market.

Dr. Barnes found six common denominators in hypothyroidism:. abnormal temperature, fatigue drowsiness, depression, female problems, and infections. The thyroid is a tiny coral-colored bow tie, weighing less than an ounce, semi-circling the windpipe under the Adam's apple. It is critical to living and the quality of life. All 5 quarts of blood circulate through the thyroid gland once every hour, depositing iodide, which is needed to make hormones, as well as a hormone from the anterior pituitary gland which stimulates production from the thyroid. When the blood level of the thyroid drops below normal, the hypothalamus gland discharges thyroid releasing hormone (TRH). This stimulates the thyroid stimulating hormone (TSH) to do its job. Once the thyroid produces sufficient thyroid hormone, the pituitary outs the thyroid on hold. A world-renowned endocrinologist, Dr. Louis Herman, summarized the critical importance of the thyroid. "Without the thyroid there can be no complexity of thought, no learning, no education, no habit formation, no responsive energy, no reproduction of kind with no adolescent expected age, and no exhibition of sex tendencies thereafter. With no thyroid gland you and I would not be human at all—we'd be vegetables."

Thyroid hormone is not a cure-all for everything that ails you. It would be too narrow to ignore the consideration of biochemical individuality—but it is a blind spot in diagnosis today. It is time for doctors to take a look at this neglected gland. It is often too late to use iodine supplements alone to correct a deficiency. Dr. Barnes and his followers have found that it takes 1/100,000 of an ounce of desiccated thyroid supplement to keep us healthy. Dr. Langer starts hypothyroid patients on ¼ to ½ grain of Armour desiccated thyroid preparation and increases the their dosage by ¼ to ½ grain every seven to ten days until the proper dosage is achieved, monitoring their temperature carefully. When it rises to normal they are kept at that level. He also advises patients to take Brewer's Yeast, rich in B vitamins, along with the thyroid supplement.

Dr. Israel has 40 years of medical practice, conducting studies with hypothyroidism. He has observed that standard laboratory tests indicated that 85% of his practice showed normal thyroid function. Yet all of them showed consistent benefits from thyroid supplementation, including a more comfortable body temperature and increased energy and vitality.

Unless hypothyroidism is corrected, the thyroid and adrenal glands can't properly operate the body's heat-regulating system: that is why so many hypothyroids are cold when everybody else in the room is warm. Experimenters have discovered that fever triggers an attack or an infection by the immune system. If heat increases our ability to fight disease, it is likely that subnormal temperatures make us more susceptible to them. One of the most common results of hypothyroidism is recurrent colds, throat and nose infections, and other respiratory ailments.

Too many risks accompany the Spartan regimen most strict vegetarians follow; there is no reason why they can't eat poultry and fish, or at least dairy products and eggs. The author feels that "the great peril of the strict vegetarian diet is the suppression of the protective and life-giving thyroid function by minimizing the intake of essential vitamins." It is possible to correct some cases of unbalanced thyroid hormone production merely by compensating for certain vitamin deficiencies, without tasking thyroid supplements.

Dr. Jeffrey Bland, Ph.D., Professor of Nutritional Biochemistry at the University of Puget Sound is a pioneer biochemist who has done original research on zinc and copper and their relationship to low thyroid function. The proper ratio for most individuals is 8 parts of zinc to 1 of copper. Zinc and copper are trace elements that are vital in many bodily functions.

Deficiencies of these two substances produce symptoms almost identical to those for hypothyroidism. There are two ways to treat hypothyroidism; to use thyroid hormone supplements, and to normalize the zinc/copper ratio of the deficient individual.

Dr. Broda Barnes feels that hypothyroidism and hypoglycemia are as closely related as Siamese twins. "A sluggish liver results from subnormal activity. During periods of stress the liver can't produce enough sugar from protein—then hypoglycemia occurs. Thyroid therapy stimulates the liver to normal function, and the hypoglycemia disappears." In more than 40 years as a medical doctor, of more than 5,000 patients he has treated for subnormal thyroid function, he has not seen one case of hypoglycemia.

Diabetes also has many of the same symptoms as hypothyroidism, and many diabetics are also hypothyroid. Common symptoms are low energy, muscle pains, high susceptibility to infection, poor wound healing, early atherosclerosis, and gangrene.

There are 18 million diabetics in the United States. The good news is that we can do something about it. Dr. Barnes noticed that a dozen diabetics he had been treating with thyroid showed no diabetic complications. His new diabetics who had high cholesterol levels, atherosclerosis, bad eyesight, and poor circulation, achieved an arrest, reversal, and sometimes complete cure of their condition. For 15 years, 43 diabetic patients who were put on thyroid supplements do not show any sign of diabetic complications. The only conclusion Dr. Barnes could draw from these results was that millions of diabetics have unnecessarily suffered pain and premature death. He stands firm in his belief that hypothyroidism is the leading cause of this condition. The key points to remember in order to prevent diabetes are:

- Avoid refined sugar and other refined carbohydrates.
- Eat chromium-rich foods like Brewer's yeast, beef liver, chicken, meat, and whole grains.
- Avoid unnecessary stress, which slows down insulin production.
- Exercise regularly.
- Eat a high fiber diet.
- Avoid obesity.
- Keep your pancreas healthy. Avoid chemicals, tobacco, alcohol, and eat raw vegetables.
- Check your temperature to see that you are not hypothyroid.
- Thyroid hormone can help to prevent the complications of diabetes.

Millions of Americans who have underactive thyroid glands are at risk for a heart attack. Most doctors in the medical establishment are not aware of this fact. Their only course of preventive treatment is to advocate the avoidance of cholesterol-containing foods which are often valuable and wholesome.   In 1977, in England, Dr. William M. Ord noticed a female patient with an enlarged, fibrous, non-functional thyroid gland. The result was myxedema, a mucin-logged swelling of all the tissues. Her arteries also showed advanced atherosclerosis. The coronary, kidney, and brain arteries were almost completely clogged. The London Clinical Society formed a task force to study and investigate the incidence of myxedema. In the next 5 years they identified more than 100 cases. A 300-page volume reported the results of experiments, autopsies, and examinations revealed that myxedema was caused by decreased function of the thyroid gland. The atherosclerosis, however, received no special attention because in those days heart attacks were a rarity.

In 1890, Viennese pathologists discovered that thyroid deficiency brought on heart attacks. Again, this discovery was little noted at the time. The knowledge that a healthy thyroid was vital to a healthy heart was a "solution for which there was no problem."

Physicians today are still married to the theory that cholesterol is the major culprit in cardiovascular ailments. A 10-year, $150 million dollar study by the National Institutes of Health (NIH) concluded in 1984 that there is a direct link between the blood serum cholesterol and heart disease, and that lowering cholesterol reduces the incidence of heart disease, and that the drug Cholestyramine can significantly reduce coronary heart disease.

Rockefeller University's Dr. Edward "Pete" Ahrens, who has conducted lipid research for 40 years, believes just the opposite. He states that "since this was basically a drug study, we can conclude nothing about diet; such extrapolation is unwarranted, unscientific, and wishful thinking." The much publicized Framingham Study of thousands of individuals has borne out Ahren's contention, failing to prove that dietary cholesterol is the enemy. Dr. William B. Kannel, the project's director stated that half the people who died of heart attacks did not have high cholesterol levels, and further, that there is "no discernible association between the amount of cholesterol in the diet and the level of cholesterol in the blood."

No thinking individual would deny the value of optimal nutrition and regular exercise. This book adds one very important thing; if you have enough thyroid hormone circulating in your five quarts of blood, you can resist infections, allergies, and a negative outlook. You can prevent debilitating degenerative diseases such as heart disease before they begin controlling your life. Remember that a normal thyroid slows down with the passage of time along with the thymus, which is the quarterback of the immune system.

CANCER
MATTHIAS RATH, M.D.

The medical world is on the wrong track with its cancer therapy. Conventional treatment involves surgery, radiation, and chemotherapy. None of these therapies has proven to extend the life of a patient. These therapies have been used for decades even though physicians know that they will not heal the disease and often even accelerate it.

President Richard Nixon declared America's war on cancer in 1971, promising to end its toll within a decade. Billions of research dollars have been spent in an attempt to conquer this terrifying disease. The number of cancer cases and deaths has continued to grow. According to the National Institutes of Health, cancer costs reached an all-time high of $18.2 billion dollars in the year 2000

The costs of cancer care are greatest during the first six months following diagnosis for treatment and therapies. The next most expensive period of cancer treatment occurs during the six months prior to death. Dr. Rath and his team of researchers have focused their research on the development of an effective, natural therapy for the treatment of cancer that enhances the body's own capacity for managing the disease. This therapy will also be safe, affordable, and accessible for all people.

Synopsis

Every year 12 million people worldwide die of heart attacks and strokes. They are the most common cause of death of our time. Cellular medicine has already found the answer to this epidemic— atherosclerosis and its consequences, heart infarction and stroke are early forms of scurvy. Based on this knowledge, coronary heart disease will be reduced to a fraction of the current figures over the next decades.

The second most common disease is cancer. There is only one plausible explanation for this—conventional medicine does not know the causes of cancer or how it spreads. The most common disease and causes of death in developing countries are infectious diseases, including the AIDS epidemic. These serious infectious diseases can only continue spreading as they do because knowledge of "Cellular Health" has not been efficiently used. This book will also provide the solution for the control of these diseases.

The Remarkable Value of Lysine

There are twenty known amino acids which compose all of the proteins in our bodies. The cells of the body can produce most amino acids themselves. These amino acids are called nonessential. However, there are nine known amino acids that our body cannot produce. They have to be supplied through the diet. These amino acids are called essential.

Lysine plays an important role within the group of essential amino acids as vitamin C does within the vitamin group. The daily requirement for lysine surpasses that of all other amino acids. Among its many functions, lysine is also the building block of the amino acid carnitine, which is important for energy metabolism in every cell.

About 25 percent of collagen, the most important structural molecule of bones, skin, blood vessel walls, and all other organs, consists of two amino acids, lysine and proline. Taking large quantities of lysine will not cause adverse effects. The body will simply excrete the molecules that are not used. Almost everyone suffers from a deficiency of lysine.

How Much Lysine can our Bodies Handle?

- A human body weighing about 155 pounds contains about 22 pounds of proteins.
- 50% of this protein mass is present as connective tissue proteins—collagen and elastin.
- Lysine forms about 12 percent (1.1 to 1.3 pounds) of the collagen and elastin mass.
- A body weighing 155 pounds contains about 1.1 pounds of lysine.

Since our bodies are used to such large amounts of lysine, taking 10 grams of lysine daily as a supplement should not be considered excessive.

An exciting discovery made by Dr. Matthias Rath using a natural approach to control cancer has been confirmed by biomedical researchers at Matthias Rath Inc. It has been found that specific nutrients are able to stop the spread of cancer cells through connective tissue, the means by which metastasis occurs. Metastasis is what causes cancer to be so deadly, and therefore, it is crucial that more be learned about this process. Conventional methods of cancer treatment do nothing to prevent the metastasis, or spread, of cancer cells from one part of the body to another.

Cancer cells develop in the body as a result of damage to cellular DNA, which destroys the control mechanism of cell replication. These abnormal cells escape destruction and begin to multiply rapidly into tumors. A tumor contained in one location of the body rarely endangers a person's life. However, approximately 90% of all cancer fatalities result from metastasis, the invasion of cancer cells into other organs and tissues.

The Spread of Cancer can be Contained

There is one crucial question that Matthias Rath's researchers sought to answer. How could we naturally inhibit the invasion of cancer cells through collagen and connective tissue in a way that would enhance the body's own capacity for managing disease? In seeking this answer, the researchers designed an experiment to investigate the ability of cancer cells to digest through a collagenous matrix and then a method to control it. The results of the experiment were remarkable. A simple combination of nutrients was able to stop cancer cells from invading the collagen matrix.

The most powerful nutrient combination contained vitamin C, the amino acids L-Lysine and L-Proline, and a polyphenol fraction of green tea known as Epigallocatechingallate or (EGCG).

The combination of Vitamin C, the amino acids L-Lysine and L-Proline, and EGCG was effective in stopping the invasion and spread of a variety of cancer cells, including those of colon, breast, and skin (melanoma)

Percentage of Cancer cells Blocked From Invading Collagen Matrix
(with vitamin C, L-Lysine, L-Proline, and EGCG)

91%	100%	100%
X	X	X
X	X	X
X	X	X
X	X	X
X	X	X
X	X	X
X	X	X
X	X	X
Colon	Breast	Melanoma

Research findings Presented at the 19th Annual Breast Cancer Conference February 27-March 2m 2002

L-Lysine and L-Proline are natural amino acids that are the building blocks of collagen and elastin fibers. In addition, L-Lysine prevents digestion of collagen by blocking sites where enzymes attach, making the nutrient critical in preventing the degredation of connective tissue. Although L-Proline is produced by the human body in limited quantities, :-Lysine is not. The health of the connective tissue depends on an optimal daily intake of these two key amino acids, as well as vitamin C.

Rath, M., Pauling, L (1991) Plasmin-Induced Proteolysis and the Role of Apolipoprotein A
Lysine and Synthetic Lysine Analogs
Journal of Orthomolecular Medicine 7: 17-23
Conventional Cancer Therapy
A Dead-End Street

"Is the medical world on the wrong track with its cancer therapy? My answer would be, yes! Constantly pressured by the pharmaceutical industry, patients are offered no options other than chemotherapy. Chemotherapy means poisoning cells. The pharmaceutical industry argues that it will damage the cancer cells. What they do not tell patients is that all the other cells of the body are damaged as well, thus, chemo-poisoning of the bone marrow- the place where red blood cells are produced. This leads to anemia and increased susceptibility to infections. Chemo-poisoning of the mucous membrane cells of the gastrointestinal tract will lead to diarrhea and internal bleeding. The damage to hair follicles leads to extreme loss of hair. Instead of strengthening the body's immune system to help fight the cancer, the chemotherapy will paralyze it. Chemotherapy's side effects require additional use of other new medications such as antibiotics, plasma replacement drugs, pain killers, cortisone and many more. The last weeks or months of life for the patients undergoing cancer therapy are an "el Dorado" for the pharmaceutical industry.

In the summary of my work I wrote, "it is foreseeable that the medical applications of Lysine and synthetic Lysine analogs, especially combined with vitamin C, will lead to a breakthrough in the control of several forms of cancer, infectious diseases, including AIDS, as well as many other diseases."

Optimal production of collagen molecules is the precondition for control of aggressive diseases. To achieve optimum collagen production three major nutrients are required.

- **Vitamin C**- controls collagen production. Collagen molecules wind around each other like a twilled rope. The optimal structure essential for biological activity and stability of collagen is not possible without the presence of vitamin C. Chemical "bridges" connect collagen strands. These bridges are formed with oxygen and hydrogen atoms- the so-called "OH groups," which anchor specific lysine and proline molecules in collagen. This "hydroxylation" process is catalyzed by vitamin C.

- **Lysine**- is a building block of the chain of amino acids that form collagen fibers. Since our body cannot produce its own lysine, every lysine molecule must be supplied through the diet or from supplements

- **Proline**- is another important amino acid component of collagen. Our body can produce it, but only in limited amounts. In people with long-term or aggressive diseases accompanied by the enzymatic disintegration of collagen, the body's capacity to produce proline can be exhausted. This often leads to a deficiency of this amino acid.

LINUS PAULING: A MAN AND HIS SCIENCE
ANTHONY SERAFINI

Serafini explores a life of brilliant achievement from the early years of Linus Pauling's poverty to the present day. Along the way science and the world are beneficiaries of the theoretical genius that has garnered two Nobel Prizes, in chemistry and peace. Chemistry, physics, biology, biochemistry, and nutrition are all part of the tapestry of this remarkable man's life. His humanitarian drive has caused Pauling and his wife Ava Helen a great deal of pain, but they continued to press their demands for a nuclear-free world.

The strides which Pauling has made in the nutrition and biochemical fields may ultimately become his most important contribution to humanity. Orthomolecular medicine, a term which Pauling coined in 1968, means "the proper amount of nutrients necessary to be in the best of health." It is his belief that megavitamin therapy and prevention can prevent colds, viral diseases, and cancer, and help solve America's costly and burdensome healthcare problem.

Synopsis

Early in Linus Pauling's childhood it was apparent that he was destined for greatness, with his limitless thirst for knowledge. His father died when he was nine years old, and young Linus, who did not get along well with his mother, withdrew into science. A high school teacher, Pauline Gabelle, said of Pauling, "he was always the intellectual frontiersman." His intellectual and intuitive powers were impressive even in 1913, when he also demonstrated a fundamental intellectual arrogance; he refused to take a course in Civics at Washington High School, which denied him a diploma until after he received the Nobel

Prize in 1962.

Pauling, fuelled by the experiments of a young friend, Lloyd Jeffries, built a laboratory in his basement as a child and "borrowed" bottles of chemicals from the Oregon Iron & Steel Company, where his grandfather was a night watchman at the foundry. The Pauling's were poor and young Linus had to work at various jobs to support his mother; when the boy insisted on going to college, she objected, saying, "no one on the street has gone to college."

In 1917 Pauling was accepted at Oregon Agricultural College where, in his junior year, he was offered a position as a full-time assistant instructor in Quantitative Analysis, a class that he had just completed. (He met Ava Helen Miller, who would become his wife, in one of these classes). Floyd Rowland, nominating him for a Rhodes Scholarship, said, "Mr. Pauling possesses one of the best minds I have ever observed in a person of his age, and in many ways is superior to his instructors."

At Cal Tech, in graduate school, Pauling taught one class per semester and met with Einstein, who was amazed when he delivered a paper in flawless German. After receiving his Ph. D., Pauling spent two years in Europe with Peter Debye and Albert Sommerfeld, the leaders in the field of chemical bonding, and in 1926 he attended a conference on magnetism in Zurich. He returned to the United States when he was offered an assistant professorship at the California Institute of Technology.

In 1931, a paper entitled "The Nature of the Chemical Bond become the basis of Pauling's most famous scholarly book. With two co-workers Pauling had worked out the structure of more than 200 substances using electron diffraction. For this work the New York Times and the Oregonian trumpeted Pauling's accomplishments, citing him as a world class scientist. He was awarded the Langmuir Prize, an award with enormous prestige, by the American Chemical Society. He had become a distinguished authority on the subatomic structure of matter.

In 1932 Pauling was the youngest person to be awarded membership in the National Academy of Sciences. He was offered a full professorship and joint appointments in chemistry and physics at M.I.T. but he stayed at Cal Tech to become chairman of chemistry and chemical engineering when Noyes died.

Pauling's intuition extended to chemistry, chemical bonding, quantum mechanics, and crystal structure. Pauling received a visit by Langsteiner, a magical name in biological chemistry and Nobel Laureate in the classification of blood types. The approach to structural chemistry outlined in "The Nature of the chemical bond" inspired Watson and Crick in their search for the structure of the DNA molecule. Pauling's growing eminence attracted students, scientists, and post-doctoral candidates to Cal Tech from all over the world.

In 1948 Pauling, as a visiting professor at Oxford, was forced by a cold to spend several days in bed and began to tinker with some folded pieces of paper on which he had drawn atoms and chemical bonds. A helix emerged and he jumped out of bed—he had discovered the Alpha Helix concept, one of the greatest secrets of life. He soon realized that all protein exists as helixes, but he needed data.

The Rockefeller Foundation supported Pauling's work in the field of molecular biology. And the structure of the hemoglobin molecule and how it takes up oxygen completely absorbed his attention. When Dr. William B. Castle described some work that he was doing in sickle-cell anemia, it struck Pauling that the disease could be caused by an abnormality of the haemoglobin molecule which might drastically reduce its capacity to carry oxygen.

Einstein and Pauling met in 1980. Their discussion was mainly about ethics, politics, and world peace, rather than science. This was an education for Pauling, and it was certain that these two great men were concerned with the threat of nuclear Armageddon. In a letter to Leo Szilard following the meeting with Einstein, Pauling states that world peace is of paramount importance.

Pauling's genius lay in his ability to project an idea to its conclusion. Jonathan Singer said that, "what was astonishing about Pauling and makes him great, was that he was willing to move a concept on the basis of certain data whose relevance was not that clear to others. Only Linus was willing to take the inductive leap." Pauling's extraordinary insight solved many problems in structural chemistry. Professor Sampson of Cal Tech compared Pauling to another scientist. "Pauling would plant a lot of seeds, basic ideas, without working them out fully... as soon as Slater gets an idea he works it out to the end before he gets a new one."

Pauling's interests ranged widely, and he often entered areas considered the domain of other scientists. Scientists are territorial about their own fields, they considered Pauling an interloper. When he entered the field of nuclear physics, theorizing about the nucleus of the atom, he was criticized.

On November 3, 1964, Pauling received news that he had been awarded the Nobel Prize for chemistry as he was giving a lecture at Cornell University. When he announced it to the audience he received a 20 minute ovation. After receiving the Nobel Prize, Pauling cut back on his research. He began to explore the area of "unorthodox medicine," culminating in his work on Vitamin C. With funding for research increased he could now turn to the chemistry of the brain, an uncharted area. He had always been curious about the effect of nutrition on mental illness, but he never had the research money, staff, and laboratory space for the more unconventional, progressive interest. Now he could explore the relationships between chemical imbalance, nutrition, and mental illness.

In 1969 Pauling accepted an appointment as Professor of Chemistry at Stanford. He exhausted all the literature on Vitamin C and the common cold, but didn't see the need for an experiment to prove its effectiveness, saying, "Everyone knows what I think about "Vitamin C and the Common Cold." I don't think I need to do any experiment." In my case there was no laboratory space at Stanford for lab work.

The medical establishment refused to accept his studies which contradicted their misconceptions, so Pauling turned to the general public. He wrote his book "Vitamin C and the Common cold" in only one month. Its thesis was revolutionary. "The natural essential food ascorbic acid (Vitamin C), taken in the right amounts at the right time, would prevent most of these colds from developing, and would greatly decrease the intensity of the symptoms in those that do develop."

Critics couldn't wait to pounce on Pauling and his views. Frederic J. Stare of Harvard said that Pauling was "lost in the woods," and Dr. K.C. Hayes also of Harvard, noted that Pauling's ideas not only "make no sense in terms of modern medicine or nutrition, but also in the irresponsible way they arouse false hopes in those who have diseases which Pauling feels can be successfully treated by his vitamin therapy." Others lined up to support Pauling's thesis; popular nutritionists Adele Davis and Carlton Fredericks echoed the virtues of Vitamin C and good nutrition in general, and Albert Szent-Gyorgyi who discovered Vitamin C added his support.

In 1971 Dr. Ewan Cameron in Scotland noted a remarkable

improvement in cancer patients given 10 grams of vitamin C per day. Pauling heard of these results and began publishing the findings. In a speech at the University of Chicago he said that, "with the proper use of ascorbic acid the mortality from cancer would be reduced by about 10 percent." The press had a field day—Pauling made good copy.

In 1978 Pauling received another setback when the results of a study at the Mayo clinic, led by the famous cancer specialist, Dr. Charles Moertel were published in the New England Journal of Medicine. They showed that "in a selected group of patients we were unable to show a therapeutic benefit of a high-dose Vitamin C treatment." Pauling pointed out the critical flaw in the Mayo Clinic's study. Many of the patients in the study had received extensive chemotherapy, while the Vale of Leven patients did not. Vitamin C energizes the immune system, and chemotherapy destroys it. Pauling contends that the vitamin C didn't work because the patients' immune systems had already been decimated.

The Mayo Clinic did another study, in which the patients were given Vitamin C for only 2 to 5 months. Again "the study failed to show a benefit for high-dose Vitamin C therapy." Pauling pointed out that the "rebound" effect when vitamin c is taken in high doses and abruptly withdrawn can lower blood Vitamin C levels drastically and even result in scurvy. Although the charge was irrefutable, the public perception resulting from the prestigious Mayo clinic studies overshadowed Pauling's claims for vitamin c. In addition, Moertel claimed that "the apparent results of Cameron and Pauling were the product of case selection bias rather than treatment effectiveness." There was certainly no evidence to support this charge, and it was equally difficult to prove that Moertel's studies at the mayo clinic were completely objective. Thus, the second Mayo Clinic study only proved that Vitamin c is ineffective when it is used for a short period of time and then withdrawn.

Pauling made an astonishing claim in a 1977 issue of Prevention; "My present estimate is that a decrease of 25% in cancer mortality can be achieved by the use of vitamin C alone, and a further decrease by the use of other nutritional measures."

Orthomolecular medicine has been rejected by the American Psychiatric Association. Most psychiatrists and physicians are either ignorant of Pauling's views or simply disregard them. However, a growing body of young medical practitioners are devoted to the concept of megavitamin therapy. They also firmly believe in the importance of good diet for the promotion of the best of health and the prevention of disease. It is becoming evident to many doctors that Pauling may have been right, and his ideas should be taken seriously.

LOVE, MEDICINE, AND MIRACLES
BERNIE SIEGEL, M.D.

If anyone doubts that there is a connection between the mind and the body. "Love, Medicine, and Miracles" will dispel them. When the rigors of a cancer surgeon's routine drained the desire to practice medicine from Bernie Siegel, he thought seriously about changing his profession. Fate stepped in and saved this remarkable person. He founded ECAP "Exceptional Cancer Patients, a non-profit organization which accepts every cancer patient regardless of his ability to pay, and provides them with a loving family and support to develop goals which give life meaning and quality. ECAP uses hope and love to prolong their lives.

Bernie Siegel proves to all his cancer patients that life is worth living. He shows how the mind and the spirit can heal the body. A patient once told Bernie, "death is not the worst thing; life without love is worse." These profound lessons are not just for cancer patients, they are important for all humanity.

Synopsis

A doctor's success is defined as saving lives. People eventually die. Dr. Siegel felt like a failure over and over again. In the 1970s, after 10 years as a surgeon, his job was getting to him. He felt that he should be more than a mechanic, but it took years of difficult growth to achieve that satisfaction.

In 1974 Dr. Siegel started a diary which eventually changed his attitude toward medical practice. It dawned on him that he'd been dealing with cases, charts, and diseases rather than people; people had been machines to repair. This distance doctors put between themselves and their patients go too far. Dr. Siegel thought of entering a new specialty, like psychiatry, so he could help people without cutting into them.

Siegel put his desk against the wall so there would be no obstacle between him and his patients, and encouraged them to call him Bernie. The change was worth it. He finally understood what it's like to live with cancer. He drew strength from his patients. In the face of their courage he wished he could do something to ease the passage, and began to feel that his profession's attempt to prolong life was one of the noblest goals of man.

At a seminar in Connecticut, where Siegel learned to meditate, he was the only "body" doctor. He was angry that his medical education never mentioned that such techniques existed. Though he was still thinking about a career change, he realized he could do more good by remaining in surgery and mobilizing the mental power of his cancer patients. If a permanent remission of cancer was possible with one patient, it must be possible for others. Why does medicine swell on failure and refuse to learn from success? Siegel used to predict when people would die, based on statistics. He longer does. Some people are too busy to head the advice, and others feel that if they are going to die, life is not worth living, so they go home and die.

Siegel formed a therapy group called, "Exceptional Cancer Patients (ECAP) to help people mobilize there full resources against the disease. Only 12 people showed up at the first meeting. It was then that he learned first-hand what patients are really like. About 15% to 20% want to die. The majority, 60% to 70% do what the physician wants them to do, passively, without question; but the last 15% to 20% are exceptional. They refuse to play the victim. They educate themselves and become specialists in their own care, question the doctor, and demand dignity no matter what the course of the disease in the world of Kathryn and Cornelius Ryan's "A Private Battle." They go out "like a tired lion, not a frightened lamb."

"Bad patients- are the ones who ask questions and are difficult and uncooperative. They live longer. Sandra levy, a National Cancer Institute psychologist, found that aggressive patients more of the protective T-cells that destroy cancer cells than do the "goog" patients. Their fighting spirit can translate into a 75% survival rate, as opposed to a 22% rate for those with "stoic acceptance."

Siegel got furious at other doctors when his patients told him what they were like in their offices. A patient might wait two hours and be refused 5 minutes of discussion. He was amazed to see many of his patients get better when they were given hope and put in control of themselves.

Siegel finally decided to remain a surgeon. He also became a healer and a teacher, working as a team with the patient. He shaved his head and people began to talk to him in a different way. Patients told him things they would never tell other doctors, sharing emotions, dreams, and premonitions. Other physicians thought he was crazy, but he was too happy about his members' improvement to care. When he wrote articles about his discoveries, however, medical journals returned them. The role of the mind in disease is only now beginning to achieve acceptance.

Science teaches us that we must see to believe- but we must also believe to see. We must be receptive to possibilities that science does not grasp, or we will miss them. It's absurd not to use treatments that work because we don't understand them. We should never say, "There's nothing more I can do for you." You can always sit down, talk, and help the patient hope and pray the physician's prognosis of how much the patient has left is a mistake; it becomes a self-fulfilling prophecy. Belief in survival can work wonders. Healing is a creative act. It takes hard work and dedication, just as in other forms of creativity. Physicians must learn to project hope at all times, even in the final hours. If a patient has decided it's time to die, Dr. Siegel sees no contradiction in aiding with that- acceptance need not take away hope. His primary task is to help patients achieve peace of mind.

Hope comes about largely as a patient's confidence in the healer. The exceptional patient wants to share the responsibility for life and treatment, and doctors who encourage that attitude can help their patients heal faster. The physician must remember that it's the patient who must make the choice and then live with it. Some surgeons insist on running the whole show—and sadly, many patients let them.

The three most dreaded words in our language are, "you have cancer." Some people refuse to accept the diagnosis, but knowing the truth and refusing to admit it prevents an effective response. If you share your fears, your body can begin the healing process. Knowing what you are fighting and how to fight are the keys. I try to convert deniers into fighters. People with cancer often feel despair for months or years, sometimes withdrawing from all human contact. Some see their impending death as a sort of sacrifice or martyrdom; they may have never done anything for themselves, or they may trade their illness for love. Patients may even die to gain love.

Many cancer patients experience a flood of self-pity. This is linked to anger. People get furious with God or their physician, but rarely express rage at the tobacco company, the nuclear-power industry, or the pesticide industry. Anger is well-founded. When Siegel began ECAP, the anger at physicians was tremendous. He left the first meeting angry too. Patients must be encouraged to express their anger, hatred, and fear. Research has shown that people who give vent to their negative emotions survive adversity better than those who contain them.

Bernie Siegel can help patients choose a treatment. He must learn their attitudes toward themselves and their disease. He asks them to answer four basic questions:

- Do you want to live to be a hundred?
- What happened to you in the year or two before your illness?
- What does the illness mean to you?
- Why did you need the illness?'

If you set a physical goal you may fail, but if you make peace of mind your goal you can achieve it. In achieving peace of mind, you may cure your cancer. The mind and the body communicate with each other on a subconscious level. You have to gain a clear conscience and accept the challenge to take control of your life, find your true path, sing your song, and decide what you want to be when you grow up,

Siegel tries to get patients to see standard medical treatments—like radiation, chemotherapy, and surgery—as energy that can buy time while the patient finds the will to live. change, and heal. In the end the body heals, not the therapy. The most important thing is to pick a therapy you believe in, and proceed with a positive attitude. It's best for patients to focus their energy on the one or two approaches they believe in most strongly. However, nutritional supplementation, exercise, and meditation are valuable and are therefore important parts of the ECAP program. Siegel won't browbeat people into radiation or chemotherapy if they think they are toxic. But he feels that about three-quarters of the side effects of radiation and chemotherapy result from patients' negative beliefs. Beliefs shape the power of the treatment as well as its side effects. Radiation can be a killing ray or a golden beam of healing energy.

ECAP is free for those who can't afford it; the modest fee only defrays costs. It's non-profit, and no one is ever turned away. It helps patients set goals for their lives, and even deal with their sexual problems. ECAP provides an instant family, in many ways more loving and supportive than real family.

Good nutrition is essential in any treatment program, but Siegel doesn't prescribe a strict regimen. If they love themselves they will eat right, exercise, and quit smoking. Vigorous exercise benefits the body in every way and offers a chance to meditate. I suggest a half-hour to an our daily, or every other day. Laughter and humor is of psychological importance. Norman Cousins has called them "internal jogging." The physical benefits of relaxation and meditation are well documented. They reduce over-competitive behavior and the threat of heart attacks. Meditation also reduces your biological age. When combined with exercise it helps you live longer and feel better, and reduces wear and tear on your body and mind.

Becoming excellent is ECAP's goal for all its members. If patients set realistic targets, their achievement reinforces feelings of competence and self-worth, and the goals themselves make the future a brighter prospect. The ultimate goal is to live for ourselves in a selfless way. We encourage people to integrate all aspects of their lives—work, physical development, spiritual and emotional needs, and to help others. Meditation and visualization are powerful tools to help you become aware of your true needs and then make them happen. Many people get well using alternative therapies because they believe in something that gives them hope. ECAP has found four faiths that are crucial to recovery from serious illness.

- Faith in oneself
- Faith in one's doctor.
- Faith in the treatment
- Spiritual faith.

Dr. Siegel believes that the healing power of love can add another dimension to medicine. "It is my fervent hope that by showing adults how the mind and the spirit can heal the body and make life worthwhile.

I can help us, as parents, raise a generation of children programmed to be loving and healthy. "Too many children get everything they want and nothing they need." When one believes in love and miracles, divine intervention can occur; the path of love will save ourselves and our universe."

LIFE EXTENSION
DURK PEARSON AND SANDY SHAW

It is now possible to do something about aging. The authors attempt to bridge the gap that usually exists between discovery and the general usage of nutrients which may be effective in extending our life span, by self-experimenting with practices that have been successful in laboratory tests of animals.

The authors advise caution and disclaim any attempt by the public to consider that this book has the answer to longevity; their own use of excessively large doses of vitamins and minerals is not an endorsement of such a regimen. Use intelligence and a physician's advice about diet and nutrient supplementation. Your family doctor's knowledge of your medical history should dictate your course of action.

Synopsis

Like extension means extending the active, pleasurable portion of one's life, not the time spent in a hospital bed. Scientific reports show that the life span of experimental animals can be doubled. "Don't let obsolete assumptions and misconceptions drive you prematurely to your grave."

The reversal of aging is a new phenomenon and we must develop a different attitude toward it. It is wise to start immediately with life extension techniques, which can only help to improve you current state of health. You may never become immortal, but you can succeed in living longer and in far better health. Life extension does not start by slowing down all the aging mechanisms at once. It slows them down one at a time until your whole system is working to maintain its integrity for an extended period.

The rate of aging depends on the relationship between cell destruction and cell repair. As time passes, the repair/destruction ratio declines and aging increases. Physiological decline varies with the individual. New research has demonstrated that aging can be slowed down and even reversed.

People live twice as long as chimps. A small number of genes may be the cause of the increased life span; we know that longer-lived species have better DSA repair mechanisms. If we can learn which genes control the life span, and how to intervene in the control systems, we can overcome the current life span limit of 110 years. Genetic engineers are now studying techniques that might be usable in a decade or two for adding more and better age control genes to ourselves.

As aging is a multi-dimensional process, there are many ways to increase your life span. One simple approach is to stop doing the things which shorten your life span such as smoking, drinking, and excessive eating. Other methods involve taking certain nutrients which have shown life-extending capabilities in clinical tests. Pantothenic acud (calcium pantothenate) has been shown to extend the life span of mice by 20%. If you can't stop smoking or drinking, sufficient doses of vitamin C and B-1 may reduce the toxic damage caused by these habits. The level of lipids (fats and oils) in the bloodstream which can cause heart attacks can be controlled by taking vitamin, E, and niacin (B-3).

You can extend your life one year for every year you apply the benefits of life extension research, as well as improving the quality of life immediately. Even a person in his eighties can do something about his aging, it is never too late. Life extension techniques allow you to spend more time youthful and healthy, not just lengthen the duration of a feeble tail end of life.

The FDA (Food and Drug Administration) and the FTC (Federal Trade Commission) have prevented vitamin, nutrient, and pharmaceutical manufacturers from making health claims for their products, and only 10% of the National Institute of Aging's research is aimed at extending life. The government may fear that an extended life span would make trouble in the Social Security System and welfare programs. This problem is remote- most people are not prepared to involve themselves in personal life extension.

The immune system, the thymus gland, white blood cells, bone marrow, the spleen, lymph nodes and ducts, and various protein and polypeptide chemicals like antibodies and interferon- can prevent the diseases of aging which kill us, including heart disease and cancer. If it is active and well-functioning good nutrition can restore your immune system to a young adult level. Nutrients which strengthen the immune system include vitamins A,C,E, the trace minerals zinc and selenium, the enzymes trypsin, bromelain and papain, and the amino acids arginine, ornitine, and cysteine.

It is known that dietary cholesterol does not determine blood cholesterol levels. The body manufactures up to 1.5 grams of cholesterol each day. The Framingham Study, which observed 437 men and 475 women for up to 10 years, found no correlation between cholesterol in the diet and cholesterol levels in the blood. Other studies confirmed these results, with additional findings that there was no clear relation between blood serum cholesterol itself and deaths due to heart disease. When the lipid hypothesis became popular, the protein link to atherosclerosis was forgotten. Low levels of vitamin B-6 show up in those who have elevated risk of cardiovascular disease. Eicosapentanoeoic acid (EPA), present in fish oils, reduces the formation of blood clots and helps in the prevention of coronary thrombosis, a form of heart attack. Vitamin C also reduces the size of atherosclerotic plaques after they have formed. Table sugar can contribute to the development of atherosclerosis; it triggers a release of insulin into the blood which is thought to cause cholesterol and other lipids to be deposited in the arterial walls.

Reducing cholesterol levels, by itself, does not lower the heart disease rate. Many risk factors in addition to high blood cholesterol contribute to the incidence of heart disease—uric acid, blood sugar, triglycerides, and unbalanced lipoprotein pattern, and sticky blood platelets caused by free radical damage. A diet to promote longevity should stress antioxidant nutrients and be sensible.

Aging is not inevitable. Science offers everyone the promise of continuing development of better methods for the control of aging and the extension of life.

GENETIC NUTRITIONEERING
JEFFREY S. BLAND, PH.D.
AND SARA H. BLENUM, M.A.

We are wrestling with one of the biggest problems our country has faced—the geometric growth in the cost of our healthcare. While our representatives in congress are struggling to find the answer, a new medical paradigm is emerging that promises to completely eliminate the problem. Our genetic destiny determines many things including our physical characteristics and our predisposition to disease. A sheep named "Dolly" may be the first step in our march to a new future. A world where we will be free of disease and able to age gracefully until we reach the maximum life span for humans, which is now 115 years.

The Human Genome project is an ongoing international collaborative project among scientists around the worlds to "decode" the genetic information locked within the 23 pairs of chromosomes called our genome. A genome is a full series of genes in an individual. Only 2 percent of the nearly 6 billion pieces of DNA that comprise human inheritance factors have been analysed. The amount of information is staggering. Some people have expressed concern that we might be better off not knowing what is locked up in our genes. These messages might tell us how and when we are going to die.

Nevertheless, scientists are learning that degenerative diseases such as cancer, heart disease, diabetes, and arthritis are not inevitable. They are the result of a poor match between genetic needs and an individual's choice of nutrition, lifestyle, and environment.

The focus of this book is the scientific revolution that is taking place around the world. As we enter the new millennium, there is promise and hope of a new way of life where an individual can achieve his maximum potential with good health, energy, and well-being.

Synopsis

A scientific revolution is taking place in university and molecular laboratories around the world. The results of this revolution will change the way medicine is practiced, and may result in the extension of life expectancy and health span, or disease-free years of life. Scientists have compared this scientific revolution to Darwin's theory of evolution.. This revolution is called The Human Genome Project.

We are living in a time of amazing paradox. Our managed care medical system delivers less and less care, and, on the other hand, a new medical paradigm is taking shape that promises to keep people healthy all through their lives. This book focuses on this new paradigm and gives you the tools to reduce your disease risk and increase your energy, vitality, and well-being. You can unlock the tremendous potential for good health that is stored in your genes. Genetic nutritioneering puts you in charge of your own health program .

Your genetic destiny is very strong. Heredity determines your eye color, predisposition to disease, your fate.—in short—your destiny. Events that would have sounded like genetic science fiction a few years ago are now daily news.

We have not only seen the cloning of a sheep named Dolly, but some scientists are working to set up a lab to clone human beings. "The fact that a lamb was derived from an adult cell confirms that differentiation of the cell did not involve irreversible modification of genetic material required for the development to term." The development suggests that all the genetic information encoded from every stage of your development from an embryo to an elderly adult and for every cell type in your body is potentially accessible to any cell in your body.

This concept is so profound that it is hard to accept. You may be able to access messages that describe as younger and healthier you. In her book, "21st Century Miracle Medicine," Alexandra Wyke points out that between 1960 and 1990 the United States witnessed an increase in healthcare expenditures from $200 million to $1 trillion annually. However, the public "are manifestly no less sick today than they were three decades ago." She predicts that the first major breakthroughs in health will come in the next few years as a result of accessing genetic information. This will allow us to express our phenotype as the best of our inheritance factors while suppressing those messages that result in premature aging and disease.

Most people assume that diseases like diabetes, heart disease, high blood pressure, stroke, arthritis, and cancer are the result of genetic inheritance factors. The Human Genome Project is proving that genes are only part of the story. More important than genetic inheritance is the phenotype- the result of gene expression and function. Your phenotype is determined by the way you have treated your genes throughout your life. When you have eaten, drunk, inhaled, surrounded yourself within your environment, endured as stresses, suffered as injury, infection or inflammation. All of these factors alter the expression of your genes and contribute in a major way to your state of health or disease.

A perfect example of nutritional modification of genetic expression is the work of Drs. Joseph and Mary Goldberger. In the early 1900s, when medicine believed that all diseases were caused by bacteria, the Goldbergers demonstrated the nutritional link to Pellagra. They proved that a deficiency of niacin (vitamin B-3) caused the disease. The old concepts die slowly, however, and it wasn't until years later, (1940_ that Linus Pauling described how a defect in genetic structure caused sickle cell anemia. In the 1950s Roger Williams described what he called "Biochemical Individuality" and "Genetotrophic Disease," a disease resulting from the suboptimal intake of nutrients necessary to meet the determined biochemical needs of the individual.

In the 1700s, the Swiss naturalist Charles Bonnet advanced an early concept of genetic inheritance. For nearly a century Bonnet's theory of evolution was a major influence on scientific thinking about the origin of acquired characteristics. The Augustinian monk Gregor Mendel, who lived from 1822 to 1884, bred pea plants and found that every pea flower had both male and female organs, and they fertilized themselves. He suggested that there was something in the pollen that determined the characteristics of the offspring. That something is what we know as genes.

The genes in our chromosomes are acquired in equal numbers from our mothers and fathers. Some genes are dominant, and others are recessive. Blue eye color is recessive to brown eye color. If you have blue eyes, both of your parents gave you their recessive genetic characteristic for blue eyes, even if they themselves did not have blue eyes. Characteristics associated with genes like the color of eyes are called "alleles." You get one from your father and another one from your mother. Homozygous characteristics are genes contributed equally by both parents. Those contributed unequally are called heterozygous.

As genetic research progressed scientists learned homozygous characteristics were often associated with a number of rare genetic conditions including hemophelia, sickle cell anemia, dwarfism, and others. Genes can undergo damage and their information could be altered. This was called a mutation. In most cases these mutations are not helpful. Occasionally, they can result in a characteristic that makes the offspring more able than his parents to succeed in the environment. Favorable mutations are what scientists feel contribute to the evolution of the species over many millions of years.

Most people, scientists and people alike, feel we have no control over our genes. They believe that when a person lives a long, healthy life he is blessed with good genes. When someone succumbs to cancer or heart disease in the prime of life, we blame his death on bad genes. When a person dies from smoking-induced lung cancer, alcoholic liver disease, or malnutrition, can we blame the death on genes alone? Certainly not. In such cases, under optimal conditions the individual's genes may have allowed him to live a long, healthy life. The deterministic view of genetics we inherited from Gregor Mendel, which would have us believe our health is predetermined by our genes, is not consistent with the revolution in the science of genetics that is taking place today. Because we believe that we could do little to influence the way our genes control our health, medicine focused on diagnosis and not prevention. This philosophy is undergoing revolutionary change as a consequence of breakthroughs in molecular biology and genetics.

The basis of the genetic nutritioneering program is the possibility of altering the expression of one's genes. Your genes are polymorphic and pluripotential. You can alter the expression of your genetic potential through the foods you eat, the lifestyle you select and the environment in which you work and live.

Regardless of your age, you can change the terms of the experiment" of your life and get different results in the way your genes are expressed. You have a lot more control over your health than you may have believed. Science is on your side. You have the chance to participate in the greatest change in medicine and healthcare since the development of the germ theory of disease, antibiotics, and immunization.

During the course of your life, many events alter the way your genetic characteristics are expressed in individual cells, tissues, and organs. These alterations are natural responses to your changing environment, such as your response to stress, cold or heat, exercise or exposure to environmental chemicals. In other cases, however, changes in gene expression may reflect changes in phenotype that indicates disease or the loss of health and vitality.

Water is an essential nutrient. If you don't drink enough water your body becomes dehydrated and an extended period of dehydration can result in altered gene expression. Water not only hydrates the body, but also provides the proper cellular environment so cells can engage in biochemical reactions associated with gene expression, protein synthesis, and metabolic function.

Nutrition also plays an important role in modulating gene expression. "You are what you eat," places the responsibility for decisions about foods. Information emerging from current scientific research strongly supports the view that the foods you eat and the nutrients they contain have the ability to communicate with your genes. Genetic messages can either be put to sleep or awakened as a consequence of alterations in your diet. Awakening those messages that enhance health and help prevent premature aging is the focus of the genetic nutritioneering program.

Chronic diseases , including heart disease, high blood pressure, diabetes, and cancer, are significant health problems in the United States. All of these diseases have lifestyle and nutrition components, reducible risk factors, that if managed properly, should lower the risk of these diseases. Yet most of us know someone who had a fatal heart attack at an early age who had moderate cholesterol and blood pressure, did not smoke, was not as diabetic, and had no family history of heart disease. We may also know someone who had a healthy lifestyle but was struck down by cancer in the prime of life.

Drs. Michael Brown and Joseph Goldstein, from the University of Texas Southwestern Medical School, were awarded the Nobel Prize in 1985 for their pioneering work on cholesterol and its relationship to heart disease. They found that families whose members have the basic genetic defect in which diet caused elevated blood levels of the "bad" LDL cholesterol occurs about 1 in 500 individuals worldwide. They determined that their bodies produced too much cholesterol because of a defect in the thermostat that controls cholesterol synthesis. This led to the development of statin drugs that could turn off the thermostat. A dietary substance called tocotrienol has the ability to help regulate the cholesterol thermostat in the liver.

In 82 percent of the 156 recently published research studies, it was found that fruit and vegetable consumption provided significant protection against many cancers. People who eat more fruits and vegetables have lower mortality than those who are not fruit and vegetable eaters. Researchers have identified a host of active substances in these anti-cancer plant foods. The following phytochemicals and their sources have been the subject of research.

- Allyl sulphides in garkic and onions.
- Phytates in grains and legumes like soy.
- Glucarates in citrus, grains, and tomatoes.
- Lignins in flax and soybeans.
- Isoflavones in soybeans.
- Saponins in legumes.
- Indoles, isothiocyanates, and hydroxybutene in cruciferous vegetables.
- Ellagic acid in grapes, strawberries, raspberries, and nuts.
- Bioflavonoids, carotenoids, and terpenoids in other plant foods.

Most of these substances influence specific aspects opf gene expression and help either to induce anti-cancer genes or put cancer genes to sleep.

More than 1,000 bioflavonoids have been found in various foods. As a class of phytochemicals bioflavonoids have important gene response modifying effects and are also antioxidants. Tea is the major source of bioflavonoids in the average diet. Both black and Chinese green tea contain high levels of bioflavonoids. Chinese green tea contains a class of bioflavonoids called catechins. They have a very powerful antioxidant and gene protective effect.

"The French Paradox," which protects the French people who consume a high-fat diet from heart disease is conferred, at least in part, by increased intake of flavonoids from fresh vegetables, as well as red wine. Red wine contains a number of phytochemicals also called phenolics, including resveratrol and quercetin, both of which alter gene expression in such a way as to protect against blood clot formation and heart disease.

Key concepts derived from genetic research over the past several decades are the following:

- Your genes don't change. Their expression does.
- Specific characteristics may differ from individual to individual as a result of genetic polymorphism.
- Each individual is biochemically unique, but family history is important in identifying general inheritance patterns.
- Your diet, and the vitamins, minerals, phytonutrients, and accessory nutrients you consume modify gene expression.
- Your genotype, which is influenced by diet, lifestyle, and environment, results in your phenotype.
- Not all genetic characteristics can be changed. Some cannot be modified by diet and lifestyle.
- Genetic characteristics are not "all or nothing."

Resisting the Aging Process

Most of us believe age is genetically predetermined. We admire vigorous 80-year olds and shake our heads over 50-year olds who look old and tired. Recent specific breakthroughs indicate that there are actually steps we can take to shape our own aging process. James Fries, M.D., a professor of preventive medicine at Stanford University Medical School, pointed out that as we age the heart and lungs ability to transport oxygen diminishes. The kidneys become less able to filter poisons from the blood. Strength declines. Short term memory is compromised. Eyesight, hearing, and skin elasticity grow poorer. However, those characteristics that we associate with aging can be modified by nutritional, lifestyle, and environmental factors. Irving Rosenberg, M.D. and William Evans Ph.D., are professors of medicine at Tufts University, in the Human Nutrition Center in Boston. They state, "You can adopt a pattern of activity and eating that maximizes your ability to age more slowly." At the turn of the century, only 4 percent of the U.S. population was over 65. Today that number is 13 percent. Life expectancy at birth has climbed from 47 years in 1900 to more than 76 years today. Gerontologists indicate it is likely to reach 83 years by the year 2030.

More and more research over the past decade has indicated that we believe a number of myths concerning aging, with the most powerful myth being that we can do nothing about it. Genetic nutritioneering and the concepts presented here can not only increase your life expectancy, but also your functional ability throughout life.

Some people believe that the secret to aging slowly is to protect against the loss of hormones that are associated with youth- testosterone in men and estrogen in women. Other hormones are DHEA (dehydroandrosterone), melatonin, pregnenolone, insulin-like growth factor (IGF), and human growth hormone (human chorionic gonadotropin). The assumption is that because younger people have higher levels of these hormones and older people have lower levels, providing these hormones in supplemental doses to older people will keep them young. The following three hormones definitely show decreasing levels throughout the aging process:

- Sex hormones (estrogen in women and testosterone in men).
- DHEA.
- Growth hormone and insulin-like growth factor (IGF)

The history of free-radical aging was first advanced by Denham Harman, M.D., Ph.D.at the University of California at Berkeley in 1956. He indicated that free radicals cause the damage we see in the aging of cellular proteins, genetic materials, and cell membranes. He pointed out that animals possess antioxidant systems to help defend against free radical damage. Antioxidants occur in the diet as essential nutrients. They include vitamin E, vitamin C, and beta-carotene (vitamin A). Animals with low antioxidant protection experienced increased damage by free radicals and had accelerated biological aging.

Enzymes work with antioxidant nutrients to defend against fee radical damage. These enzymes include superoxide dismutase (SOD), glutathione peroxidise and catalase, each of which is manufactured in cells from a message taken from the genes.. A diet rich in antioxidants including vitamn E and C, carotenoids and flavonoids, plus trace minerals like zinc, manganese, and copper, can defend against free radical induced oxidative stress.

After several years, free radical-induced organ damage can result in the appearance of "twisted molecules." These unnatural molecules can activate the body's immune system to combat foreign invaders, resulting in damage to organs like the thyroid from autoimmunity. Excessive skin wrinkling is related to accelerated free radical production. Medical studies have shown that skin wrinkling occurs many times faster in smokers. The same phenomenon occurs with sun-induced damage to the skin. Free radicals create damage to collagen and elastin, the proteins that hold skin together.

Beyond Cholesterol

Cholesterol has gotten a bad reputation because of its presumed role in heart disease. We seem to have forgotten that cholesterol is a valuable substance. It helps cells maintain their structure and function. It is also the material from which sex hormones are produced in the ovaries, testes, and adrenal glands. Medical investigators in the U.S. Department of Agriculture Human Nutrition Center on Aging recently reported that cholesterol plays an important role in protecting against aging of the brain and heart by serving as an antioxidant, retarding the effects of oxidative stress. Proper cholesterol control can result in good health, whereas too little or too much can increase the risk of disease.

In older people, oxidative stress and free radical aging present a greater concern, higher blood cholesterol levels may have a protective effect against brain and heart aging. Recent studies from Leiden University Medical Center in the Netherlands indicate that in people older than 85 years, high blood cholesterol levels are associated with longevity and good health, owing to a lower mortality from both cancer and infectious diseases. According to a medical report from these studies the presumed protective effect of elevated blood cholesterol in the elderly indicates that we should reevaluate the use of cholesterol-lowering therapy after a certain age. Lowering cholesterol may actually be increasing rather than decreasing the risk of disease. The authors wrote, "Our study shows that a high serum blood cholesterol concentration is not a risk factor for cardiovascular disease in people over 85 years and over. On the contrary, it is associated with longevity.

On the evidence of our data, cholesterol-lowering therapy in the elderly is questionable."

Dr. Earl Bendit, a pathologist at the Washington University School of Medicine, believes that the initial stages of heart disease may be caused by exposure of the arteries to mutagenic substances that alter gene function. We might consider atheroma to be a wart on the inside of the artery, a benign tumor that becomes inflamed, irritated, and later infiltrated with cholesterol and calcium to cause heart and artery diseases. In addition to inflammation, elevations in C-reactive protein, and serum amyloid A protein, elevated LDL cholesterol in the blood and oxidant stress factors, scientists have identified another heart disease factor. Nearly 30 years ago, Kilmer Mccully, M.D. suggested that an amino acid called homocysteine, which is found in the blood of some individuals, triggers heart disease. Dr.McCully recounts his discovery of the role of homocysteine in his book, "The Homocysteine Revolution."

Elevated levels of homocysteine in the blood are now universally accepted as a strong predictor of death from heart disease. Since standard medical exams did not measure homocysteine blood levels, elevated blood levels of homocysteine have been a "silent killer" for yeas. Many other investigators have confirmed the observation that elevated blood homocysteine is a marker for a number of genetically determined risk factors for accelerated biological aging and an important determinant of risk for heart disease and dementia. Fortunately, Dr. McCully found that elevated homocysteine levels could be reduced by increasing the intake of folic acid, B-12, B-6 and the B complex substance betaine which communicated with the genes in such a way as to reduce homocysteine levels to zero.

It is worth noting that even Victor Herbert, M.D., J.D., an outspoken critic of vitamin supplements, recently urged his medical colleagues to petition the FDA to increase levels of B-12 and folate in the RDA to protect against homocysteine disease. This advocacy for nutrient supplementation is a remarkable change in position for Dr. Herbert. He acknowledges the safety of these nutrients when given at increased levels.

We are once again reminded that our bodies work not as a collection of individual organs but as a collection of organ systems operating synergistically. The concept of genetic nutritioneering requires that we consider the web-like patterns in which interacting organ systems give rise to the function of the individual.

Increasing evidence indicates that diet plays a major role in the development of cancer. More than 30 years ago, Carlton Fredericks Ph.D. discussed the important role of B vitamins and antioxidants like vitamin E in reducing the risk of hormone-related cancers and cancers of the breast and endometrium. Dr. Fredericks' observations now appear prescient given the advancing understanding of cancer genes and how the expression can be modified through improved nutrition.

Pharmaceutical companies are racing ahead in their research on new drugs to combat cancer. This research is trying to find natural, biologically based substances that alter gene expression in cancer cells, arrest their growth, and give the body's immune system an opportunity to kill them. It is important to understand that cancer is an unusual event. Our cells undergo hundreds of perfectly normal divisions throughout our lifetime. When the gene of a specific cell, at a moment in its cycle of divisions, undergoes change or alteration in expression, including cancer, it is an unlikely event. Even when it does develop, a cancer is a very weak cell. Its metabolism is not nearly as vital as that of as normal cell. A healthy immune system can take advantage of this weakness, selectively killing the cancer cell and leaving the body's normal cells intact. Diet and nutrition play an important role in supporting the defense against cancer and are fundamental tools in modifying genetic risk of cancer. A striking example of the relationship between dietary patterns and cancer incidence is that the incidence of prostate cancer in American men is 30 to 50 times higher than in Asian men who eat a traditional Asian diet.

In the healthcare of the future, patterns and health practitioners will work together to understand how the patient's genes can best be expressed into full function and healthy aging. Let your diet and lifestyle speak gently but firmly to your genes throughout your lifetime to promote optimal expression of healthy aging. Your genetic inheritance has given you this potential by making appropriate decisions about what to eat and how to live.

OVERDOSED AMERICA
JOHN ABRAMSON, M.D.

The Vigor Trial, published in the NEJM in the fall of 2000, raised the possibility that Vioxx increased the risk of heart attacks and other cardiovascular complications. The NEJM review article (August 2001) reported that Vioxx caused twice as many heart attacks, strokes, and cardiovascular deaths, and four times as many heart attacks as people who took Naproxen. The authors dismissed the results with the comment that the finding "may reflect the play of chance." The two authors of the review article had financial ties to the manufacturers of Celebrex and Vioxx, even though financial relationships between authors of review articles and drug companies were prohibited by the NEJM at the time the article was published. Drug companies spin their scientific evidence, and when necessary, keep the results of their studies secret. I was determined to find out the real story.

Synopsis

The FDA's internal analysis of the research data that the manufacturers of Celebrex and Vioxx had submitted to the FDA from the Class and Vigor studies was an eye-opener. I could not believe what I was seeing. The "Not-yet-spun" data revealed a very different picture of the safety of these two drugs than had been presented in the JAMA and NEJM articles. Physicians were encouraged to prescribe drugs that provide few benefits and possibly cause harm. Safety of the two drugs kept growing and my patients kept requesting and demanding that I prescribe there "better" new drugs for their aches and pains.

Pharmacia (Celebrex's manufacturer) has continued to engage in false and misleading promotion of Celebrex. The JAMA article was biased in the manufacturer's favor. It was incomplete, and presented an inaccurate picture of the so-called safety advantage over other less expensive (NSAIDS).The NEJM review article didn't even mention the warning label issued to Pharmacia.

People in the Vigor Study who took Vioxx were 24 times more likely than those who took Naproxen to experience a serious cardiovascular complication. The Vigor Study showed that for every 100 people with cardiovascular disease treated with Vioxx there were between 7 and 11 additional serious cardiovascular complications each year (on the FDA website). The most important finding in the NEJM article (which was not even mentioned), was that overall, including GI, cardiovascular, and all other serious complications, the people who took Vioxx had 21 % more "serious adverse events" that usually lead to hospitalization or death than the people who took Naproxen. There is something wrong with a system that leads people to demand that their doctors prescribe a drug that causes more serious side effects.

Vioxx costs $100 to $134 a month vs $18.9 for Naproxen or $7.50 for OTC Naproxen. One month after the NEJM article that dismissed the increased CVD risk as a "play of chance," and failed to mention the significantly increased risk of serious complications in people who took Vioxx, the FDA sent a warning letter to Merck, citing it for "marketing that was false, lacking in fair balance, and otherwise misleading."

Can we Trust our Most Respected Medical Journals?

Unlike the article about statins and strokes that I investigated, this went beyond spin. The frightening part of this story is that all this information is publicly available. Why hasn't the FDA spoken up more publicly about the misleading journal articles? Dr. Janet Woodstock, director of the FDA"s Center for Drug Education and Research, explained that the FDA" could not constrain communications" in a scientific journal. "This was a first amendment right of commercial speech issue."

By the end of 2001, 57% of all the money spent on arthritis prescriptions was spent on Vioxx and Celebrex. They were among the top ten selling drugs in the United States. My research into statins and now Celebrex and Vioxx showed that what our most trustworthy sources of the best medicine was often quite the opposite—and that commercial distortion of medical knowledge had become a major impediment to good medical care.

The United States healthcare system is expensive, yet it doesn't produce better results. "Marketing a disease is the best way to market a drug (Dr. Love). Drug companies place ads in medical journals showing wheel chairs, x-rays of crooked spines, and they fund lectures about osteoporosis . They turn a "normal spectrum of skeletal aging into a feared disease." The National Osteoporosis Foundation was started with drug company money in 1996. Doctors (including me) feared that hip-bones would suddenly snap, with minimal trauma. In more than 20 years as a family doctor I never saw such a thing.

Hormone Replacement Therapy

A New England Journal of Medicine article cites the Framingham Study-women on Estrogen were 50 % more likely to develop heart disease. By 1992, Premarin sales topped its 1975 peak. One out of five postmenopausal women in the U.S. were taking hormones. HRT is recommended by the American College of Obstetrics and Gynecology and the American College of Physicians. They state that all women should consider preventive hormone therapy. The truth about HRT came out slowly and was difficult for most doctors to accept. JAMA in the year 2000- an 8% increase in the risk for breast cancer. By 20012 Premarin was still the most frequently prescribed drug in the U.S. July 2002- The American College of Physicians and the American College of Obstetrics and Gynecology had made a big mistake. 16,000 women in the Women's Health Initiative was to run through 2005, but women received letters telling them to stop taking the study medication because the risk of breast cancer, heart attack, stroke, and blood clots was found to be greater than the benefit. There was a 15% increase in adverse events.

The final nail in the coffin was the million woman study in the Lancet (3 months later). Women taking hormones had a 68% higher chance of getting breast cancer. 30% of those taking Estrogen, 100% for those taking Progestin and Estrogen, than the women who were not taking hormones. 20 million American women have taken hormone replacement therapy. They unwittingly exposed themselves to breast cancer, heart attacks, stroke, Alzheimer's disease, and blood clots. 100,000 cases of breast cancer developed. The fundamental lesson to be learned from the HRT debacle is that therapeutic decisions must be based on solid and unbiased scientific evidence. The trend is going in the opposite direction. My ideals and personal goals now call on me to investigate, full time, just how the mission of American medicine was being undermined-and how we might begin to fix it.

In 1991, drug companies spent $55 million on advertising. Over the next 11 years spending increased 50 fold to $3 billion in 2005. By 2002, one out of five medical students chose primary care as their first choice (21.5%) Only 3 out of a 1000 thought good students were being encouraged to go into primary care. It takes commitment and idealism to choose a career that is not supported by role models in training, and it pays far less than other specialties, making it difficult to pay the $100,000 debt they usually incur.

The threat of malpractice litigation is also increasing the cost of American healthcare. 3/5 of doctors in the U.S. admit they do more diagnostic testing than is necessary. And why not! Those extra tests often set off a cascade effect requiring even more tests to follow abnormal results, many of which turn out to be normal.

The FDA has fallen under the influence of the drug and medical device industries. The FDA is understaffed, underfunded, and under pressure. The Los Angeles Times reported that approved drugs caused more than 1,000 deaths (although the number of deaths could actually be much higher, because reporting of adverse events to the FDA is voluntary). All told 22 million Americans, 1 out of 10 adults, had taken a drug that was later withdrawn from the market. (1997 and 2000)

The Rezulin Story

In June 1996, Rezulin was selected as one of the two drugs in a diabetes study. Dr. John L. Gueriguian, a 19-year veteran at the FDA, in his review, recommended Rezulin not be approved. It offered no advantage over other drugs on the market. It also caused inflammation of the liver. Warner-Lambert complained to the FDA higher-ups and Dr. Gueriugian was then removed from the approval process for this drug.

The advisory committee met to decide on the approval of Rezulin. They were not informed of Dr. Gueriguian's concerns about liver toxicity. The FDA approved Rezulin on February 1997 and it became a "blockbuster" drug. Reports of liver toxicity began to appear. Despite deaths in the U.S. and Japan and the withdrawal of the drug because of liver toxicity on December, 1997, Dr. Eastman and his colleagues continued to treat volunteers in the Diabetes Prevention Program Study with Rezulin.

Audrey LaRue Jones, a 55-year old high school teacher died of liver failure in May, 1998. Rezulin was no longer given to volunteers in the study. Warner-lambert maintained that Rezulin was not responsible for the liver failure that led to her death. Despite mounting reports of liver problems in the U.S., Rezulin was not withdrawn from the market until March, 2000. $1.8 billion dollars of the drug had been sold. The Los Angeles Times reported that Rezulin was suspected in 391 deaths and 400 cases of liver failure. Looking back on his experience, Dr. Gueriguian told the L.A. Times "either you play games or you're going to be put off limits—a pariah."

Dr. Eastman received at least $200,000 in consulting and related fees, and the L.A. Times reported that no fewer than 12 of the 22 researchers who were overseeing the $150 million dollar government-sponsored diabetes study as "principal investigators" were receiving fees or research grants from Warner-Lambert.

Health care costs are rising with no improvements in our health. The American health care system is getting closer to the breaking point. Medical research has become big business. Billions of dollars are involved. The search for scientific truth is unpredictable. From a business point of view, there is too much at stake to leave this process to the uncertainties of science. The role of the drug and medical-device companies are no longer the things they make. Now their most important product is "scientific evidence." This is what drives sales. The standards of good science has been radically weakened, and in some cases abandoned. Here's how it works.

As government funding declined, the medical industry was more willing to step in and lend a hand. Universities had no choice but to accept commercial funding. By 1991, 4 out of 5 commercially sponsored clinical drug studies were being conducted by universities and academic medical centers. Medical research companies emerged in response to commercial funding opportunities. By 200, only one-third of clinical trials were being done in universities and academic medical centers. The rest were being done by for-profit research companies that were being paid directly by the drug companies.

The drug companies now killed two birds with one stone. They could now call the shots on most of the studies that were evaluating their own products without having to accept input from academics who were grounded in traditional standards of medical science.

In 1999, Dr. Drummond Rennie, Deputy Editor of JAMA characterized the response of academic institutions to the changing climate. "They are seduced by industry funding, and frightened that if they don't go along with these gag orders, the money will go to less rigorous institutions. It's a race to the ethical bottom."

There is nothing illegal or unethical about these commercial arrangements. Certainly, commercially sponsored research has produced important findings. However, research is manipulated, misrepresented, or withheld, with the goal of maximizing sales.

The drug companies pour billions of dollars each year into medical research, and they need to have a few successes in order to stay in business. In a JAMA editorial, Drs. Bruce Psaty and Drummond Rennie said, "medical research, even if it is conducted by the pharmaceutical industry, is not solely a commercial enterprise destined to maximize personal gain or company profits. The responsible conduct of medical research involves a social duty and moral responsibility that transcends quarterly business plans or the changing of chief executive officers."

From the moment doctors enter medical school to the moment they retire, drug companies and medical-device manufacturers attempt to influence their medical decisions. Company salesmen schmooze and muscle their way into doctors' offices, leaving behind a trail of freebies emblazoned with their products' names. Doctors are invited to conferences in tropical paradises. Some companies lure doctors into becoming paid consultants, or lecturers to hawk their companies' products to their peers

Dr. Richard Smith, editor of the British medical journal said, "The major journals try to counterbalance the might of the pharmaceutical industry, but it is an unequal battle, not least because journals themselves profit from publishing studies funded by the industry."

I've turned down more offer than I can count for "educational" dinners, sporting events, golf and ski outings, and even weekends in the best hotels, plus $500. And, I must confess to have given in to temptation on several occasions.

The quid-pro-quo, of course, comes from subtle pressure to prescribe the company's product to the threat of withdrawing future funding for research, and, of course, to being cut off from future freebies. The number of reps making sales pitches in doctors' offices has tripled over the past ten years. In 2001, drug companies spent $4.7 billion "detailing" to the 400,000 office-based doctors in the United States, or about $10,000 for each doctor per year, and that doesn't include the cost of drug samples the reps left.

Statin Drugs

In 2001, the expert panel on detection, evaluation, and treatment of high blood cholesterol in adults issued perhaps the most influential document in the history of modern American medicine. It increased the number of Americans taking statin drugs from taking 13 million to 36 million.

Dr. Claude Lenfant, the Director of the National Heart, Lung and blood institute (NHLBI), under whose auspices the NCEP does its work, told the New York Times that if the new guidelines were followed, coronary heart disease, "would no longer be the number one killer in the United States.

The lead author of the guidelines, Dr. Scott M. Grundy, said, "these statins are amazing drugs--- when you say you can't put that many people on drugs, you've got to balance that against the tremendous devastation of coronary heart disease." Largely as a result of these guidelines, cholesterol control has become the main focus of preventive health care in the United States.

The Framingham Heart Study, starting in 1948, enrolled 5,000 residents of Framingham, Massachusetts, with the goal of identifying the factors that contribute to coronary heart disease. In 1957, the study reported that high cholesterol levels increased the risk of heart disease.

CHD results from the occlusion of one or more arteries, reducing the flow of blood to the heart muscle. The build up of plaque on the inside of the artery walls is a slow process. Then, like a garden hose that is being stepped on, when a coronary artery is completely blocked by plaque, muscle cells die. This is known as a heart attack.

Most heart attacks are caused by a thrombus, or blood clot that can obstruct the flow of blood through the artery. Lowering total and LDL cholesterol, with medication, the theory goes, lowers the risk of CHD. From the 1960s to the 1980s, fibrates were used to lower cholesterol, but after many years of use the World health organization (WHO) found Clofibrate (brand name Atromid-s) increased the overall risk of death by 47 percent (about half the excess deaths were due to cancer). A study by the National Public Health Institute at the University of Helsinki, Finland showed that the death rate among people taking another fibrate, Gemfibtozil (brand name Lopid) for 8.5 years was 21 percent higher than for people taking a placebo. Enter statins in 1987. The first statin, Mevacor, is now available as a generic called Lovastatin, which costs less than half as much as the brand name statins. The best-selling statins in 2003, were Lipitor, Pravachol, and Zocor. Crestor was approved by the FDA in August, 2003.

Cholesterol is the most common organic molecule in the brain (this may explain why statins have a negative effect on cognitive function). It is also an essential building block of the body's most important hormones, such as stress hormones, blood sugar regulating hormones. And sex hormones. Cholesterol is an integral component of nerve cells. The cholesterol-lowering frenzy has ignored the essential role that cholesterol plays in many of the body's biological functions.

In 1993, an article in the Archives of Internal Medicine analysed data from the Framingham Study that showed higher total cholesterol in people over 60. An alarming finding from this study is that the risk of death from causes other than CHD increases significantly with lower total cholesterol levels for men and women after they reach age 50. 4 of the 5 experts writing the guidelines, including the chair of the panel, had relationships with all three manufacturers of the best-selling statins. If the guidelines are followed, sales of statins will increase by $20 billion to $30 billion per year.

AFCAPS/TEXCAPS_ 100 people in this study would have to be treated with a statin drug for 25 years to prevent one death from cardiovascular disease.

WOSCOPS- 100 men in the study had to take Pravachol for two full years in order to prevent a single heart attack. The cost- $336,000 for the drugs alone. The bottom line- the case for prescribing statins for men with moderately elevated cholesterol is not compelling. JAMA-1995- "There is no evidence from primary prevention trials that cholesterol lowering affects total mortality in healthy women." It is hard to justify putting millions healthy women on statins.

Framingham warned, "Physicians should be cautious about initiating cholesterol-lowering treatment in men and women above 65 to 79 years of age." There is not even an increase in the risk of heart attack associated with higher cholesterol levels once the age of 65 is reached.

The CARE and LIPID studies showed that statins lower the risk of recurrent CHD in women with CHD, but do not appear to lower their overall mortality.

The ALLHAT Study-10,000 patients at risk for CHD. Equal numbers of men and women age 55 and older. 90% of men and 75% of women qualified for statin therapy under the new 2001 guidelines. The study found that tripling the number of people on statins neither prevented heart disease nor decreased the overall risk of death. These findings were major news, but there was a virtual press blackout. Only the Wall Street Journal carried the story.

The 2001 cholesterol guidelines were reassuring about statins not causing cancer. However, JAMA-1996- "Carcinogenicity of lipid-lowering drugs: "pointed out that statins caused cancer in laboratory animals. The authors (Newman and Hulley) state, that the risk of cancer caused by statins could take many years. Most studies are too short.

The medical industry has convinced most Americans that the answer to almost every health problem can be found in a brand-name pill or high-priced medical procedure. The challenge in determining optimal medical care is to identify the boundary between effective care that truly improves health and commercially driven care that can be harmful.

The drug companies have no more responsibility to oversee the public's health than the fast-food industry has to oversee the public's diet. Controlling medical costs in this near free-for-all commercial grab is a contradiction in terms. Does it make sense to talk about reducing national expenditures for cars, clothes, or beer? Medical care, by far the largest consumer commodity in the United States, is no different.

"Quality of care" is now defined largely in ways that best serve the financial interests of the drug and other medical industries, rather than the health needs of the American people. Drug companies earn higher profits when more people use expensive drugs, not when more people achieve better health.

As individuals we have the opportunity to reclaim responsibility for much of our health through intelligent lifestyle decisions and informed use of medical care. Courageous leadership is urgently needed to redirect American health care. I chose to leave my practice to write this book, and I hope that I have helped to improve the health of more people than I might have otherwise. I also hope that I will have inspired some to become more critical consumers of scientific evidence. I will have succeeded in my task if I have motivated some readers to be more regular about exercise, adopt a healthier diet, and stop smoking. My greatest hope is that this book will inspire readers to consider the responsibility of citizenship- in this time of excessive medical profiteering and corporate influence.

We have come to a critical juncture, and our future depends on our willingness to act on our country's highest ideals. In this sense, the health we seek for ourselves, for our families, and for all Americans is a metaphor for something greater even than physical well-being- that extends beyond the narrow confines of the biomedical-commercial paradigm of medicine.

DR. KATZ'S GUIDE TO PROSTATE HEALTH
AARON E. KATZ, M.D.

Prostate cancer is the second leading killer of men. 31,000 of the 220,000 men diagnosed with prostate cancer this year will die of the disease. Lung cancer is number one. 9 million men are living with prostate cancer and nearly 100 percent of them can survive if it is detected early.

Men of any age can develop prostate cancer. However, 8 out of 10 men who are diagnosed are 65 or older. Diagnostic techniques and testing have advanced in the last 15 years. Treatments are better than ever. There is still a lot of work to do so that men who are afflicted can live a long and healthy life.

Enlarged prostate, benign prostate hypertrophy (BPH), affects every man after age 50. It is not cancer, but it can be very annoying. I have written this book to help guide you to the effective use of nutritional therapies for prostate disease.

Synopsis

Most doctors treat prostate disease with drugs and surgery. They don't use herbs, diet, and lifestyle changes or supplements. Our research at Columbia has found that natural substances such as saw palmetto and pygeum can help. Older men with early stage prostate cancer, with a Gleason score of 6 or less and PSA values of 10 mg/ml, is to "watch and wait."

I don't use watchful waiting in my practice. I actively use targeted nutrition and herbal medicines. My practice uses holistic and allopathic treatments. They enjoy an excellent quality of life, maintain low PSA values, and have a renewed sense of hope- a new lease on life. My purpose in writing this book is to increase awareness in this area.

When I started my academic practice at Columbia University, I worked with Dr. Robert Atkins at his famous Atkins' Center in Manhattan. He advised patients to use herbs and nutrients. I thought, "This is a bunch of (mild expletive)" It's not going to work. In 1998, I convinced myself that integrative, natural therapies could hold an important place in urology. I opened the Center for Holistic Urology at Columbia University Medical Center. I had a feeling that my colleagues would receive it with great suspicion.

Today, I am one of the few urologists involved in clinical and laboratory studies of natural formulas. I am in a unique position to help you make a thoroughly informed decision on how best to support the health of your prostate. We can tell our patients about all of the treatment options, and we're honest about the risks and benefits of each option.

The Prostate

The prostate is a gland that wraps around the upper part of the urethra that carries the urine from the bladder out through the tip of the penis. It is the source of the semen that transports and nourishes the sperm on its journey towards attempted procreation. It is about the size of a walnut, and it is located below the bladder and in front of the rectum.

The prostate needs male hormones to function. Testosterone is made mainly by the testicles, and in small amounts by the adrenal glands. The prostate plays a key role in man's sexuality, providing 90% of his ejaculate, including semen that is required for fertilization of the ovum.

There are three ways in which the prostate can become diseased: 1. Benign enlargement 2. Chronic inflammation. 3. Cancer.

BPH (benign prostatic hypertrophy) is the abnormal non-cancerous growth of prostate cells. 90 percent of men between 70 and 90 have symptoms of BPH.

Prostatitis- is inflammation of the prostate gland.

Prostate cancer- is the most common type of cancer (excluding skin cancer)

Taking care of your prostate can extend your longevity, and can enhance your potency and virility.

It is important to work with your urologist to get an accurate diagnosis that will ensure the condition is only an enlarged prostate, and not prostate cancer. As the prostate gets larger, the gland presses inward against the urethra like a clamp on a garden hose. Prostate enlargement is as common a part of aging as gray hair. BPH may occur because estrogen within the gland promotes cell growth. The cause of BPH is not well understood. We don't know much about the risk factors for the disease.

The PSA Blood Test

The PSA measures the blood levels of a protein made in the cells of the prostate. Most urologists agree that a level between 4 and 10 is a strong indication that cancer is present. If cancer is suspected, the only way to definitely confirm the diagnosis is to perform a biopsy of the suspicious tissue.

There are two drugs that can shrink your prostate, Proscar and Avodart. They do so by inhibiting the enzyme that converts testosterone into DHT. These drugs actually shrink the gland. Unfortunately, they haven't earned rave reviews. Some doctors say they're a bust. The improvement in urinary flow is "not impressive." Sometimes we get decent results with a combination of Proscar and an alpha-blocker like Flomax.

The Prostate Cancer Prevention Trial results were published in the NEJM. 18,000 men took Proscar or a placebo for seven years. The trial was terminated early because Proscar had a 25% reduction in the evidence of prostate cancer. Unfortunately, the men who did develop prostate cancer had more aggressive cancers than the men taking a placebo. At this point in time, taking into account all of the data, I would personally not take the medication to prevent prostate cancer.

The FDA has approved four alpha-blockers (smooth muscle relaxants) Hytrin, Cardura, Flomax, and Uroxatral. All drugs in the alpha-blocker class have side effects of a drop in blood pressure, dizziness, possibly leading to fainting. Men who take an alpha-blocker should avoid driving for 12 hours after the first dose. Other adverse reactions to alpha-blockers may include weakness, headache, nasal congestion, heart palpitations, nausea, blurred vision, etc.

The transurethral resection of the prostate (TURP) is the gold standard urological procedure for men who need to have obstructing prostate tissue removed. Today the TURP is used for 90 percent of all BHP surgeries. A laser procedure was approved by the FDA in 2001. It appears to have the same success rate as the TURP in alleviating symptoms, with less bleeding and a shorter hospital stay. This is clearly an advance in technology and can be performed even on very large prostates. Surgery usually offers relief from BPH for at least 15 years. Although some of the signs of BPH and prostate cancer are the same, having BPH does not seem to increase the chances of getting prostate cancer. No causal relationship between the two has been found. Tissue removed during BPH surgery is routinely checked for hidden cancer cells. In 1 out of 10 cases, some cancer tissue is found, but often it is limited to a few cells of a nonaggressive type of cancer, and no treatment is needed.

I learned about the benefits of alternative therapies from the patients in the Atkins' Center. It takes a while for the supplements to "kick in" and i have yet to see any unpleasant side effects from the herbs I will discuss:

Saw palmetto- this plant extract is effective in improving the urinary flow and decreasing urine volume.

Pygeum Africanum- this substance is derived from the bark of an African evergreen tree. It is the drug of choice in France and other European countries.

Beta Sitosterol- this product relieves the symptoms in BPH. One study with 200 men given 200 mg. of Beta Sitosterol 3 times daily for six months increased urinary flow significantly. The placebo group had no improvement.

Vitamin B-6- produces picolinic acid which helps in the utilization of zinc. Both zinc and vitamin B-6 work together to rebalance the body's hormones and build testosterone.

Amino acids- Glycine, Alanine, and Glutamic acid have been found to improve BPH symptoms.

Pumpkin seeds- are widely used in Europe to heal prostate problems.

Essential fatty acids- (EFAs)- proper amounts of fatty acids and nutrition can help to reduce the size of the prostate by reducing inflammation.

Exercise- a higher level of physical activity appears to be protective against BPH. In some men, BPH can lead to prostatitis due to the retention of prostatic fluid, which can then become calcified and form stones or serve as a breeding ground for infection. We don't know what causes it. Some patients try a number of different drugs, but they may not work. In a study of men who abstained from sex, a prescription of twice daily masturbation provided moderate relief for 78 percent of the 18 subjects.

Prostate Cancer

Nearly 31,000 men die each year of prostate cancer in the United States. The median age at which a prostate cancer diagnosis is made is 72. However, due to widespread PSA screening I have treated men in their early 40s with early stage prostate cancer. Unfortunately, mortality from prostate cancer has not declined much in recent years. We are making headway, but we still have a lot of work to do on behalf of the men who are at risk.

There are risk factors that are strictly out of your control, such as age, race, and family history. If your father or brother has the disease the risk of developing prostate cancer is doubled. Your risk is greater if you are diagnosed while young (under 50). Over 80 percent of prostate cancer patients are over 65, and the risk spikes in men over 50. Prostate cancer incidence is highest in North America and Western Europe. Countries with diets higher in animal fat tend to have higher rates of prostate cancer.

Men with prostate cancer have histories of greater sexual activity and more venereal disease. Other risk factors include BPH and prostatitis , obesity, physical inactivity, pesticide exposure, and others. Cancer is not a single disease. It is a group of many diseases, but all of them have a few important things in common. Finding cures for cancer is an "excruciating" tough task. The best thing to do is to prevent it, and barring that, catch it early and get rid of it with the most advanced methods in our possession, and then do all we can through integrative medicine to try to prevent as recurrence.

Normal cells grow and divide, producing new, healthy cells as the body needs them. Old cells are destroyed to make way for the new. Sometimes, cells keep dividing despite the fact that no more new cells are needed, and the excess cells end up forming a mass called a tumor. Some tumors are benign, which means they are not cancerous, and will not spread. When a cancer has spread, it is named for the organ in which it began its formation. If prostate cancer has spread to the bones, we will identify these cells as prostate cancer cells, and it is called metastatic prostate cancer.

Early prostate cancer causes no symptoms. However, some men do experience symptoms. They may include:

- Frequent urination, especially at night.
- Difficulty starting urination.
- Inability to urinate.
- Weak flow of urine.
- Painful or burning during urination.
- Blood in urine or semen.
- Frequent pain in lower back, hips, or upper thighs.

PSA Testing

The PSA test has limited ability to distinguish cancer from benign prostate conditions. A Stanford University study that was published in the Journal of Urology concluded that the PSA exam causes many men who have slow-growing prostate cancers to have their prostates removed, even though they would most likely never have died from their cancer. According to the American Cancer Society, only 1 in 32 m2n who get prostate cancer ever die from the disease. Some radical experts believe that the PSA is not a useful test, because it leads to too many men having unnecessary, invasive treatments. There are a lot of false positives. When it comes to the PSA, it can be elevated in men with large prostates, but without cancer. A man with a high PSA doesn't always have cancer, and a man with a low PSA isn't always cancer free.

I'm in favor of PSA screening. Men aged 50 to 65 benefit most from screening, and those over 70 to 75 the least. If we find prostate cancer in a man over 80, it is not likely to grow large enough to cause his death.

Diagnosis

The following list of procedures are used to diagnose prostate cancer.

1. Blood tests
2. Digital rectal exam
3. Urinanalysis
4. Trans-rectal ultrasonography
5. Intravenous pyelogram
6. Cystoscopy
7. Biopsy

The number of prostate cures-thin conical samples of prostate tissue-has risen over the past few years. It is now almost the standard to take 12 biopsies, 6 on the right and 6 on the left. There is still a chance that the biopsy can miss an area of cancer.

Staging

Stage T1- The cancer isn't palpable by a rectal exam.
Stage T2- The tumor is felt in a rectal exam.
Stage T3- The cancer has spread to tissues near the prostate.
Stage T4- The cancer has metastasized to the rectum, the bladder neck, or levator and muscle(T4b).

Treatment

Radical Prostatectomy- preferred route if the patient is under 65 and otherwise healthy. It requires a hospital stay.

Laparoscopic and Robotic prostatectomy- makes the surgery safer, less bleeding, and it reduces incontinence and impotence afterwards. It shortens recovery time to a few days.

Cryotherapy/Cryoablation- targeted Cryoablation is a promising, minimally invasive therapy. It has a 89% to 92% success rate for localized cancer.

Cryosurgery- It is performed in the hospital. We freeze cancer cells to death, protecting the healthy tissues from damage.

Nerve-Sparing Radical Prostatectomy- There is a bundle on each side of the prostate. We remove the prostate without damage to the nerve bundles, necessary for erection.

Men with heart disease, especially those who use nitrate drugs, cannot use Viagra. A man who has had a complete prostatectomy, will no longer produce semen, and will have dry orgasms. Viagra, Cialis, and Levitra are designed to bring on a hard erection in response to stimulation.

Chemotherapy

Some cancers are treated with chemotherapy. The side effects are many. Patients may experience hair loss, vomiting, nausea, and diarrhea. Don't be alarmed if your doctor uses the term remission instead of cure. This does not mean that your cancer will definitely return; it means that it may. Chemotherapeutic measures will help maintain your health once you are in remission, but natural health measures support your healing and recovery.

If every man who was told to "watchfully wait" entered into a chemoprevention program we would see a major shift in their health in the ensuing years. It involves the use of nutritional supplements and herbs, but it also involves dietary changes.

Nutrition

America's diet kills because it makes you fat. Obesity has been found to dramatically increase your risk for prostate cancer. It clogs your arteries, thickens your blood, and exposes you to high levels of carcinogens. Cancer-causing chemicals are found in the meat because farmers use estrogenic drugs to fatten livestock. Plastic packaging can also migrate into the food that it contains. The typical American diet is heavy on fried food, sugar, and simple starches. "I'm a doctor, not a chef, I got most of my ideas from nutritionists."

Essential Fatty Acids

Omega-3 fats appear to protect the prostate. Omega-6 fats have been shown to have either no effect or a disease-promoting effect. The American diet is high in Omega-6, inflating the Omega-6 to Omega-3 ratio to almost 40 to 1. The best ratio should be 1 to 2 Omega-6 to 1 Omega-3. You can improve your ratio with the following diet:

- Eat more salmon, sardines, and codfish.
- Eat fruits and vegetables.
- Add flaxseed, walnuts, and pumpkin seeds to your diet.
- Avoid saturated fats (meat, dairy, and butter).
- Don't eat hydrogenated fats and use extra-virgin olive oil.
- Avoid processed flour and sugar.
- Eat fermented soy-based foods such as Tempeh and Miso.

You don't have to go totally vegetarian. Greens and crucifers are highly protective. Epidemiological studies show an inverse relationship between soy consumption and deaths from prostate cancer.

With this book, my aim is to advance natural healing methods like herbs, nutritional supplements, and acupuncture into the mainstream. It is my belief that these two kinds of medicine added together have much more to offer than either one alone.

Respect what your doctors have to say; they want the best for you and they know a lot. Share the information in this book with your doctor and discuss how it can help you return to wellness. If you are a man who has been through prostate cancer treatment, your job is to do all you can to ward off a recurrence.

Even if you don't have prostate disease, but want to live a long and healthy life, natural therapies strengthen the body's ability to maintain its own total balance. Herbs, supplements, a balanced diet, avoiding toxins, exercise, and stress reduction support not only prostate health, but also cardiovascular and nervous system health. They'll improve your energy, your brain power, and keep your digestive tract running more smoothly. Research suggests that the changes described in this book will aid in the prevention of more than one kind of cancer.

THE RISE OF TYRANNY
JONATHAN W. EMORD

Our federal government has become a bureaucratic oligarchy scarcely resembling the federal republic the founders created. George W. Bush gave the pharmaceutical industry an enormous degree of political control over the U.S. government. I did not appreciate how extensive big pharma influenced the FDA's decisions until I read John Abramson's eye-opening "Overdosed America and interviewed him on my radio program. Dr. John Abramson chronicled the drug industry's influence over medical school, education, physician's prescription practices, and big pharma's control of the FDA and Congress.

I now lay before the reader the terrible corruption and loss of principle that I have found along the way. I pray for the day when our country may once again become the best hope on earth. This book is an expose of industry's takeover of the government. I do not hold back the truth. I identify the steps to bring down the regulatory state and return the nation to its constitutional moorings, and to a constitution of law, not of men. My hope is that Americans will resurrect the constitution and remove from office those who use the instrumentalities of government to build fortunes and political fiefdoms at public expense. Our nation is too grand and majestic to suffer such a lowly fate.

Synopsis

There are now over 180 independent regulatory commissions and agencies. They have the power to create law through regulation without obtaining the consent of congress. Their budgets range from hundreds of millions to billions of dollars. They have the power to prosecute those whom they charge with violating their regulations.

Throughout history powers (legislative, executive, and judicial) in single hands has been defined as tyrannical and despotic. Our founding fathers fought a revolution, created a constitution that vests these powers in separate branches of government replete with checks and balances to disable encroachments of power. They warned about concentration of those powers because they believed it would spell the end of liberty and the rise of tyranny.

James Madison wrote, "No political truth is certainly of greater intrinsic value, or is stamped with the authority of more enlightened patrons of liberty than the principle of separation of powers." Jefferson wrote, "That the concentration of the three powers in the same hands is precisely the definition of despotic government."

We now live in a country where three-quarters of all laws are the product of unelected officials, oligarchs, appointed to rule administrative agencies and commissions, possessed of combined legislative executive, and judicial powers.

Agencies and commissions have virtually no check from the American people, the congress, the executive, or the courts. The federal agencies are all powerful, outlive presidents and members of congress, and are largely unaccountable for their actions. Those who run them are more powerful than the president, the congress, and the courts. They have absolute powers within the areas of their jurisdiction, not unlike English monarchs who ruled before the Magna Carta in (1215).

This book reminds us of our legacy of liberty. It reminds us of the founders' design, and of their warnings that if we allowed power to be concentrated in single hands we would soon see our liberties sacrificed in favor of tyranny.

This book calls for a return to the founders' constitution, and in defense of liberty. It calls on us to vote out of office those responsible for the delegation of power that is destroying our republic.

The founding fathers admired 18th century philosopher Montesquieu. They adopted his view that political liberty results from the separation of powers, and incorporated that principle into the constitution of the United States.

The constitution was meant to serve as a counterweight to the formation of a despotic government, just as the bill of rights was meant to provide a barrier against government exercise of power in ways that would transgress the people's liberties.

The Supreme Court has found no delegations of power from congress to the federal agencies unconstitutional since 1935, ignoring the founders' demand for separation of powers and non-delegation. Congress has delegated the power to make laws affecting every area of popular concern to independent regulatory agencies and commissions. The transfer of power is an abdication by Congress of the central constitutional duty to make laws. The politician's lust for permanent office and power has won out over constitutional sensibilities. In that way, Congress has avoided the need to account directly for unpopular actions, deflecting public outcry toward the agencies despite Congress's ultimate blame for having relinquished decision-making power to these agencies in the first place.

John Locke warned against delegation of legislative power, explaining that it would violate the social compact by which people consent to be governed. Franklin Delano Roosevelt instituted the first major experiment in delegation. The NIRA (the National Industrial Recovery Act) (193 3). It granted the NIRA the power to enforce price-fixing and production restrictions. The powers were so extensive that Benito Mussolini said, "Ecco un Ditatore." "Behold a dictator."

When Roosevelt commenced his campaign to transfer power, he was stymied by the Supreme Court, unwilling to countenance the broad delegation of power. The court said that "Congress is not permitted to abdicate or transfer to others the essential legislative functions with which it is vested." In his second term, Roosevelt nominated 5 pro new deal justices. Each was confirmed by the senate. The change became the death knell for the non-delegation doctrine.

Within the span of 74 years, 180 federal regulatory agencies and commissions have come into existence, with vast new powers to create laws. They regulate everything from the air we breathe when born to the drugs we last receive when we die. Today there is no matter of any economic or political import that is not regulated by a federal agency or commission. We have created the concentration of powers that our founders described as tyranny.

When an agency head is possessed of independent power, the threat of self-interest to the public must be acute. Today's bureaucratic lawmaker, prosecutor, and judge wields those plenary powers with virtually no sanction, after the fact, for the abusive exercise of discretion.

The pharmaceutical industry enjoys monopoly status through the FDA approval process and through long-lived patents. They enjoy 13.9

and 15.4 years of monopoly protection for their FDA approved drugs. The regulatory costs of new drug approval are astronomical (over $860 million in 2004 dollars per drug).

Monopoly protection from governments all over the world has allowed the pharmaceutical industry to amass great wealth (over $286 billion in U.S. prescription drug sales in 2007 alone). That has allowed them to invest part of that wealth in a sophisticated, comprehensive, and increasing program of influence peddling, affecting:

• Education in medical schools and among practitioners (through gifts to medical schools' faculty, teaching hospital staffs, and prominent scientists who write for medical journals, and through an army of 66,000 attractive sales representatives who shower physicians with free drug samples and gifts).

• Medical research and the content of medical journals, and advertising in those publications.

• Prescription decisions of practitioners.

• Regulations, policies, and decisions of the FDA commissioners.

• Actions of members of Congress and the president (through campaign contributions, gifts, and lavish junkets).

In the past decade the industry's lobbying expenditures exceeded $1 billion. There is no other industry in the history of the United States that has enjoyed more largesse in the form of federal dollars from the U.S. treasury than the pharmaceutical industry.

The passage of the Medicare Drug Improvement and Modernization Act (establishing Medicare part D) reveals just how far Congress will go to answer the call of the drug industry. It involves a massive transfer of wealth from the taxpayers directly to the pharmaceutical industry. The bill went into effect with President George Bush's full endorsement. The bill includes a remarkable provision that prohibits the federal government from negotiating reduced drug prices. Under Medicare part D taxpayers pay 58% more for drugs, on average, than the Veteran's Administration, according to a study by Families USA.

The drug price no-negotiation provision was secured at the behest of the drug industry and the President by a key point man, a former congressman Billy Tauzin. Tauzin steered the bill through the house. In appreciation for his efforts, Tauzin was named president and CEO of the Pharmaceutical Research and manufacturers of America, the drug industry's chief lobbying organization, with a salary of over $2.5 million a year.

The cost of Medicare part D is estimated to reach the staggering figure of $724 billion by 2015. The runaway healthcare crisis threatens to bankrupt America.

The prescription drug bill, a massive 1,000 pages in length arrived at legislators' offices in the morning before the 3 a.m. vote on it, leaving little time for members to read its contents, let alone debate it. Walter Jones (RNC) described the evening as "the ugliest night I have seen in 22 years in Congress." In all, at least 15 congressional staffers and federal officials left to go to work for the pharmaceutical industry, whose profits were increased by several billion dollars.

The FDA, DEA, and CMS have fulfilled the dire prediction of the founders, that the union of the three governing powers in single hands would beget tyranny. Each of these agencies is ruled by one all-powerful leader-a veritable dictatorship. The FDA commissioner can promulgate any rule, and can override any judgment of agency medical reviewers, and can approve for marketing, any drug, regardless of the scientific evidence that may exist against the drug's safety and efficacy.

The Congress of the United States has vested in one person the enormous power to regulate everything we consume and use for our sustenance and health-all food, drugs, cosmetics, biologics, medical devices, and dietary supplements. There is little real check on the exercise of the FDA commissioner's discretion, not from the courts, the Congress and the President. The same is true for the DEA administrator and the administrator of the Center for Medicare and Medicaid Services.

The FDA commissioner has repeatedly approved drugs that the agency's own medical reviewers have deemed too unsafe to enter the market, thus favouring the pharmaceutical company proponent of the drug over the American public. The results have been catastrophic, leading to tens of thousands of deaths and injuries.

On September 23, 2005, Lester A Crawford resigned as commissioner of the FDA. He had sworn that he did not own stock in companies that did business before the FDA. In point of fact he did. He resigned only 2 months after being confirmed as FDA commissioner. He copped a plea and avoided jail time. He was a key figure in defense of the pain killer Vioxx before its removal from the market for causing over 140,000 heart attacks, including 60,000 deaths. He was rewarded with a lucrative position with the Washington lobbying firm Policy Direction, Inc. a firm that represents drug firms, including Merck & co., maker of Vioxx.

FDA Approval of Unsafe Drugs

The FDA is a regulatory leviathan. It employs over 12,000 people and regulates products worth $1.5 trillion dollars in annual sales. This amounts to 10% of the American economy. The FDA is beholden to the drug industry. It approves drugs that are unsafe (even to the point of condoning death and serious injury). The FDA silences scientific criticism, eliminates evidence of dissent, and hides critical reviews of drugs from the public. These forms of corruption recur without substantive response from Congress or the President. The FDA commissioners have "literally gotten away with murder."

Redux

Dr. Leo Lutwak, the lead medical reviewer for the diet drug Redux, objected to the approval of the drug. He felt thast the drug had low effectiveness and very high risk for pulmonary hypertension. Despite Lutwak's findings, the FDA approved the drug. An estimated 1.8 million Americans consumed it. On September 15, 1997, the drug was withdrawn from the market. The drug was implicated in 123 deaths. American Home Products paid approximately $4.83 billion to settle 11,000 lawsuits involving the drug.

Rezulin

In 1997, the FDA approved Rezulin. Dr. John L. Gueriguian was removed from the review panel and his alarm about serious liver and heart toxicity was purged. The drug was given fast track approval on January 29, 1997, over staff objections. Lutwak, Gueriguian, and Mishin were all made subjects of a criminal investigation. Lutwak told CBS News"In my own agency I'm treated like----. I'm treated worse than a criminal. I'm accused, I'm threatened, I'm taken away from my work." Lutwak, Mishin, and Gueriguian all eventually resigned from the agency.

Rezulin was implicated in 391 deaths, including 63 from liver failure. The drug was removed from the market on march 22, 2000. Dr. William L. Isley, an endocrinologist who helped develop Rezulin for Warner-Lambert said, "the drug should never have gotten on the market-the whole thing is a travesty."

Avandia

Avandia appeared to increase the incidence of congestive heart failure in study participants. Mishin warned about the long-term effects on the heart. His recommendations were rejected by agency managers. On May 25, 1999 the FDA granted Glaxo Smithkline approval to market Avandia. On May 21, 2007 the NEJM published a meta-analysis which found that Avandia increased the risk of heart attacks by 43 Percent. In June 2007, 8 years after approving Avandia, a black box warning is included on Avandia labels. The FDA's Dr. David J. Graham recommended that Avandia be removed from the market. The committee voted 20 to 3 that Avandia increases cardiac ischemic risk in type 2 diabetics, but nevertheless voted in favour of keeping the drug on the market.

Vioxx was approved on May 29, 1999 with labelling to warn physicians that the drug would increase heart attack risk. A study by Merck was submitted to the FDA. It revealed a seven-fold increase in the risk of heart attack from low-dose Vioxx. Another study by Merck showed a five-fold risk of heart attack. The FDA took no action based on the information.

In 2004, Dr. Graham presented to his FDA superiors a huge epidemiologic study he had performed with Kaiser-Permanente in California. The study revealed that high-dose Vioxx significantly increased the risk of heart attacks and sudden death. Senior FDA officials ordered Graham to change his conclusions and recommendations and threatened that if he did not, he would not be permitted to present his findings at a conference in Bordeaux, France. In their E-mails the FDA said, "it was not contemplating a warning against the use of high-dose Vioxx and Dr. Graham's conclusions should be changed.

In mid-August 2004, despite the evidence of high risks of heart disease, the FDA announced that it approved the drug for use in children with rheumatoid arthritis. The FDA medical reviewers were incredulous. How could the FDA approve Vioxx for use in children in the presence of evidence that the product increased the risk of heart attacks in adults?

On the eve of Graham's senate testimony, Commissioner Crawford offered him a policy position in the commissioner's office (with a higher pay grade). He would leave drug safety and be director of a new center for product safety. It has been estimated by Graham that 88,000 to 139,000 Americans had heart attacks and strokes that were due to Vioxx.

The list below is just a small sample of the drugs that the FDA has approved over the safety objections of its own medical reviewers. Others that have been withdrawn from the market after the FDA approved them as safe and effective are:

Trovan- is an antibiotic that caused acute liver failure and death.
Omniflox- is an antibiotic that caused hemolytic anemia.
Lotronex- is a treatment for IBS that caused ischemic colitis.
Baycol- is a cholesterol-lowering drug that caused severe muscle injury, kidney failure, and death.
Bextra- is an NSAID for arthritis that caused painful menstruation, heart attacks, strokes and death.

Dr. David Graham testified before the Senate finance Committee that other drugs still on the market were unsafe including Acutane and Arana (for rheumatoid arthritis) that cause "an unacceptably high risk of liver failure and death, and Crestor (a cholesterol-lowering drug that causes myopathy and rhabdomyolysis). There are many others. The FDA has betrayed the public trust and violated the constitution, they have sworn an oath to uphold. They have created a tyrannical bureaucratic oligarchy that sacrifices the lives and property of the many to support the riches of a few.

In 1999, the FDA took the position that only a drug could be accompanied with claims of disease treatment. Following the Supreme Court's denial of plaintiff's petition for a writ of certiorari, the FDA had a legal predicate for unravelling the health claim regime. The FDA now had a precedent that would help censor truthful information concerning nutrient-disease relationships.

In May, 2003 the agency received a health claim petition concerning the benefits of Glucosamine and Chondroitin Sulfate. The evidence supporting the claims was successful. The FDA management formed an expert advisory panel to review the science. 11 of the 17 experts had conflicts of interest. They had direct and indirect financial ties to the NDAID industry, answering the call of the drug industry for a monopoly on therapeutic claims. The FDA has led consumers to regard drugs as their only therapeutic options. The FDA operates outside the constitution. They are unanswerable to the Courts, the Congress, and the American people. They are possessed of so much power that they are never made to account for constitutional law violations or for the many lives they choose to sacrifice.

The Way Back to Liberty

The following reforms must be constituted. WE MUST:

- Vote the corrupt members of congress out of office.
- Prevent congressional relinquishment of of law-making power.
- Prevent industry capture.
- Require meaningful federal judicial review.
- Punish officials who violate the constitution, agency rules, or commission-enabling statutes for personal gain.
- Protect the public from unsafe drugs.
- Eliminate FDA jurisdiction over health claims and establish new anti-fraud protections.
- Mandate due process to Medicare part B reimbursement cases.

We are at a critical point in our history. Government corruption is pervasive. The founders made preservation of liberty a solemn trust to be passed from generation to generation. Our nation has been brought low by actions that sacrifice the lives, liberties, and property of the many to benefit the few in power. It will take a vigilant public willing to throw out the rascals in Washington and out in place patriotic souls who will do what is necessary to restore the republic.

THE FOUNTAIN
JACK CHALLEM

This book contains the work of 25 experts who offer their recipe for a long and healthy life. Ponce de Leon, the Spanish explorer discovered Florida while searching for the mysterious fountain of youth. In 1866, F.C. Havens published the "possibility of living 200 years." He summarized the advice of other authors and experts.

Sixty years later, Denham Harman developed the Free Radical Theory of Aging which holds that excessive oxidation leads to disease and aging. That is why we take antioxidants such as vitamins C and E.

In The Lost Horizon by James Hilton, The Hunza Valley in northern Pakistan people were supposed to live exceptionally long and healthy lives. The truth is that Hunza Valley residents did not enjoy long lives. Malnutrition was common, so was disease. So much for an earthly paradise.

The Fountain's contributors base their recommendations on solid science and their own personal experience. Most are physicians, researchers, and health experts. We asked our contributors to write from their hearts. Some emphasize natural foods, others recommend nutritional supplements. They tell us what worked for them. You can choose the ideas that appeal to you. We hope this book leads you to your own fountain of youth. Unfortunately, we can't cover all 25 experts because of space requirements.

Synopsis

Robert Abel Jr., M.D.

My mother chided doctors for their ignorance about nutrition. Carlton Fredericks and Adele Davis pioneered the use of nutrition as a basis for wellness. When I took biochemistry in medical school, I learned that essential nutrients prevented scurvy, beriberi, and pellagra. I realized that operating cataracts was treating a symptom and not treating a cause

As an ophthalmologist I have found that the eye is not only the window of the soul, but also the window of the body. Supporting eye health is akin to supporting total body health.

I use the acronym NEWBARS for healthy eyes. It stands for nutrition, exercise, water, breathing, alternative options, relaxation, and socialization.

NUTRITION-the healthy choices include vegetables, fish, grapes, seeds, berries, and some red wine. Reduce the five white thieves- white rice, white flour, white sugar, lard, and salt.

EXERCISE- Use it or lose it. This includes walking, jogging, running, biking, and yoga.

WATER- Drink 6 glasses a day.

BREATHING- It is called inspiration for no reason!

ALTERNATIVE OPTIONS-Use arm massage for carpal tunnel syndrome, neck massage for headaches, magnesium for restless leg syndrome, and saw palmetto for urinary frequency.

RELAXATION /SOCIALIZATION- Be sure to enjoy nature, walking, yoga, and the company of others.

MY DAY

I get up at 5 A.M. I have a small cup of coffee, a bowl of whole-grain cereal with nuts, berries, and pomegranate juice. I eat little dairy, drink two glasses of water, and take 1,000 mg. of vitamin C, 1,000 mg. of MSM, 1,000 of quercetin, and 50 mg. of B-complex vitamins.

After a shower and stretching and Qi Gong I have a second breakfast—usually eggs, multivitamins, 400 iu vitamin E, 500 acetyl-l-carnitine, 500 DHA and 6 mg. of lutein.

At lunchtime, I have a salad, a large portion of leafy green vegetables. Dinner consists of a sweet potato, a green vegetable, and fish or organic beef. I take 1 or 2 grams of vitamin C with many glasses of water.

Night time is devoted to calling patients, writing, and getting to bed by 10 P.M. I take 500 mg. of magnesium to relax the muscles and the mind.

Lyla Cass, M.D.

Death is inevitable. Our goal should be to have a joyous, fulfilling, and healthy life. There are no magic pills. Death can happen at any time. Don't take anything for granted. Here is a checklist which is useful.

1. A positive attitude
2. Good relationships
3. A healthy lifestyle

Don't indulge in alcohol, drugs, or overeating. Have regular meals of fresh organic food. This includes lots of fruits and vegetables and a moderate amount of protein- fish, chicken, and lean meat. Use high potency multivitamins and multi-mineral combinations. They should include B-complex vitamins, vitamin C, D, and E, calcium, magnesium, potassium, zinc, chromium, and manganese, plus boron, vanadium, and molybdenum. Essential fatty acids, fish oil and flaxseed oil are important for brain health, hormone function and smooth skin.

Get enough sleep. Take fewer prescription drugs. Exercise aids circulation, boosts oxygenation, helps us maintain our weight and other benefits. Drink 8 glasses of water to allow for proper hydration.

In conclusion, for mental and spiritual health combine prayer and meditation. Nutrition and supplements, exercise, water, and sleep will provide a buffer against aging.

Jack Challem

Healthy eating and supplements are synergistic. As we age we have to work harder to stay in good health. Quality protein-fish, chicken, turkey, eggs, and lean meats, vegetables and fruits are the core of a good diet. Eat salads, broccoli, cauliflower, raspberries, blueberries, cherries, kiwis, and others.

Limit starchy grains including breads, cereals, bagels, muffins, pastas, and most sugary energy bars. Although many people tout the benefits of whole grains, they are nutritionally weak compared to vegetables.

Water is important. Other healthy beverages include sparkling mineral water, green and black tea, herbal teas, organic coffee, green drinks, and coconut water.

Vincent C. Giampapa, M.D., FACS

We are the first generation of human beings to directly take charge of how we age, and to be personally responsible for their ongoing health and longevity. Sampling your DNA and utilizing this information to create a personalized anti-aging program. Over the coming decades stem cell therapies, nanotechnology, and new drug delivery systems will add another dimension of health and longevity to our lives.

There are 5 processes that are essential to optimize cellular health and are directly related to aging.

- Glycation-cross-linking of proteins.
- Inflammation- molecules released as a result of free radical damage.
- Methylation-genetic activity that turns genes on and off in the correct order.
- Oxylation-The amount of free radical damage.
- DNA Repair- the efficiency of repairing damage to DNA from free radical attacks

Caloric restriction offers a number of amazing effects, all documented in the scientific literature. These include:

- A reduction in free radical production.
- A de crease in DNA damage.
- A decrease in the loss of our stem cells.
- A decrease in insulin production.

Metformin is a prescription medication for diabetes that not only lowers blood sugar by improving insulin receptor sensitivity, but also interacts with the same group of genes that are positively altered by caloric restriction. Cox-2 inhibitors in a natural form from a hops extract can improve inflammatory gene function.

Our newfound ability to extract and store adult stem cells will revolutionize the anti-aging industry in the future. Why? Because we can utilize these stem cells in large numbers as we grow older. GEMS, or gene expression modifiers are naturally occurring compounds that are produced in the liver. They turn off oncogenes and improve skin texture and quality, plus cholesterol levels. I have combined all of the above information into the new anti-aging program that I follow, as do many of my patients.

- Personalized genetic health gene testing.
- The use of a core nutrition supplement program.
- The use of category-specific prescriptions.
- Four months of GEMS to repair DNA damage.
- The harvesting and storage of adult stem cells for future use.
- An environmental lifestyle modification program which focuses on diet, exercise, and state of mind.

We have the science, technology, and laboratory diagnostic testing to markedly improve the quality of our health and our longevity. For the first time in our history we have the ability to maintain our health at the level of our DNA, and to maintain our DNA function

Ann Louise Gittleman, Ph.D., CNS, ND, MS

My personal health odyssey transformed me into a vegetarian, vegan, raw food aficionado and macrobiotic devotee—only to learn that the right way to eat for vitality and longevity never seemed to work for my type a personality.

As director of nutrition for the Pritikin Longevity Center in Santa Monica, California in the early 1980s I met many distinguished individuals who casually mentioned Dr. Ana Aslan's procaine therapy, known as Gerovital H-3 or (GH-3)

World leaders like Charles De Gaulle, Ho Chi Minh, Mao Tse Tung, and John F. Kennedy were purported users. Throughout the 1960s Gerovital was kept off the U.S. market. I was offered the opportunity to research and design the next generation GH-3, which was named Ultra H-3. It is a patented procaine product which is considered 100% bioavailable. It is a powerful product which seems to provide whatever your body needs.

Each tablet of Ultra H-3 contains 100 mg. of procaine hydrochloride. It releases PABA (paraaminobenzoic acid) and DEAE (dierthylaminethynol). Both act like muscle relaxants and have antihistamine properties. In addition, Ultra H-3 contains ascorbic acid, citric acid, niacin, folic acid, biotin, and magnesium- all in a base of gingko biloba and bilberry extracts to optimize circulation throughout the body.

Whatever path you take to find the fountain, it is my fervent hope that you will find it.

Robert Goldman, M.D., Ph.D., DO, FAASP

I consider fitness to be a universal and leading anti-aging intervention. My concept of anti-aging medicine considers the specialty to be the next generation of sports medicine. The hallmarks of anti-aging include the following:

- Not smoking.
- Eating 5 or more servings of fresh fruits and vegetables a day.
- Moderate alcohol consumption.
- Regular aerobic exercise

My program for quality sleep:

- Practice good sleep hygiene.
- Eat for sleep-starchy foods like breads, pastas, potatoes, and milk help promote sleep.
- Herbs help.
- Avoid certain medications- caffeine, blood pressure medicines, diet pills, and decongestants.
- Lower your body temperature. Take a power nap-just 20 minutes.

Fitness as a Universal Anti-aging Intervention:

- Exercise two or more days a week.
- Dumbells, weights, machines, or no weights at all.
- Start with one or two pounds and increase over time.
- Exercise-involve all major muscle groups.
- 8 to 15 repetitions.
- Do not hold your breath.
- Rest between sets.
- Avoid locking the joints in your arms and legs.
- Stretch after completing all exercises.
- Stop if you feel pain at any time.

The American Academy of anti-aging medicine projects that the human life span will reach at least 125 productive, healthy, and beyond by the year 2049. I expect to live at least 125 productive, healthy, and vital years. Adopt the anti-aging lifestyle, get quality sleep, engage in regular physical activity, and you might accomplish the same.

Abram Hoffer, M.D., Ph.D., FRCPC

I never thought I would search for eternal youth-nor do I think it will ever be found. The United States mandated the fortification of flour with a few B vitamins. Within a few years a major pandemic called pellagra was brought under control. Small amounts of vitamin B-3 cured psychosis and death. No action has ever equalled this amazing public health measure. Vitamin B-3 has two forms-niacin and niacinamide. Are they safe? I have been taking niacin for the past fifty-two years. There are no toxic side effects. It is the world's gold standard for lowering total cholesterol, for elevating HDL, for decreasing triglycerides, for decreasing Lp(a) as a major anti-inflammatory substance, and not surprisingly-in decreasing mortality and extending life.

Avoid any foods that make you sick. A good rule is to avoid any food that contains added sugar, if possible. Eat three meals each day starting with a healthy, protein-rich breakfast. I do not consider a doughnut and coffee a healthy breakfast. I avoid dairy products, eggs, wheat, oats, peanuts, coconut, pecans, and sugar because they make me sick. This is my personal program. I do not recommend it for everyone. It is based on the principles of orthomolecular medicine, a wonderful, accurate term presented to us all as a gift by Linus Pauling, a two-time Nobel Prize- winner. It is best to start as early as possible, but it is never too late:

Vitamin A - 30,000 daily
Niacin- 1 gram three times a day
Vitamin C- 1 gram twice daily
B-Complex- 100 mg. once daily
Folic acid- 5 mg. daily
Vitamin D- 6,000 daily
Vitamin E- 400 iu twice daily
Selenium-200 mcg.daily
Calcium Citrate- 600 mg. daily
Magnesium- 300 mg. daily
Zinc Citrate- 50 mg. daily
Salmon Oil- 1 gram three times daily
Co-Enzyme Q10- 100 mg. three times daily
N-Acetyl Cysteine-1 gram three times a day
Alpha-Lipoic Acid-200 mg. three times a day

You and your health advisor are partners in keeping you well. Don't leave all the responsibility up to them. Learn about orthomolecular therapy. Adhere to its tenets and protocols, and you will enjoy the best of health.

Ronald L. Hoffman, M.D., CNS

Here is the Core Program for Optimal Health. Start with a good multi. Forget those that contain token amounts of critical nutrients just to create the false impression that they are comprehensive. Antioxidants work. Thousands of studies support their efficacy for the prevention of degenerative diseases.

Add: mixed carotenoids-10,000-15,000 IUs.
Vitamin E- mixed tocopherols, high gamma 400 IU.

Vitamin C- 500 mg. three times a day.

Chelated zinc-30 mg. a day.

Chelated selenium-200 mcg a day.

Alpha-lipoic acid-300 mg. twice a day.

NAC- 500 mg.twice daily.

Oils- Pharmaceutical-grade fish oil. (2.8 teaspoons a day).

Greening- EGCG (Epigallocatechingallate)—Polyphenols found in green tea.

SGS- (Sulfuraphane glucosinolate) – Indole compound from the cabbage family

Pycnogenol- A French pine bark- get 85-90 percent or 1 or 2 100 mg. capsules a day.

Curcumin- a powerful antioxidant derived from the curry spice turmeric.

Add Probiotics

Vitamin D- the 21st century story- essential for everyone for the following: Metabolism, bones, hyperparathyroidism, cancer, body aches, autoimmune disease, immunity, and mood.

Add: Lutein and zeazanthin-for eye health 10 mg. and 2 mg. respectively

Glucosamine sulphate or hydrochloride-1,200 mg. and 1,500 mg. respectively.

MSM- 2-4 grams.

Heart problems-CoQ10- 200-500 mg. a day. L-Carnitine-2,000 mg. a day.

Expert help from an experienced and trusted professional is valuable. May you reap major health dividends

Beatrice Trum Hunter

My quest for knowledge about nutrition and health has centered mainly around books. They have served as the source of my understanding about the vital role played by good foods and nutrition as they relate to good health. Books have influenced the direction of my life. My early years were dominated by white bread, Crisco, and sugar. Up to my college years, my body reflected this dreadful diet. I developed dental caries. I had acne, lustreless hair, frequent headaches, and a low level of energy.

One book changed my life, "100,000 Guinea Pigs." It pointed out the dangers in everyday foods, drugs, and cosmetics. I limited sugar, cut out lunch meats and frankfurters. I began eating fruits and vegetables. MY skin cleared up, my hair shone, the headaches disappeared, and I had more energy. The dietary changes were responsible for the improvements.

In my heart I was eager to learn more about foods, nutrition, and health. I was an avid reader. My conclusions:

Choose basic foods such as eggs, poultry, muscle and organ meats, marrow bones, fin fish, and shellfish. In addition, eat vegetables, legumes, fruits, nuts, and seeds. If you are not allergic, eat dairy products and whole grains.

Nutrition is not the whole answer to good health:

- A healthy diet.
- Low stress.
- Economic security.
- Pleasant living quarters.
- Accessibility to services.
- Social connections.
- Meaningful work beyond self.
- Hobbies.
- Mental stimulation.
- Take time to relax.

Smell the flowers. Enjoy the spectacular sunset while you munch a pear.

Ronald Klatz, M.D., DO

Anti-aging medicine is the fastest growing medical specialty in the world. It is based on sound principles, is scientifically based, and well-documented in leading medical journals. Cutting-edge therapies for life enhancement and potential life extension include the following:

- Exercise and lifestyle: add 5-15 years

- Anti-aging drugs: add 55-20 years
- High-tech biomedicine: add 10-30 years
- Fasting and caloric restriction: add 20-70 years

Technologies of tomorrow

- Advanced prospective diagnostics: add 3-10 years
- Genetic screening and interventions: add 3-10 years
- Stem cell therapeutics: add 6-15 years
- Nanotechnology: add 7-20 years
- Artificial organs: add 8-20 years

We are ushering in a new reality in which 75 year olds may well be considered middle aged. We must bridge the gap between today and 2029. If medical knowledge doubles every 3 to 5 years or less, by 2029 we will know at least 256 times more than we know today. By 2029, we anticipate that science will enable us to achieve "practical immortality"- a healthy human life span of 150 years and beyond.

I submit that the leading causes of death could be eliminated in the immediate future. I predict the following timetable for major medical breakthroughs:

- Aids and infectious disease-eliminated 2015
- Alzheimer's disease- eliminated 2015
- Cancer- eliminated 2021
- Diabetes- eliminated 2017
- Heart disease eliminated 2016

Kilmer S. McCully, M.D.

My discoveries concerning the biomedical origin of disease were the culmination of my lifelong interest in biochemistry, genetics, molecular biology, etc. In 1968, I discovered the relation of homocysteine to vascular disease. It was not acceptable to the promoters of the conventional cholesterol hypothesis. I was forced to leave Harvard Medical School after 11 years of teaching, practice, and research. Immediately, I was able to continue my work at the VA Medical Center in Providence, Rhode Island, and since 2001 in Boston.

I published "The Homocysteine Revolution" and "The Heart

Revolution." Optimal nutrition is achieved with a lifelong diet that provides abundant B-vitamins, folic acid, and B-6 to keep homocysteine levels in the optimal range (6-8 micromoles per liter). The heart revolution diet includes fish oil, vitamins D and A, CoQ10, vitamin k2, beneficial phytochemicals, and the minerals magnesium, potassium, calcium, selenium, and other trace minerals.

It eliminates processed foods and provides little or none of the deleterious nutrients that contribute to aging. Some of these are soy, fluoridated water, and trans fats from hydrogenated oils. Soy foods contain toxic proteins and phytoestrogen substances that cause hypothyroidism, infertility, poor digestion, and poor absorption of minerals.

Richard A. Passwater, Ph.D.

I am not just interested in living longer, I want to live better longer.. The goal is to increase the quality of life. We want to add more life to our years. Slowing the aging process is all about living better and longer.

Here is a short list of advice on how to live better longer:

- Live a healthy life. Don't smoke, drink in moderation, and wear your seat belt.
- Watch the calories. Eat fruits and vegetables and avoid animal and saturated fats.
- Be active. Exercise 30 minutes a day.
- Be positive. Stay engaged in life and make new friends.
- Challenge your brain. Along with a good diet, supplements can affect pronounced additional improvement in living better longer.

The following is my daily supplement program:

- A good multivitamin/mineral
- Vitamin C 2,000-4,000 mg. (divided doses)
- Pycnogenol- 50-100 mg.
- CoQ10 30-100 mg.
- Alpha-lipoic acid- 25-100 mg. (divided doses)
- Acetyl-l-carnitine 500 mg.

- Resveratrol-500 mg. or more
- Fish oil-1,000 to 3,000 mg. (divided doses)
- Phosphatydylserine-500 mg.
- Magnesium-400 mg.
- Selenium-200 mcg.
- Vitamin D 2-500 IU
- Vitamin K2-50 mg.
- L-Arginine-500 mg.
- Silicon-10-25 mg.

Fred Pescatore, M.D., MPH, CCN

"Diabesity" was coined by Dr, Robert C. Atkins 14 years ago. I was associate director of his center in New York City. It was there, at the start of my medical career, that I saw people taking charge of their own health. For the first time, they got well the use of harmful prescription drugs.. In this short essay I'm going to show you how to prevent obesity and its devastating side effects.

Obesity is responsible for 4 of the top 10 leading causes of death in the United States: heart disease, cancer, stroke, and diabetes. Obesity affects one in three Americans and one in four children. If this continues, everyone in the United States will be overweight or obese by the year 2025.

Diabetes affects 40 million Americans-and 20 million more are undiagnosed. Diabetes is the leading cause of blindness and amputation in the United States. It can lead to high blood pressure, kidney disease, gangrene, and impotence.

We are literally eating ourselves to death, and encouraging our children to do the same. The consumption of too many simple carbohydrates causes the pancreas to secrete too much insulin. This leads to insulin resistance. This puts you on the road to diabetes. As you continue to eat pasta, white bread, cake sugar, pretzels, soda, and fruit juice your system will break down. Sugar is sugar, is sugar, no matter how it is disguised. Honey, molasses, and anything that ends in ose and ol are all forms of sugar. We eat ourselves into the problem and we can eat ourselves out of it. Unfortunately, we have a health care system that is solely based on treating illness, not preventing it.

The program I recommend is outlined in my books. We need to eat like our ancestors and more like people in Mediterranean lands.

- Lean proteins- fish, pork, and some red meat
- Vegetables, nuts, seeds, and healthy fats and oils
- Whole grains, beans, legumes, and fruits

These are the foods we should eat.

If you want something done right, you have to do it yourself. This especially includes your health care. There are various roads to health. One is taking vitamins and other nutrients in the great super highway. I have no financial association whatsoever with the health products industry. Vitamins in appropriately high doses are both preventive and therapeutic.

If you have a cold- a gram of vitamin C every five minutes will do the trick. If you are stressed or anxious- a few hundred milligrams of vitamin B-3 will make you feel better in a few minutes. You may have a flush, but you must read about the work of Robert Cathcart III, M.D., Fred Klenner, M.D., and Abram Hoffer, M.D.

My Supplement Regimen

Vitamin C- 15,000-20,000 mg. (hourly doses)
Vitamin E- (Natural mixed tocopherols) 600-8000 IU
Lecithin- 1-2 tablespoons (inositol, choline, EFAs)
Vitamin D-1,500 IU
Fish oil-2,000 mg. (300 EPA, 240 DHA)
Zinc-100 mg.
Magnesium- 300 to 400 mg. with some calcium
Chromium- 200 to 400 MCG
Orthomolecular nutrition has served me well so far. I think it will help you too.

Stephen T. Sinatra, M.D., FACC, CNS

As a physician for 35 years I have learned about healthy and graceful aging. The way to achieve it is basic. A Russian gerontologist examined

20,000 healthy people aged 80 and older, many of whom were over 100.

They had the following in common:

- They worked outside- getting sunlight, fresh air, and physical activity.
- They ate a diet of grains, fresh fruits, and vegetables.
- They enjoyed good relationships, rich in love, intimacy, and support--from cuddling and kissing to intercourse. The intimacy meant the most to them.
- They were optimistic about life.

MALIGNANT MEDICAL MYTHS
JOEL L. KAUFFMAN, PH.D.

When your physician tells you that you need a test, a prescription drug, or an operation, he could be wrong. There are many false positives and false negatives. Aggressive diagnosis is not prevention, merely early detection.

There is considerable evidence that prescription drugs do not prolong life or improve its quality. This includes cholesterol-lowering drugs, blood pressure drugs, and most anti-cancer drugs used for chemotherapy. At least a dozen drugs were recalled by the FDA in the 1990s just a few years after the FDA approved them. The FDA has sometimes been an obstructor of effective, non-toxic alternative treatments, while accepting toxic drugs based on surrogate outcomes in RCTs (randomized trials).

One reason for the poor performance of the FDA is that one-third of the committee's nine members had financial ties to the drug manufacturers who submitted new drug applications.

Research at the NIH ($30 billion a year) is far from independent. Since 1980, staff members could engage in consulting deals. Can university or medical school faculty or researchers be trusted? Researchers who go ahead and publish findings unfavorable to the sponsor have been threatened with the loss of all funding, lawsuits, blacklisting from future contracts, or even employment.

Synopsis

Myth #1
The use of low-dose aspirin can no longer be supported.

If you give 81 mg. of "baby" aspirin to 1,000 people, 25 of them will likely bleed excessively. Another 25 will have no observable effect on platelets whatsoever. The FDA reaffirmed its position on aspirin in December, 2003. "Aspirin is the drug of doctors' dreams. It is highly effective. It is likely to remain the only heart attack preventive sold in grocery stores for years to come. Aspirin and other drugs can and do prevent clots, but they can also cause side effects and lead to hemorrhagic stroke or sudden cardiac death due to arrythmyia.

Studies have shown that vitamin E, magnesium, certain Omega 3 fatty acids, and CoenzymeQ10 provide much greater long-term benefits than aspirin. All of these supplements have fewer side effects. Despite all the evidence for the value of these supplements, your mainstream physician will continue to recommend aspirin. Why? Because Bayer is advertised more than all four supplements put together.

Myth #2
Low-Carbohydrate diets are unsafe and ineffective
for losing weight.

Because the USA adopted the high-carbohydrate/low fat diet for the past fifty years, we are now faced with an epidemic of obesity and type 2 diabetes. We were instructed to emphasize a diet which was high in carbohydrates in the form of bread, potatoes, pasta, and rice. Dr. Paul Dudley white, president Eisenhower's cardiologist claimed, "I began my practice as a cardiologist in 1921 and never saw a myocardial infarction patient until 1928. Back in the MI-free days before 1920, the fats were butter, whole milk, and lard and I think we would all benefit from the kind of diet we had when no one had ever heard of corn oil." (Duane Graveline, M.D.)

For 50 years government agencies were telling us to restrict our intake of animal fats because of their content of cholesterol and saturated fats. This meant eliminating most meats and eggs. Then, 25 years ago anything containing polyunsaturated oils were touted for better health.

These oils were mainly corn, cottonseed, safflower, soybean, and sunflower. The partially hydrogenated versions were the source of the ubiquitous trans fatty acids, the ones found in Crisco, Oreo cookies, Triscuit crackers, pie crust, cake icing, and a zillion other products. They became as common as classic Coca Cola, a high-carbohydrate drink.

The extent of the evidence for the benefits of low-carbohydrate diets is so great as to invite questioning of the motives among all the government agencies and private foundations still recommending high-carbohydrate diets and presently coordinating a world-wide attack on low-carbohydrate diets despite the obvious result of weight loss among at least 40 million Americans alone (based on book sales) who use low-carbohydrate diets. It is simply resistance in defense of an entrenched position that should not have been adopted originally.

Myth #3
Using Cholesterol-Lowering Drugs, Especially the Statins Would Benefit Everyone

The pharmaceutical industry's profits from the statin drugs depends a great deal upon your insurance and compliance with your physician, who may have been paid up to $2000 to start you on Crestor, Lipitor, or Zocor.

Space doc Duane Graveline experienced Lipitor-associated amnesia. He thought it was just old age. Statin drugs, while lowering cholesterol levels, have several side effects. They inhibit the production of Coenzyme Q10. Doctors should be better informed about the true legacy of statin drug side effects. Despite the mounting evidence for cholesterol's irrelevance, the public is still focused on cholesterol. Statin drugs have never been more aggressively marketed. The only thing we can be absolutely certain of is that lowering everyone's cholesterol produces the incredible profits for the pharmaceutical industry-money absolutely wasted because of the harm done.

TV ads for Lipitor showing a man with high cholesterol collapsing in the street, or a body in the morgue to symbolize death from high total cholesterol have no basis in fact. The Federal Trade Commission and the FDA are derelict in allowing those ads to run anywhere.

Cholesterol is always present in our blood, and is necessary for life. Cholesterol is an essential component of our membranes, of nerve junctions, and of brain functions, and as a source of hormones.

Dangers of Low Cholesterol

Very low levels of cholesterol are a serious danger. A large number of clinical studies show that total cholesterol levels less than 188 are associated with depression, accidents, suicide, homicide, etc.

In 2001, the FDA ordered Pfizer to stop promoting Lipitor as a treatment for cardiovascular disease, noting that it had not been established as effective in reducing the rates of myocardial infarction. It may only be promoted as a cholesterol-lowering drug.

The serious side effects of statins are cancer, erectile dysfunction, myalgia, polyneuropathy, rhabdomyolysis, l;iver and kidney damage, congestive heart failure, and amnesia. That is why in 1996, the editor-in-chief of the American Journal of Cardiology reported that 50% of the patients prescribed a statin drug quit in one year, and only 25% continued for 2 years.

Tom Scherer, a civil rights activist, was started on Zocor and developed myalgia and chronic fatigue. He E-mailed me on July 28, 2004 that he had obtained data from the FDA under the Freedom of Information Act (and congressional intercession proved necessary) on adverse events reports actually reported from Nov. 1997 to may 14, 2004 on Zocor. The data showed 11,589 individual adverse events reports of which 416 resulted in death. It is believed that only 5% of the adverse effects of frugs are actually reported to the FDA

Statins are the drug class most likely to bankrupt Medicare, Medicaid, and other insurance plans without any significant benefits. It is up to you not to ask for them, not to take them if offered, and to inform your loved ones to do the same.

Nearly Everyone over 50 Should Take Drugs for High Blood Pressure

The drug industry liked it, the doctors liked it, and the public liked it. So began our national focus on lowering blood pressure. The evolution of hundreds of drugs designed to lower blood pressure,, and the beginning of a still-growing, multi-billion dollar business. Mainstream medicine ignores the fact that the side effects of the drugs are so bad that 20% to 60% of the people taking them stop within 3 years.

Elevated blood pressure is called hypertension, low blood pressure is called hypotension. There are no symptoms of high blood pressure unless it is very high (200 over 100). This is seen in only 8% of old people. Blood pressure tends to rise naturally with age in both men and women. Acceptable blood pressure levels are now 140 over 90. Uffe Ravnslov, M.D., Ph.D. does not prescribe blood pressure drugs with blood pressure lower than 200/100 (malignant hypertension).

Only 1 out of 5 people who lower their salt intake show any benefit. Drug use should be considered for extremely hypertensive people (to 20%). After a low carbohydrate diet and supplements such as L-Arginine, Magnesium, and fish oil success has been achieved this allows you to take much lower doses of drugs, minimizing side effects.

Myth #5
A Drink a Day keeps the Doctor Away

Moderate drinking can't harm you, but if you have any perceptions of health gains-forget about it. Doctor Barnard, the doctor who performed the world's first successful heart transplant, believed that red wine would reduce heart disease by 40%. However, none of the studies cited the all-cause death rate for various levels of alcohol consumption.

A Stockholm county, Sweden, 26-year follow-up study in 2001 concluded that moderate drinkers do not live significantly longer than low-level and non-drinkers.

In sum, there is no evidence that moderate drinking of any common alcoholic beverage has worthwhile health benefits overall. Even Nobel Prize winners may fall victim to common dogmas. Any overall benefit of moderate drinking is minor to non-existent. At least, no harm is done.

Myth #6
Exercise! Run for Your Life. No Pain, No Gain!

Dr. Duane Graveline (Space Doc)-Having lost several of my apparently healthy, young colleagues to sudden death during stress exercise, I realize that sudden death is the price paid for our running shoes hitting the pavement. Progrddive deterioration of cartilage, ligaments, and tendons is a problem of major proportions.

Christian Barnard—"There is a great deal of evidence to support the fact that exercise is good for the heart."

Exercise does not reduce blood pressure (Myth#4). The goal of this chapter is not to debunk exercise altogether, but to show the adverse effects of strenuous exercise as compared with mild to medium or moderate exercise. Most authors caution that a stress test should precede strenuous exercise. Dr. Henry Solomon's evidence shows that it is not good advice to press part pain to obtain the vaunted "runner's high."

The complete story of the marathon run of Phidippides is rarely told. After his run of 26 miles from marathon to Athens, and delivering his message, he dropped dead. (Solomon) James F. Fixx (The Book of Running) died of a massive heart attack at age 52.

Henry A. Solomon, M.D. cardiologist at Cornell University medical college, New York—"There is about the same relationship between activity and longevity as you might find if you were to compare the amount of chocolate pudding children eat with the likelihood of their coming down with chicken pox. There is no relationship at all."

It is clear that moderate activity such as fast walking, slow swimming, slow dancing, Yoga, light weight lifting, mild calisthenics-will make those who enjoy activity feel better and possibly live a little longer.

Myth#7
EDTA Chelation Therapy for Atherosclerosis is a Fraud.

Imagine 20 million intravenous infusions of EDT, no ill effects when properly done. "Chelation doesn't work!" says the medical establishment. Yet an extraordinary 87% success rate based upon very reasonable objective indicators of benefit. "There is no money to be made with such a simple and therapeutically safe procedure." "We should feel deeply indebted to Dr. Kauffman for the immense effort he has expended in reviewing this difficult subject." (Dr. Duane Graveline)

Chelation is the Greek work for claw. A safe and effective procedure first used to treat heavy metal poisoning, and then to open up atherosclerotic blood vessels. EDTA chelation therapy has been attacked and vilified by mainstream medicine. The attacks have led to disbarment and delicensing of physicians who used EDTA chelation to treat patients by state medical boards. Chelation is an excellent alternative to bypass surgery in 80-85% of cases and should be tried first. Long term studies show almost no benefit from bypass surgery in mortality after 10 years. Balloon angioplasty may be somewhat safer, but its effects last only a few weeks or months.

Discouraging sick people from undergoing an effective treatment such as EDTA chelation therapy is despicable. It is estimated that by the year 2000 more than a million patients will have received more than 20 million infusions of EDTA. There were no ill effects when the procedure is correctly done. About 88% of patients improved. (Dr. Elmer Cranton).

Myth#8
Annual Mammograms Prolong Life

Mass cancer screenings is big business. A 50 year old woman's chance of contracting breast cancer is under 2% and the chance of the same woman dying is 0.3%. If 1,000 women of ages 40-50 had periodic mammograms we know that 8 to 8.9 of these women will actually have breast cancer. Seven of these positives will be found by mammography. The other will be missed. Of the 992 women who do not have breast cancer, 70 will be identified as falsely positive. Of the 77 positives, only 7 will be correct. It is mind boggling to try to fathom how this has come about. (Space Doc Duane Graveline, M.D.) (Dr. Kauffman's story is a true public service)

The media says 1 in 9 women will get breast cancer. The chance of dying from breast cancer is 4%,1 in 25, or 0.3%. For this reason, mass screening of women under 50 for breast cancer would not achieve much beyond profit for the cancer industry and plenty of anguish for women.

The "1 in 9" dramatics is a scare tactic used by the American Cancer Society to coerce women to get mammographic screenings.

Summary—Undergoing annual mammograms does not improve all-cause mortality. After a diagnosis of breast cancer expenditures on screening, mammograms are a serious waste of money.

Myth#10
Cancer Treatments are Better Than Ever
and Have Cure Rates of 60%

Cancer experts claim current treatment approaches achieve a 60% "success rate." The 5-year survival rate is the function of patients alive after 5 years from diagnosis. Even the modest progress will be seen as a product of early diagnosis, with very little improvement due to the benefit of mainstream types of treatment.

Oncologists usually mislead patients about benefits of mainstream treatments and minimize the delayed effects and the side effects. They disparage alternative treatments regardless of the evidence. Most alternative cancer treatments are of no value, but many are non-toxic, so that a higher quality of life can be enjoyed whole one is hoping for a remission.

Another term that is used by oncologists to encourage or confuse cancer victims is the response rate. When a patient asks, "what are my chances with chemotherapy?" The answer is likely to be 60%. The patient thinks that means a cure rate, the odds of a cancer disappearance. Response rates to standard treatments for common cancers range from 60-90%, yet cancer-free survival is 0.20% (Ralph Moss, 200 pp 56-57).

With few exceptions oncologists will exaggerate the benefits of mainstream treatments including tumor removal and beyond to minimize the side effects. If a patient refuses to follow the oncologists advice, or suggests an alternative treatment, the first response is often a death threat from the oncologist. If the patient is persistent, the oncologist may refuse ri serve the patient any longer. (Fulder "How to Survive Medical Treatment."

"The medical profession and the media applaud the introduction of every new "miracle drug" that appears on the scene. The process has gone on since at least the start of the "War on Cancer in 1971. We are told of increasing response rates with some of these agents. But whether improvements in "responses," "active," "disease-free," or "progression-free" survival convey any real survival is still a matter of debate. If there is a survival advantage (even ignoring quality-of-life), it is generally so small that it is undetectable through the normal route of clinical trials." (Ralph Moss, 2000)

Summing up

You can be sure that cancer cure rates are not 60%, and that here has not been much change in 40 years. The 5-year survival rate is 60%, and has appeared to improve only because of earlier detection and some adjustments. A patient in a clinical trial dying just before a treatment program of even 6-12 months duration has been completed is not counted as a failure on the grounds that the patient has not completed the treatment program! A control patient dying of any cause is counted as a failure of non-treatment.

Early detection is not prevention. When treatments are so poor, as the mainstream ones beyond surgery are at this time, there is almost no point in screening for cancer. Certainly, it is beyond dispute that mammography in women and the PSA test for prostate cancer in men with no symptoms have no overall benefit.

Claimed reductions of mortality from cancer are of no use if the all-cause mortality rate remains the same or worsens, yet the first is usually the only sort of claim made for most treatments.

The highly toxic chemotherapeutic drugs developed in the 1950s and up to the present time kill all rapidly dividing cells in the body, which means not only cancer cells, but also many kinds of healthy cells. Unfortunately, the immune system, the body's natural defense system against cancer, is itself composed of rapidly dividing cells. So both the disease and the protection against disease get zapped. (Pert, 1997)

New treatments may appear at any time; find out whether your cancer is a candidate for one of them. Determination to survive, willingness to travel for a treatment, and supportive family or friends will make a great difference to the outcome.

DEATH BY MEDICINE
GARY NULL, PH.D., ET AL

Statistics show that the real hazard to your health is government sanctioned medicine. Health care in America is not as safe as it should be. Adverse drug events, surgical mistakes, etc. take a great cost in human lives. The FDA says that "ADRs are one of the leading causes of morbidity and mortality in health care. The irony is that safer (and less expensive) preventive alternatives are often attacked and ridiculed by regulatory powers.

In "Death by Medicine," we will present compelling evidence that today's health care system frequently causes more harm than good. This book reveals the following astounding number of facts:

Synopsis

- 2.2 million adverse reactions to prescribe unnecessary antibiotics prescribed drugs in hospitals.
- 4.5 million unnecessary antibiotics prescribed annually.
- 7.5 million unnecessary surgical procedures performed every year.
- 8.9 million unnecessary hospitalizations each year.

The most stunning statistic is that the total number of deaths caused by conventional medicine is nearly 800,000 per year. By contrast, heart disease in 2005 (the most recent statistic) was 652,091, and cancer 565,650 men and women died in 2008.

Dr. Graham of the FDA has said, "The American public is virtually defenceless if another medication such as Vioxx proves to be unsafe after it's approved." Yet the FDA prevents us from taking dandelion root.

Natural medicine is under siege. The FDA interferes with those who offer natural products that compete with prescription drugs. Studies at the Institute of Medicine estimate that 2,216,000 ADRs in hospitalized patients cause over 106,000 deaths annually. It is also estimated that over 350,000 ADRs occur in nursing homes each year. The Institute estimates that nearly 100,000 patients die in hospitals each year due to medical errors. This is three times as many who die on the highways.

The CDC claims that American hospitals account for an estimated 1.7 million infections and 99,000 associated deaths each year. In the U.S. at least 794,936 deaths are iatrogenic-that is, induced by a physician or surgeon. The mortality costs alone exceed $282 billion a year.

Health care costs are growing at an unsustainable rate. Annual health care spending was $2.4 trillion in 2007 and 2008, or $7900 per person-17% of the gross domestic product. The total was projected to reach $3.1 trillion in 2012. One estimate shows a ten-year total of 7.95 million iatrogenic deaths. The figure is more than all the casualties from all the wars fought by the U.S. throughout its entire history. Medically induced deaths are the equivalent of six jumbo jets falling out of the sky each day.

This book is the first time all the statistics on the multiple causes of iatrogenesis have been combined in one book. Medical science amasses tens of thousands of papers annually. To look at only one piece "is like standing an inch away from an elephant and trying to describe everything about it. You have to step back to see the big picture."

When health care spending rose to $2.4 trillion dollars per year in 2007, it represented 17% of the gross domestic product. With this enormous expenditure (which occurred in 2008 as well), we should have the best medicine in the world. However, we aren't preventing and reversing disease, and doing minimal harm.

Medicine is not taking into consideration the following aspects of a healthy, human organism:

1. Stress
2. Insufficient exercise
3. Caloric intake
4. Highly processed foods grown in chemically damaged soil
5. Exposure to tens of thousands of environmental toxins

A recent article states, "The U.S. spends $700 billion on unnecessary medical tests." It appears on the "healthcare economist" website. As little as 5% and no more than 20% of iatrogenic events are ever reported. If medical errors were completely and accurately reported, we would have an annual iatrogenic death toll much higher than 794,936.

At a 1997 press conference, Dr. Lucien L. Leape noted that medical errorscould be as high as 3 million could cost as much as $200 billion. He used a 14% fatality rate in 1994 which led to 180,000 deaths. In 1997, Leape's base number of 3 million errors would increase the annual death rate to as high as 420,000 for hospital inpatients alone.

Medication Errors

A 2002 study shows that 20% of hospital medications had dosage errors. The error rate in this study was 24%, intercepted by pharmacists. This made the potential minimum number of patients harmed by prescription drugs 417,908.

Adverse Drug Reactions

The Lazarou Study in 1994 estimated that 106,000 deaths occur annually due to adverse drug reactions. The costs for the Lazarou Study's 2.2 million patients with serious drug reactions amounted to $12 billion.

Reuters reported that nearly 5% of hospital admissions (over 1 million per year) are the result of drug side effects.. In 2004, the world pharmaceutical market did $550 billion in sales. 48% of that total, or $248 billion was sold in the U.S., one-half of the world's prescription drugs.

Underreporting of Side Effects

Only one in twenty side effects is reported to hospital administrators or the FDA. Jerry Phillips, of the FDA said, "the 250,000 reports received annually represent only 5% of the actual reactions that occur. Dr. Jay Cohen notes that there are 5 million medication reactions each year.

Direct to Consumer Advertising

In 2004, pharmaceutical manufacturers spent an estimated $415 billion on direct-to-consumer advertising, according to IMS Health. There are those who surmise that consumers are [paying for these expensive ads when they buy medications that cost more than they are worth.

Problems with Specific Classes of Drugs

30 million pounds of antibiotics are used in America each year. 2.5 million pounds are used in animal husbandry- 23 million pounds are used to try to prevent disease and promote growth. Only 2 million pounds are given for specific animal infections. Antibiotics are measurable in many of our foods and in various waterways around the world, much of it seeping in from animal farms. The pharmaceutical industry claims it supports limiting the use of antibiotics. The CDC also is involved in trying to minimize antibiotic resistance, but nowhere in its publications is there any reference to the role of pharmaceuticals in boosting the immune system.

NSAIDS (Non-Steroidal Anti-inflammatoryDrugs)

In ten years NSAIDS kills 165,000 people. This amount is about 2.5 times as many people in a ten year period as were killed in the ten years of the Vietnam War. In 2003, the British Medical Journal warned who took Advil, Motrin, and Naprosyn that they had an 80 percent higher risk of miscarriage than women who avoided these medications.

Vioxx was withdrawn on September 30, 2004 by Merck. The Lancet questioned why the manufacturer did not withdraw it several years earlier. Vioxx was withdrawn after evidence came to light that it doubled the risk of heart attacks and strokes in people who had been taking it for 18 months. Dr. David Graham, testifying before the U.S. senate, estimated that 88,000 to 138,000 Americans had heart attacks and strokes as a side effect of Vioxx. "Of these, Graham said, "30% to 40% probably died." That would be an estimated 27,000 to 55,000 preventable deaths attributable to Vioxx.

Graham said, "If there were an average of 150-200 people on an aircraft-it would be the rough equivalent of 500 to 900 aircraft dropping from the sky. This translates to 2 to 4 aircraft every week for the last 5 years.

Ulrich Abel, Ph.D. wrote a monograph which was published in a peer-reviewed medical journal. His exhaustive review of 3,000 articles concluded that there is no direct evidence that chemotherapy prolongs survival in most patients with advanced carcinoma. According to Abel, "many oncologists take it for granted that response to therapy prolongs survival, an opinion which is based on a fallacy and which is not supported by clinical evidence."

Unnecessary Surgical Procedures

In 2004, 75 million unnecessary surgical procedures were performed resulting in 37,136 deaths at a cost of $122 billion (1974 dollars)

X-Rays

In 5 scientifically documented books Dr. John Gofman provides strong evidence that medical technology (x-rays, CT scans, mammography, and fluoroscopic devices) are a contributing factor to 75% of new cancers. Dr. Gofman predicts that ionizing radiation will be responsible for 100 million premature deaths over the next decade. David Brenner, Ph.D., professor of radiation oncology and public health at Columbia University in New York estimated the dose from a single full-body CT scan to be 14 to 21 million g-rays. The exposure is equal to 100 chest x-rays or 100 mammograms.

Conclusion

The office of technology assessment was perhaps the U.S. government's last honest agency that critically reviewed the state of the nation's health care system. Shortly after the OTA released a report that exposed how entrenched financial interests manipulate healthcare practice in the United States, congress disbanded the OTA

For years our nation has avoided the responsibility for expanding the major healthcare crisis, to our own mounting peril. Now we have an iatrogenic epidemic. More Americans are dying each year at the hands of medicine than all our American casualties in the First World War and the Civil War combined.

The physician is rewarded for his efforts, not for his results. The patient signs away his or her rights before surgery, so that the surgeon and the hospital are protected even if they are negligent.

There is currently a systematic program to defame every natural vitamin, supplement, and health food throughout the world. Corruption is rampant. Honest scientists are unable to get grants, unable to publish, possibly unable to work. The medical environment has become a labyrinth of interlocking corporate, hospital, and governmental boards of directors and advisors, infiltrated by the drug companies.

Drug companies pay our legislators, our scientists, and the NAS. Drug companies have propaganda campaigns launched through the CDC, such as a rush to vaccinate as soon as "bird flu" appears on the horizon.

The media, scientists, professors, universities, hospitals, government agencies, such as the FDA and the CDC are having a banquet at the pharmaceutical table. This is not the way to practice medicine. This is not a scientific community; instead of objectivity and compassion, our medical system is powered by weakness, greed, envy, and fear.

The cumulative daily effect of steaks, colas, pizzas, pollution, computers, cell phones, and pesticides, place us in a toxic soup environment. Instead of cleaning this up, many turn to medication for help. Drug companies are paying our legislators, television and radio stations, schools, and news outlets to keep this information from you. Big pharma is paying the quack busters to attack anyone who tells you the truth about what is really making you sick enough to seek expensive "care" from the number one source of fatalities in America, care that might readily making you sick enough to seek expensive "care" from the number one source of fatalities in America, care that might readily kill you and your loved ones-DEATH BY MEDICINE.

VITAMIN C THE REAL STORY
STEVE HICKEY AND ANDREW SAUL, PH.D.S

"Just about everything doctors have been telling us about vitamin C is wrong."

The controversy over vitamin C stated when Nobel Laureate Linus Pauling, Ph.D. advocated megadoses to prevent and treat diseases such as the common cold. Pauling suggested that people need 100 times greater than those recommended by doctors and other nutritional experts. The medical profession labelled him a "quack."

Synopsis

When Albert Szent-Gyorgyi, M.D., Ph.D. first isolated vitamin C and identified it as ascorbic acid he did not want it to be called a vitamin because he suspected that for optimal health, people might need gram levels of vitamin C. Orthomolecular scientists believe that vitamin and nutrient intake is woefully inadequate to achieve optimal nutrition. Linus Pauling coined the term "orthomolecular" in 1968.

Mainstream medicine ignores clinical observations on high-dose vitamin C to the detriment of people's health. Most animals do not need to consume vitamin C because they manufacture it within their bodies. However, humans have lost the ability to synthesize vitamin C. Without it—they die—the deficiency in humans, apes, and guinea pigs causes a fatal disease-scurvy.

On early sea voyages scurvy killed many sailors. Pauling estimated that early humans probably had an intake of 2.5 to 9 grams of vitamin C a day. We can reasonably assume that our early ancestors were largely vegetarian. The loss of the gene to make vitamin c did not create the lack of evolutionary fitness.

An optimal intake of vitamin C is the amount that prevents disease while minimizing the potential risk. To get an accurate estimate of the optimal intake would be necessary for studies to include intakes of vitamin c ranging from 50 mg. up to at least 10,000 mg. per day. And this has not been done.

After James Lind's 1747 finding that consumption of citrus fruit could prevent scurvy, the British Admiralty delayed the edict to consume Citrus fruit. In that intervening period, thousands of sailors died. A review of nine studies, covering 290,000 adults, found that those who took more than 700 mg. of vitamin C per day had a 25 percent lower risk of heart disease.

Some stage, almost every chronic disease has been related to an insufficient intake of vitamin C. However, it may take centuries to determine which chronic diseases are related to a shortage of vitamin C. In the meantime, the debate goes on. It is time for medical science to realize that attacking and demeaning vitamin c and other nutritional therapies can no longer be tolerated.

Dr. Claus Washington Jungeblut demonstrated that ascorbic acid inactivates the polio virus. At high doses, vitamin C acts as a broad-spectrum anti-viral agent.

Dr. William H. McCormick appears to have been the first person to connect scurvy with a predisposition to cancer. He reported that cancer patients typically had very low levels of vitamin C. McCormick cited mortality tables from as early as 1840 and suggested that death from tuberculosis, diphtheria, Scarlet Fever, whooping cough, rheumatic fever, and typhoid fever were primarily due to inadequate dietary vitamin C.

A few milligrams a day will prevent scurvy. In the 1990s, Dr. Mark Levine, M.D. at the NIH found that an adult needs at least 200 mg. a day.

Government values do not consider long term effects of deprivation. For example, atherosclerosis and heart disease could be the result of chronic subclinical scurvy. If that is true, we will all suffer the consequences of doses that are too low.

The NIH suggests 700 mg. a day was the saturation level. Dr. Levine claims that doses above 400 mg. a day provide no additional benefit. At this level, most of the tissues of the body are in a state of depletion. 18 grams a day are required to provide maximum sustained blood levels. (Pauling)

Abundant glucose competes with vitamin C. When glucose (blood sugar) is high less vitamin C is transported into cells. "Take more vitamin C and eat less sugar and carbohydrates" might replace the old adage, "starve a cold, lest you feed a fever." One explanation for the long term symptoms of diabetes is that the person's cells are chronically short of vitamin C.

Nutritional intakes are required to maintain optimal health. Dr. Robert Cathcart III, M.D. and others have used 40 grams, 60 grams, and even 200 grams a day in divided doses to treat a variety of diseases with apparently great success

What is the Optimal Intake?

The optimal intake has not been established. The government RDA is flawed and the recommended intake of vitamin C is woefully inadequate. Low intakes may cause much of the world's chronic diseases. Recently the NIH experiments caused a revision of the daily RDA of vitamin C from 60 mg. to 90 mg. for men and 75 mg. for women. Smokers should take an extra 35 mg. per day.

People need far more than previously assumed. The intake for a healthy adult should be in the range of 500 mg. to 20 grams (20,000 mg.) or even more. Some people would require low doses and would not tolerate higher intakes; others need higher levels, above 10 grams.

One needs to determine his bowel tolerance level. To do this, start with a low dose and increase your intake until unpleasant bowel effects are observed. This level is the optimal amount that you should take every day.

Forms of Vitamin C

There is no advantage to supplementing with "natural" vitamin C over synthetic L-Ascorbic Acid. A large dose of liposomal Vitamin C can deliver a gradual increase in blood levels. The peak level may be far higher and the response is sustained compared to that obtained by a tablet.

Are High Doses Safe?

Vitamin C is remarkably safe. It is unusual in that it can be taken in massive doses, for long periods, without apparent harm. Vitamin C is far safer than commonly used drugs such as aspirin, antibiotics, tranquilizers, sedatives, etc.

"We have not found a single validated report of a healthy person dying from a vitamin C overdose in the scientific literature-not one." To put the safety of vitamin C in context, we consider that it might be easier to commit suicide by overdosing on pure water than by eating too much vitamin C.

The U.S. Poison Control Center reports that from 1983 to 2005, (23 years) vitamins have been connected with the deaths of only 10 people. In 16 of 23 years the AAPC reported there was not a single death due to vitamins.

Does vitamin C Cause Kidney Stones?

Vitamin C does not cause kidney stones. In fact, it has been proposed and used as a treatment for kidney stones. Dr. Cathcart says, "this theoretical difficulty concerning C is typical of how orthodoxy will expand a theory into a fact without any evidence." The only side effect for high doses of vitamin c is diarrhea. It is a natural laxative. One reason for the abundance of vitamin C and antioxidants in both animals and plants is resistance to cancer.

Vitamin C and Cancer

After Vitamin C was identified, William J. McCormick, M.D. anticipated a relationship between cancer and a shortage of vitamin C. In his view, malignant cancer was a disease of inadequate collagen, resulting from a lack of vitamin C. Irwin Stone, Ph.D. also documented a relationship between a shortage of vitamin C and cancer. His early research work led Linus Pauling and Ewan Cameron to perform their influential studies of vitamin C and cancer. A number of Dr. Cameron's patients were cured. Pauling reported that "the ascorbate-treated patients have lived, on the average, over five times as long as the matched control patients. Vitamin C, acting as an oxidant, is selectively toxic to cancer cells, inhibiting their growth or killing them outright. This is good news about cancer and ascorbate.

A Typical redox-synergy therapy based on vitamin C is given here:

- Vitamin C- 3 to 5 grams 6 times a day- 20 grams total
- Alpha-Lipoic Acid- 200-500 mg.-with each dose of Vitamin C-total 5 grams
- Vitamin D3- 4,000 units a day
- Selenium- 800 mcg. A day (maximum safe level)
- Absorbable Magnesium- 400-2,500 mg. a day (citrate or chelate)
- Very low carbohydrate and low-calorie diet
- Lots of fresh raw vegetables

Vitamin C is crucial for a healthy heart. People need not die of heart disease or stroke because evidence suggests that an adequate intake of Vitamin c and other antioxidants would prevent and potentially eliminate these conditions. Orthomolecular physicians have claimed that the cause of heart attacks and strokes is low-grade scurvy. Ignoring these suggestions may have made these diseases the biggest killers of the western world.

The Real Cause of Heart Disease

Conventional medicine's infatuation with dietary fat and cholesterol has stifled research into vitamin c and heart disease since the middle of the twentieth century. The cause of heart disease involves numerous pathways that end in a shortage of Vitamin C, inflammation, and oxidative damage, smoking, high blood pressure, and a high fat diet may contribute to atherosclerosis. But they are not the cause. Some people will live a long life despite being at high risk from all major lifestyle risk factors. Others will die early from rampant atherosclerosis, but be non-smoking vegetarians who have a particular aversion to animal fats. The key feature linking the main risk factors is that they produce free radical damage and increase the requirement for vitamin C.

The human requirement for Vitamin C is one of the most ubiquitous genetic abnormalities for our species. The loss of the ability to synthesize vitamin C appears to be an explanation for the human susceptibility to cardiovascular disease.

One of the most important local hormones regulating vascular tone and blood flow is nitric oxide (NO), which is released by the endothelial cells. It typically acts to dilate blood vessels and increase blood flow. Nitric oxide is dependent on adequate amounts of Vitamin C. NO is an essential early part of the defense mechanism of the arterial wall. Prevention of heart disease requires a minimum of 3 grams of vitamin C. Dr. Pauling and others have proposed the addition of several amino acids.

We have followed the story of Vitamin C from its evolutionary beginnings to its identification as ascorbic acid. In the early years of the 20th Century its classification as a vitamin confused conventional medicine into a rigid paradigm, in which only milligram amounts were deemed "necessary." However, since its isolation, some doctors and scientists have been arguing that people need larger amounts. These doctors were ignored despite reporting effects for large doses of vitamin C.

Soon, healthcare without high-dose nutrient therapy will be considered to be like childbirth without sanitation or surgery without anaesthetic. But, can we afford to wait?

THE LONGEVITY FACTOR
JOSEPH MAROON, M.D.

In the beginning...

The story of discovery may well begin with the formation of the universe 14 billion years ago. "The Big Bang" in which space expansion and particles of the embryonic universe coalesced to fotm the billions of galaxies that now make up the universe, including our own Milky Way, with its billions of stars. After the big bang, heat and radiation were released and subatomic particles were formed-including protons, neurons, quarks, and baryons-all of which became the building blocks of life as we know it. This material cooked until 1.5 billion years ago. When the earth was formed, initially recorded ion Genesis, water completely covered the globe. There was no oxygen- only intense cosmic radiation, turbulent seas, volcanic eruptions and frequent meteoric bombardments from outer space. During the next billion years primary elements needed to support life were formed, including carbon, oxygen, nitrogen, phosphorus, sulphur, magnesium, calcium, copper, and iron.

Synopsis

The Origin of Life

It was from the primordial soup that life developed. RNA (ribonucleic acid) may have been the first complex molecule on which life developed. RNA is the common ancestor that has given rise to major cell lines of life. The first of these belong to a type of bacteria called prokaryotes, which lack a cellular nucleus. 2 to 3 billion years ago bacteria found in ancient rocks from Australia have survived through the millennia.

The second cell line is eukarote. These cells contain a nucleus. This is where the cell's DNA is housed. Eukarotic cells are the basic building blocks of all animal life, from single-celled amoebas to complex human beings.

Cells of the third type, the archae bacteria inhabit hot springs, extremely alkaline or acidic waters. They live in the mud at the bottom of the ocean, and in other hostile places.

The first animal cells appeared 1.5 billion years ago, single cell organisms that were able to reproduce. These cells were protected by a cell membrane formed of protein and fats. They were also able to use raw materials that could be converted into energy. These reactions were facilitated by enzymes.

Enzymes are proteins and act as complex proteins and nucleic acids that make up RNA and DNA. They are critical to the function and survival of all living beings. Yeast was formed 900 years ago . 600 million years ago the first animals, invertebrates such as sponges, jellyfish, worms, and insects made their appearance. Plants-400 million years ago. Vertebrates animals-300 million years ago- 65 million years ago dinosaurs were eradicated. Humans have only a 15,000 year recorded history.

Molecular biology begins in 1859 with Charles Darwin. He explained that life is a competition for survival. Some species were better able to adapt to their environment. His concept of evolution, driven by natural selection was incomplete. Gregor Mendel in 1856 provided the framework for the "code of life." In 1902, Walter Sutton isolated chromosomes in the nucleus of a cell. They are arranged in pairs of 23 in humans. In plants and animals each parent provides half of the pairs, thus mixing different traits from different parents. Wilhelm Johannsen, 20 years after Mendel assigned the name Gene (origin-giving birth to) to the physical and functional unit that controls heredity. In the 1920s, Hermann Muller noticed anatomical changes in fruit flies after blasting them with radiation. In 1946 he won the Nobel Prize for the discovery that x-rays can induce general mutations. Beadle and Tatum shared a 1958 Nobel Prize. They discovered the relationship between enzymes- the protein catalysts responsible for all chemical reactions essential for life.

The brilliant Austrian physicist, Irwin Schrodinger, won the Nobel Prize in physics in 1933. He published a book in 1933 titled "What is

Life?" He wrote, "In these chromosomes, DNA strands formed into paired genes found in the nucleus of a cell, that contain in some kind of code the script for the entire pattern of the individual's future development, and of its functioning in the mature state."

In February, 1953 Watson and Crick stood on the shoulders of giants who preceded them, and launched the modern era of molecular biology.

Causes of Aging

Why do we age? The giant tortoise can live more than 170 years. Moses lived 120 years. Jeanne Calment in Arles, France lived 122 years. She recommended walking and two glasses of red wine a day. The average American born today lives 77.9 years. That's respectable, but it is not as long as citizens of 41 other countries.

What is Normal Aging?

Satchel Paige once asked, "How old would you be if you didn't know how old you were?"

Starting with Clive McKay in the 1930s caloric restriction has been proven to extend one's life span. Ancel Keys, at the University of Minnesota, the Japanese at Okinawa, the biosphere 2 experiment in Tucson, Arizona, and Dr. Leonie Heilbronn, who reported in JAMA (2006) –all demonstrated the effectiveness of caloric restriction in prolonging life.

While the reasons why restricting calories work are still not clear, caloric restriction definitely was able to prolong the healthy, disease-free period of life and postpone rapid decline near the end of life.

Longevity Genes

Sydney Brenner received the Nobel Prize in 2002. In the early 1960s he pioneered the research that studied how genes direct the production of specific proteins. Leonard Guarente studied for 10 years to find the gene that would be the holy grail of aging. He used the lowly yeast- the same form used to make bread, beer, wine, and other spirits for thousands of years. It turned out that by reducing the amount of glucose the yeast fed on – they lived 50% longer. Another observation was that under stress the yeast became sterile. Following international acclaim, Guarente hired a doctoral student in Australia, and David Sinclair became a star researcher. Guarente and Sinclair showed for the first time how caloric restriction increased longevity ion yeast was related to the function of the SIR2 gene. Their findings were confirmed by other researchers. Their conclusions can be summarized as follows:

- Caloric restriction stresses the organism.
- Mechanisms within the cell promote survival.
- SIR2 enzyme levels rise creating an environment in the cells that promote longevity.

Sinclair's team discovered another longevity gene PNC1 which was also activated by restricting calories. SIR1 is the counterpart of SIR2 in mammals. Experiments identified 19 compounds that stimulated SIR1 activity-all of them were found in red wine grapes or other plant sources. All of these but two were polyphenols.

Polyphenols

Polyphenols are the most abundant antioxidants in our diet. They give the red to red wine, the dark brown to chocolate, and the green to green tea. Grapes, apples, onions, soy, peanuts, berries, and other fruits and vegetables are loaded with polyphenols.

Xenohormesis

Hovitz and Sinclair asserted that certain molecules in our food have significant health and longevity-enhancing effects that may turn out to surpass anything current medications can achieve. Remember that Hippocrates, the father of Western medicine said, "let food be your medicine and medicine be your food."

The French Paradox

French people eat more cheese, and nearly 3 times more pork, yet they have about half the amount of heart attacks the Americans suffer. CBS's 60 minutes in 1991 suggested that the French people's consumption of red wine was the reason for the lower rate. How did Resveratrol and the polyphenols in red wine lower cardiovascular risk in the French? The French weren't restricting calories. Was it the antioxidant effect of the polyphenols?

Resveratrol, Quercetin, and Catechins have powerful beneficial biological effects including prevention of heart attacks, cancer, and strokes.

A 2003 paper by Hovitz and Sinclair confirmed that these polyphenols activated the SIRT1 gene, so the French Paradox appeared to have been solved. Xeno factors like Resveratrol are also found in grape juice, berries, peanuts, pistachios, pomegranate juice, and dark chocolate. Resveratrol is found in red and white grape skins. Italian researchers demonstrated that Resveratrol-fed fish increased their swimming activity by one-third. Their experiments proved that muscle and brain function, and increased longevity was the result of Resveratrol treatment.

Raphael de Capo and David Sinclair reported dramatic findings in July, 2008 in "cell metabolism." In summary, Resveratrol showed the following benefits:

- Despite a high-fat diet, the treated mice did not gain weight.
- It prevented diabetes.
- It increased mitochondria in muscle cells.
- It burned body fat.
- It increased aerobic activity.
- It maintained cell sensitivity to insulin.
- It transformed muscle fibers.
- It improved the animals' coordination.
- There were no adverse effects on the liver or other organs.

Dr. Klatz recently stated, "We're looking at a life span for baby boomers of 120 to 150 years of age." In April, 2008 David Sinclair told Barbara Walters that the science of aging has split the atom, "and imminent scientific discoveries will allow us to live 120 to 150 years. Richard Miller at the University of Michigan stated that "if we can produce drugs that can slow down aging in mice or rats, the average person would live to 110 to 115 years."

What Should a Person do?

- Drink wine-two glasses for men-one glass for women.
- Drink grape juice-for non-wine drinkers.
- Drink green tea- EGCG (epigallocatechingallate) protects against inflammation.
- Eat dark chocolate-polyphenols in cocoa have catechins similar to green tea.
- Apples- high in procyanadin and phloridzin.

There are many Resveratrol supplements. It takes 5-7 years to move a pill through the FDA at a cost of about $1 billion dollars. Natural Resveratrol has benefits and it is wise to add it to your supplement regimen. Beware of exaggerated claims from unscrupulous companies.

KNOCKOUT
SUZANNE SOMERS

The trillion dollar cancer business has been nourished by the medical establishment's insistence on treatment. The ultimate solution according to Nobel Laureate Otto Warburg is prevention. His research proved that once a cell becomes cancerous it will never be normal again.

Suzanne Somers' book spotlights the futility of the current treatment modalities of surgery, radiation, and chemotherapy. Her celebrity will help spread the message of some of the outstanding practitioners who are achieving amazing results with alternative protocols.

Unfortunately, the monolith that controls the cancer industry is very powerful and the glacial movement of acceptance in medicine will provide a formidable barrier to the new modalities that are currently being developed.

Synopsis

Julian Whitaker

"Conventional medicine's approach to cancer is a debilitating, often deadly fraud. It is a faulty paradigm." A paradigm is a belief system. Cancer cells proliferate rapidly. All you need do is to stop the cells from dividing, and the cancer will disappear. "I believe cancer can be cured." We are not winning the war on cancer. There is hope. Not everyone survives.

Suzanne Somers

I woke up at 4 A.M., November, 2008. Every inch of my body is covered with welts except my face. We race to the emergency room. I am suffocating. Breathing is all I can think about. They inject Decadron, a powerful steroid. They inject Benadryl for the rash. They put me on oxygen and slowly life returns.

"We have to do a CAT scan." I know that there are large amounts of radiation. This is the first time in 8 years that i have had drugs in me. There are times when drugs and CAT scans are necessary-as a last resort. This was one of those times.

I was wheeled into the CAT scan room. Three more rounds of oxygen and I'm starting to feel normal again. Drugs have been my life saver this time. I'm hopeful that this will be the only time I have to resort to drugs. The radiologist injects dye into me.

"Have you had breast cancer?"

"Yes," I answer.

I'm wheeled into the ER- I want to go home

The doctor says,

"We have very bad news."

"You have a mass in your lung. It looks like cancer. It has metastasized to your liver. Your liver is so enlarged it is filling your entire abdomen. You have so many tumors in your chest we can't count them, and they all have masses in them, and you have a blood clot, and you have pneumonia." We are going to treat the blood clot because that can kill you first."

"Heparin for the blood clot, Levaquin, an antibiotic for the pneumonia, and Ativan to calm me down,

ME-the non-drug advocate. We had so many drugs this morning that my head is spinning.

"My oncologist has the bedside manner of a moose."

"I've never seen so much cancer-It's everywhere."

My children and grandchildren call. I will never see them grow up. I start to cry. This is the most devastating day in my life. Alan is choosing to die with me.

Barry Manilow walks into my hospital room. He can't believe that I have cancer.

I have a biopsy to see if I have cancer. When I come out of the fog of anaesthesia, Alan is talking to me.

"You don't have cancer."

Meet the Doctors

There are pioneers who cure cancer. They are attacked, ostracized, and ridiculed because they are courageous enough to think outside the box.

Dr. Stanislaw Burzynski has found that in the absence of sufficient amounts of antineoplastons, a peptide that is produced in the liver and controls cell multiplication, cancer develops. His theory is that if the peptide is replaced, cancer is knocked out. Many patients have recovered. He has been treating patients for 30 years

The Texas medical board tried to take away his medical license. The FDA tried to put him in jail. There were two trials. Scores of patients passionately supported Dr. Burzynski. He was acquitted on all charges after two federal criminal trials. Throughout this ordeal, Dr. Julian Whitaker was a tireless advocate of Dr. Burzynski's work. His newsletter, "Health and Healing" raised many hundreds of thousands of dollars and helped the Burzynski clinic survive the government attacks. Ultimately, Dr. Burzynski fought the U.S. government and won!

Dr. Nicholas Gonzalez is another maverick. He lives in Manhattan and treats all types of cancers. He offers an aggressive nutritional program and his patients swear by his therapy. His protocol involves diet, supplementation, and intensive detoxification. Dr. Gonzalez is known for his work with advanced cancer. He believes that it is the pancreatic enzymes that target and kill cancer cells.

Dr. James Forsythe's protocol emphasizes good nutrition, a balanced lifestyle that includes exercise, rest, sleep, emotional harmony, detoxification, and treatments that ensure efficient working of the body's organs. On February 16, 2005, the government tried to close his office, put him in prison, and ruin his reputation. He prescribed human growth hormone to a government shill posing as a patient. He was treated like a criminal, ordered to kneel, with a gun at his head. After his false arrest it took 14 months for the acquittal. The jury deliberated for only a few hours

The Birth of a Big Business

When it was announced on Larry King's show that I had breast cancer, I received a phone call from a person in the cancer industry. He said, "The truth is that we want to find a cure for cancer-it's too big a business." Cancer is the disease that keeps hospitals open, and adds an extra $100,000 dollars a year to oncologists' income (a modest estimate).

The doctors you will meet in this book have taken a big financial hit. Rolling in money is not their driving force. What they care about is making people well. Not all patients have the same degree of success. Some will die. I believe cancer is preventable, manageable, and curable, in many cases.

As a nation we are taking pharmaceutical drugs and chemicals at an unprecedented rate. We have a drug for every single human ailment. By the time seniors reach their golden years they can't think from the toxicity, chemicals in our food, preservatives, artificial sweeteners, high fructose corn syrup, etc. They are on a sure route to cancer.

Ralph Moss, Ph.D

Ralph Moss, Ph.D. cut his teeth in the cancer industry as a public relations director for New York's Memorial Sloan-Kettering. He was fired because "I had broken ranks with the party line which had declared that laetrile was completely ineffective. In fact, Laetrile had proven to perform excellently in our animal studies."

Over the last 30 years Dr. Moss has written many books on cancer. His "Cancer Industry" is a classic. His books provide a wealth of information on health and healing. He cites statistical evidence that reveals the shocking truth that chemotherapy is mostly inappropriate, ineffective, and dangerous for most people who receive it. Up to 600,000 Americans every year get chemotherapy at their doctors' recommendations.

Speaking to him was fascinating. His frankness was refreshing. He is a scholar who is not driven by the almighty dollar. " the FDA has never approved any nontoxic drug, herb, vitamin, or any nonpatentable substance for cancer." It's quite enough to know that the FDA acts like a local enforcer for the drug industry. That's what they are.

A study was done in Canada relative to lung cancer and

chemotherapy. When asked, 75% of the doctors said they would not take the platinum-containing therapy themselves. Suzanne-here are two sets of facts. Ten years ago stage IV colon cancer treatment cost $500. Ten years later the cost is around $250,000, and that's only for parts and labor.

Oncologists make money four ways off a drug. First of all they get paid by the patient. Second, they have the chemotherapy concession. They buy the drug wholesale and sell it retail. The third way is to promote a drug and receive an honorarium or a speakers' bureau fee.

"I have looked at the cases of Drs. Gonzalex and Burzynski. They are doing exciting work. They have made advances in cancer and they've helped a lot of people. But their successes are not 100 percent."

Suzanne- "I can't think of anybody in the country who has the ear of more people than you do. I believe that we are seeing a little bit of sunlight. I do see that the system is crumbling. I get going every day for 35 years. I pull up the facts and do not go overboard with my enthusiasm or endorsement of alternative treatments.

Stanislaw Burzynski , M.D. was born in Poland in 1943. He has pioneered the use of peptides (antineoplastons) in preventing and treating cancer since 1967. Burzynski's clinic in Texas has effectively treated fifty types of cancer. I met Dr. Burzynski at the ACAM (American College for Advancement in Medicine) in November, 2008. It was only one week before I was misdiagnosed with full body cancer. His successes are a threat to the orthodox cancer protocols. Those who discredit him ask, "if the treatment is so good, why don't other oncologists jump on board?"

According to Dr. Julian Whitaker, "the paradigm that governs all conventional cancer treatments is "purge the body of cancer cells." If there is an approach that doesn't work, this is it. The death rate for cancer has doubled over the last 50 years. However, the cancer establishment is firmly entrenched and universally accepted.

The chemotherapy business is $200 billion dollars a year. A cure would force all present protocols to halt. Dr. Burzynski arrived in America with $15 dollars in his pocket. He is living his dream of doing the work he loves and living free. His answer to cancer is antineoplastons, but our government tried to put him in jail. He does not have a free hand and the FDA limits him to clinical trials. He has worked within these limits and his patients speak about him with exuberant reverence. In spite of everything, he has carried on.

The Interview

SB   There is a system of peptides which are deficient in cancer patients, which can inhibit the growth of cancer cells. Replacing these peptides kills cancer cells without killing the normal cells.

SB   We are now in phase 3 studies and hope to have FDA approval for marketing soon.

SS   Tell me, what exactly is a peptide?

SB   A peptide is a molecule which is composed of two or more amino acids. If you combine two amino acids through a special chemical bond called a peptide bond, you have a peptide. Protein is a large peptide.

SS   What is a protein?

SB   When you have more than 50 amino acids in a molecule it is called a protein. A molecule with 50 or fewer amino acids is called a peptide.

SB   We can't live without amino acids. 8 amino acids are essential. You would die if you don't have them. Proteins are the building blocks of life.

SS   How many people responf to your treatment?

SB   About 85 percent for whom we have the proper gene signature. About 15 percent don't respond.

SS   You talk about gene-targeted therapy Is that chemotherapy?

SB   No. Antineoplastons are natural compounds. They exist in our blood and form a protective system against cancer.

SS   If a patient comes to you who has been ravaged by chemotherapy and radiation, does that make your job harder?

SB   The majority of patients we see come to us after being told that there is nothing that can be done for them. They have tried everything and we hear horror stories.

SS   I have to ask again. You are saying the cancer doesn't just shrink, it goes away?

SB   Yes. In many cases the tumors go away completely.

SS   How many patients have had a complete response?

SB   It depends on the type of cancer. 58% response in breast cancer. There are types of cancer where mortality rates are 100 percent.

I must say that for pancreatic cancer chemotherapy is doing practically nothing.

SS Why are doctors prescribing it?

SB they are brainwashed.

SS What about liver cancer?

SB There is no reason to use it. Lung cancer is the main cancer killer. Last year there were about 1.3 million deaths worldwide from lung cancer. Last year there were 600,000 deaths. This year we are expecting 700,000 deaths from liver cancer.

SS Do you have the cure for cancer?

SB it is difficult to say I have the cure for cancer, but I have cured a good number of them. It's great to see these people in good shape, leading normal lives.

Dr. Nicholas Gonzalez

Dr. Nicholas Gonzalez is a renegade. He graduated Phi Beta Kappa and Magna cum Laude from Brown University. His honors are numerous. As a medical student he met Dr. William Donald Kelley. He was an eccentric dentist who developed an intensive program for treating advanced cancer with great success utilizing pancreatic enzymes and nutritional approaches. Dr. Gonzalez's treatment protocol is controversial.

Interview

I met Dr. Kelley when I was an immunology fellow under Dr. Good. I turned down a job at Sloan-Kettering and opened up a practice to start using the therapy.

SS This program mainly involves pancreatic enzymes, right?

NG Yes, but Dr. Kelley's program had three basic components. There are ten basic diets and ninety variations. 107 years ago Dr. Beard, a Scottish embryologist said that pancreatic enzymes are our body's main defense against cancer. He put his thesis in a book in 1911. People thought he was insane. He died in obscurity-angry and bitter. Dr. Kelley resurrected the enzyme theory.

NG Diet, supplements, large doses of enzymes, and the third component is detoxification. Routines like the infamous coffee enemas, juice fasts, liver flushes, and other things. It's a three-pronged approach, but essentially it's about pancreatic enzymes.

The first year is most expensive. You buy a juicer, a water filter, and all the supplements. Then there are the enzymes. The whole cost is $12,000, including the office visits and initial valuation which takes four to five hours. It gets less expensive after that. Chemotherapy runs $50,000 to $70,000 easily, and radiation $25,000 easily. You can't patent enzymes –there's no incentive for a drug company to do what we do. They know about my work but hope I get hit by a bus.

SS   Are you affecting their bottom line?

NG   No. last year chemotherapy brought in $100 billion.

SS   Add doctors' fees and hospitalization and it's actually $200 billion.

NG   A stage IV patient who has metastasis, has had no chemotherapy and radiation, and has been diagnosed within two months of seeing us has a 50% chance of doing real well. Chemo and radiation reduces their chances of success.

NG   We turn away patients we don't think we can help because there's no point. There's no benefit to them.

NG   When I met Dr. Kelley I started going through the records whatever my career path was to be. I knew that the guy was reversing cancer. In spite of the fact that Kelley was considered a lunatic, I kept seeing patient after patient with advanced cancer who got well. For me there was no choice. As a scientist you can't walk away from that.

NG   The fact of the matter is that for the major cancer killers-metastatic breast, lung, prostate, and pancreatic- chemotherapy does absolutely nothing...zero.

NG   "These people come to me half dead because they were promised that these treatments work. These people were given regimens that never could have worked, and so often they're dying and we cannot help them because it is too late. They have lost their window of opportunity.

SS   Why is there so much cancer?

NG   It's usually the wrong diet. Electromagnetic contamination is another problem and it's everywhere.

SS   You mean cell phones?

NG   Yes. cell phones. There are thousands of towers giving off electromagnetic fields. Twenty years ago they didn't exist. Computers give off electromagnetic radiation. The food supply for most people, unless you eat organically, is only decreasing in its nutritional content.

SS Tell my readers about diet soda.

NG Richard Wurtman at MIT says aspartame is neurologically toxic. A non-diet soda has ten teaspoons of sugar. The average American eats 160 pounds of sugar annually. The accelerating rate of diabetes is now a clear indicator that we are killing ourselves.

SS Some people think that ketchup is a vegetable.

NG I love that. We treat our cars better than we treat our bodies. No one would think about putting the wrong fuel into their expensive car, but they will go out and put the biggest pile of junk into their mouths.

NG I love coming to work. It's not easy. I treat mostly advanced patients, and not all of them make it. I spend two hours each night returning phone calls. It's an enormous amount of work and there are other ways of making a living.

SS Did you do it for the money?

NG (laughter) if I wanted to make money I'd be a cardiovascular surgeon making $60,000 an operation. They do two a day.

NG The drug companies control medicine and they are very powerful. There are 1,000 full time paid drug industry lobbyists in Washington D.C., that's not counting state capitals. They all get six figure salaries. But I think the truth is powerful and I also believe that truth always comes to the top.

SS What's all this hoopla about the new wonder cancer drug Gemzar?

NG They have compared Gemzar to the previous "best" chemo for pancreatic cancer. Median survival improved from 4.2 months to only 5.7 months—about one extra month of life for this expensive drug. Not a single patient out of the 126 in the study lived longer than 19 months. But Gemzar has been considered such an advance that the FDA approved it, and now it's a billion dollar industry.

SS I am deeply moved by you. Thank you and God bless you.

Dr. Russell Blaylock

Dr. Blaylock is an oncologist, a brain surgeon, and a neuroscientist. He attended Louisiana State University School of medicine and the Medical University of South Carolina in Charleston. After 26 years of practicing neurosurgery, in addition to having a nutritional practice he now devotes his full attention to nutrition and research.

Interview

SS Are most of the treatments for cancer ineffective?

RB If you look at the major cancers, the real killers- like lung, breast, and prostate- they've made no significant inroads in reducing mortality. They've had real success with leukemia. They are overdosing cancers-meaning they are diagnosing a lot of cancers that never would have spread in the first place because they are slow-moving and invading.

SS Why are they doing this?

RB Part of it is they are making a lot of money. Like mammograms, for instance, which all hospitals use- you've got doctors who specialize in this technology. All these things become big money-makers, and then it feeds on itself.

There is evidence that mammograms are not really that diagnostic and may be inducing breast cancer. But so much money is being made that no one wants to admit the truth. Defenders say mammograms are the greatest. As an oncologist, I think to myself, why? You can't cure it. Your chemotherapy is ineffective. And radiation doesn't work so well. So all they can talk about is early diagnosis.

But what these tests are telling us, that the diagnostics are not really accurate, and they are causing a lot of women to have chemo and radiation for no reason at all. This is a big discussion in oncology journals, but the public never hears about it.

SS I've heard that smashing a woman's breast between the plates of the mammogram machine can be damaging. Is that correct?

RB We were taught in medical school and I know long ago that a woman with a lump in her breast every time you squash it, the cells are pushed out into the lymphatic system and the blood vessels, and you are more likely to cause metastasis. But they never tell this to women and women don't know what doctors are saying among themselves.

RB   If I were a woman, I'd never have a mammogram.

SS   What if an MRI scan does find cancer?

RB   If it were me, I would say I'm not having chemotherapy or radiation.   I would have a simple lumpectomy and treat the rest with nutrition

SS   So once again it comes back to nutrition.

RB   the final theory of cancer causation is that it is a disease of chronic inflammation. The number one link is aging. Most cases affect older people. Before age forty it's a very low risk. After 50 it becomes a disease of concern, and at 60 or 70 it increases a lot faster.

SS   What about sugar?

RB   feeding cancer patients sugar is really a cause for malpractice. If you do-they will die sooner.

SS   What's wrong with our medical schools?

RB   medical centers get most of their funding from drug companies. When you give tens of millions of dollars to universities such as Harvard, Yale, Columbia or Duke you're not going to have physicians who are dependent on the drug money criticizing chemotherapy.

SS   What would you give a cancer patient?

RB   I recommend turmeric, flavonoids, and other plant-based nutrients.

SS   Do drug companies want to find a cure for cancer?

RB   The problem is that it is such a big business, if we found the cure the impact would be hundreds of billions of dollars. hospitals, drug companies, and physicians would be impacted enormously.

SS   What other foods protect us from cancer?

RB   berries are very important-blueberries, raspberries, and blackberries. Drink purified water, a little red wine is good, and avoid MSG.

SS   Soy is always surprising. Explain why soy is bad.

EB   avoid all soy foods. Soy products have a high concentration of fluoride, glutamate, and manganese-they are terrible.

Dr, Michael Galitzer

Michael Galitzer is an integrative-anti-aging doctor. He has brilliant instincts and is a proponent of the triad that body, mind, and spirit work together toward the goal of optimal health.

MG   Let's talk about what causes cancer. Healthy cells utilize oxygen to create energy, but, with cancer, instead of utilizing oxygen, cancer cells revert to a primitive way for creating energy by fermentation of sugar.

SS Is this called anaerobic metabolism?

MG   Absolutely, you got it. Anaerobic metabolism is occurring. You want to limit sugar intake. No sugar for any cancer patient. Number two, you must increase the oxygen supply to the cell.

MG   This was discovered by Otto Warburg in the 1920s. He won the Nobel Prize

SS   How do you do that?

MG   Joanne Budwig, a German biochemist in the 1950s discovered that if you combined cottage cheese with flaxseed oil in the diet you could increase the oxygen supply to the cells. The Budwig diet is a mainstay of a lot of therapies. You can look it up on the internet.

SS   What exactly is it?

MG   It's two-thirds of as cup of cottage cheese and six tablespoons of flaxseed oil. You mix them in a blender with berries or nuts. No peanuts.

SS   How would you take this?

MG   Once a day divided into two doses. For maintenance you take half.

SS   What does this do. Why do I want to eat this?

MG   This combo gets to the cell membranes, increases the oxygen level in the cell and can cause increased cellular energy production.

INTELLIGENT MEDICINE
RONALD HOFFMAN, M.D.

The kind of medical care Americans receive today is hardly intelligent. For one thing most orthodox physicians treat the disease, and not the patient. For another, they treat the symptoms of the disease and not the cause.

Dr. Ronald Hoffman has astutely titled his book, "Intelligent Medicine." Since intelligence can be defined as the ability to learn, I assume that the author's credo is to use everything we've learned in his attempt to cure his patients' ailments. His book describes a paradigm shift in medicine-prevention is worth more than the cure.

The comprehensive coverage in this book of the human condition is done with flair and daring. Dr. Hoffman displays the same attention to details as he does on his syndicated radio program on WOR in New York. Healthcare is a dynamic field. We learn more every day. Holistic practitioners are few in number compared to the 600,000 or so orthodox physicians in America. We should therefore appreciate the effort that went into the writing of this book, and learn the valuable lessons of what truly is "Intelligent Medicine."

Synopsis

Let's face it, America's healthcare system is facing unique challenge as we enter the new millennium. But we have far greater knowledge than we've ever had before. We know more about diet, illness, nutrients, etc. We know that physical activity can increase our resistance to disease and prolong life, more than any other time in the past. We have the tools and the knowledge to pursue excellence in health, maximize longevity, and prevent unforeseen crises.

The generation of baby boomers have led a sheltered existence, except for Vietnam veterans. Their first health crisis is somewhat of a shock. Your body has let you down. I personally experienced this feeling when I fell really hard and fractured my shoulder. It was my first confrontation with mortality. I fortunately recovered nearly all of my function. I can swim and play tennis, albeit with a trace of stiffness now and then.

What is it about my parents' lifestyle that has them encountering cancer in their fifties, or heart attacks in their sixties? The American way of life: smoking, drinking, the high-fat, high-sugar diet, sedentary, inactive routine. Their parents, with the same genetic strain, were farmers, poor, physically active, and often lived into their nineties.

Our immune system is under attack. Pasteur developed the germ theory of infection and showed that killed cells from an infected animal can immunize another animal. It is one of the great triumphs of research, from diphtheria to polio. Researchers are looking for new vaccines against Lyme disease and AIDS.

The immune system weakens with age, starting about age thirty. The thymus, which produces T cells, is the size of a walnut in children, a pea in puberty, and almost disappears by the age of fifty. Malnutrition conjures up images of starving children in famine-ridden parts of the world. Yet, so-called well-fed Americans can suffer from malnutrition. Our diet has seen a steady decline in nutritional content over the past forty years. Processed foods have important vitamins and minerals removed from them. Good nutrition turns out to be the best way of strengthening the immune response.

Sugar is an immune suppressive food. A rise in blood sugar can paralyse our immune system. We see this in diabetics. Sugar also inhibits Vitamin C absorption. Refined sugar is not the only culprit, alcohol, simple carbohydrates, or a big plate of spaghetti will rapidly raise the blood sugar. Complex carbohydrates such as whole grains and beans are better for you. They release sugar more slowly, so that blood sugar levels don't swing wildly up or down.

Excessive caloric intake seems to impair immunity. The biggest source of excess calories in the American diet is fat. There is evidence that high-fat diets increase the risk of cancer. The most harmful type of fat is trans-fat, saturated, or hydrogenated artificial fats, normally found in margarine and vegetable shortening. The ideal immune-supporting diet is low-fat, low-cholesterol, and low-sugar, with plenty of complex carbohydrates. Protein is important, since protein deficiency can suppress immune function. The best immune-supporting diet is the salad and salmon diet. It is good for cardiovascular health and the immune system. Studies show that supplements of vitamins and minerals can play an important role in maximizing immune health.

The effect of regular exercise (30-40 minutes, three or four times a week) is just as powerful as the effect of good nutrition in supporting the immune response and slowing its decline with age. Mental attitude is also related to health. Morman cousins showed the world that he could recover from cancer by taking a daily dose of funny movies. We may be approaching the end of the antibiotic age as we know it. There are many new strains of antibiotic resistant diseases. It is imperative to avoid unnecessary antibiotic use. Many Americans demand antibiotics from their doctors when they get a cold or the flu, but antibiotics are useless against viruses.

This is an exciting time for immunologists. New discoveries and breakthroughs are happening yearly. The immune system provides a whole array of natural killer cells, macrophages, and the compounds called gamma interferon, and tumor necrosis factor (TNF). The immune system does decline with age, and the number of cancers rise. But it is tragic that there is a high incidence of mid-life cancer. Immunology is a wide-open field and we are continually learning more about the impact of nutrition on the immune system. It is a low-tech approach that offers exciting new developments in supporting immune health for baby boomers. The field of psychoimmunology treats the nervous system and the endocrine system, and the immune system as one complex interactive field.

50 million Americans are suffering brain and nervous system disorders at a cost of $300 billion dollars annually. Research has been aided through new imaging techniques such as MRI and CAT scans. We can now watch the brain at work with a SPECT scan. While our brain mapping and monitoring activity has become more sophisticated there has been an increasing assault by environmental toxins on all body systems. 60,000 new chemicals have been released into the environment, and the brain and nerves are the tissues most sensitive to them.

Headaches cause 50 million doctors visits and cause $50 billion dollars in lost productivity. Four billion dollars are spent each year on pain relievers alone. Many over-the-counter drugs are not effective and some have harmful side effects. Aspirin, ibuprofen, and naproxen carry the risk of gastrointestinal bleeding. Acetominophen burdens liver function and depletes the crucial antioxidant glutathione. It is more important to find the origin of the pain than to mask it with palliatives and drugs. Headaches arise from many causes, but a common one is a low level of magnesium, which is essential in controlling muscle spasms. A good general magnesium supplement would be 200 milligrams twice a day of magnesium citrate. Diarrhea is a possible side effect.

The brain uses 20% of the body's oxygen and is extremely sensitive to a deficient blood supply. In fact, there is some speculation that most age-related senility is linked to decreased blood flow to the brain. Atherosclerosis (hardening and narrowing of the arteries) reduces the flow of blood and in cases of severe cerebrovascular disease can result in a stroke. Ginkgo biloba increases blood flow in the brain and improves memory in elderly patients.

Alzheimer's disease was first described in 1906. It now affects 10 percent of the United States population over the age of 65 and 20% of those over 75, about 4 million victims in all. More than half of all Americans in nursing homes are suffering from Alzheimer's, a tremendous cost to families and insurers. We don't know enough about the risk factors, preventive factors, or effective treatments. We must take the same proactive approach to Alzheimer's that we now use to prevent heart disease. "Mens sana in corpore sano"- a sound mind in sound body- is not just for the young.

Few people know that the hormones of the endocrine system regulate the function of nearly all the organs and tissues of the body. More than one hundred hormones are secreted by the glands of the endocrine system. Thyroid disease is so common that even conservative estimates claim that it affects 15% of the population. Women are particularly susceptible to thyroid disease. Thyroid hormone is one of the least invasive medications. Thyroid specialist, Dr. Stephen Langer lists over one hundred known symptoms of thyroid deficiency in his book, "Solved: The riddle of Illness." Barnes Basal Temperature Test detects hypothyroidism. As soon as you wake up in the morning, insert the thermometer in your armpit for ten minutes. If your temperature is below 97.4 degrees F for three consecutive days you have a hypothyroid condition.

The adrenal glands sit on top of the kidneys. The adrenal hormone cortisol counters the effects of insulin. When Cortisol is low, insulin may lower blood sugar excessively causing sugar cravings. Weak adrenals may cause blood sugar abnormalities and "sugar disease." Our high carbohydrate sugar-laden diet leads to sugar disease in its extreme form-diabetes. The incubation of this disease is 20 to 30 years. The diet will eventually damage the system. The pancreas, which produces insulin in the Isles of Langerhans, is the key element of health and energy.

We eat such an obscene amount of sugar and other simple carbohydrates it is not surprising that so many Americans succumb to hypoglycaemia (low-blood sugar), diabetes, heart disease, and chronic fatigue. Keeping your blood sugar and insulin level balanced is an important part of maintaining good health in mid-life and beyond. When blood sugar is low, brain cells are starved. To maintain optimal health your body needs to keep a constant balance between glucose and oxygen in the blood stream. When you eat refined sugar (sucrose or table sugar) or even honey, maltose, and maple syrup, it is quickly absorbed into the blood and converted to glucose, upsetting the balance between glucose and insulin.

As blood glucose soars, flooding the body, adrenal hormones sound the alarm and insulin streams out of the pancreas to hold down the blood sugar level. The blood glucose level crashes and results in a second crisis. You feel exhausted, listless, and irritable. This roller-coaster ride leads to powerful mood swings. An individual may succumb to sugar cravings a million times in a lifetime, which leads to an overproduction of insulin and is a precursor of syndrome X resulting in diabetes and heart disease.

Americans love carbohydrates .Our surgeon general's office claims that our eating habits account for two-thirds of all deaths from five of the killer diseases-and diabetes is one of them! Hypoglycemia (low-blood sugar) is increasingly prevalent in our country. It can cause an array of symptoms such as headaches, tremors, hot flashes, fatigue, and panic attacks. Low-blood sugar triggers hunger-especially carbohydrate craving because the brain is starved for glucose. Sugar perpetuates a cycle of craving and hungering. It is best to switch to a diet emphasizing protein and complex carbohydrates which provide the body with a slow and steady release of blood sugar.

Heart disease is America's "number one killer." In 1996, sixty million people had some form of heart disease. In 1993, nearly one million people died of heart disease, 42% of all deaths. Heart disease is listed as the cause of death for four out of five Americans over 65, but more than one-sixth of all people who die of heart disease are under 65. There is a good side to these scary statistics.. Heart disease has started a steady decline since its peak in the 1950s. Lifestyles have changed. We eat a lot of fat. We have changed our attitude toward smoking, and we exercise more.

The most common indicator of heart disease is hardening of the arteries or arteriosclerosis. When the walls of the arteries get thicker and lose their elasticity they can't expand to permit the blood flow needed for the muscles and other organs. This leads to a build up of a porridge-like growth, a fatty substance on the interior walls of the arteries. The inner walls become sticky and attract clots which can grow large enough to completely block a blood vessel. A stationary clot is called a thrombus. In the heart, the death of a tissue is called a myocardial infarction. If a clot occurs in the brain it is called a stroke. This kind of damage will cause the heart and brain tissue to die, it's gone forever. The fear of a heart attack and stroke is enough to scare patients into all kinds of tests from angiograms to bypass operations. There are some people who benefit from these procedures, however, there are other ways of dealing with this problem.

Let us now turn to the subject of cholesterol. When we think of heart disease today, we invariably think of cholesterol. The barrage of media hype bias has established cholesterol as the culprit in heart attacks. It has been drummed into our heads that we should watch our cholesterol level and avoid eating anything high in cholesterol. The food industry has engineered low-cholesterol and cholesterol-free foods with the goal of lowering the incidence of heart disease. Guess what! The cholesterol level in the United States has been about the same for the last one hundred years. But the food industry has prospered. So has the pharmaceutical companies that manufacture the cholesterol-lowering drugs.

Cholesterol is a yellowish, waxy, fat-soluble substance that is found in animal tissues, meats, dairy products, egg yolks, and some oils. Cholesterol is manufactured in every cell in the body, because it is part of the structure of cell walls. 80 percent of its use is the manufacture of bile, the liquid that breaks down foods in the intestine. In sum, cholesterol is indispensible-we couldn't live without it. Most of it is manufactured in the liver. Only a small amount comes from our diet. The total cholesterol is less important than the amount of HDL (high density lipoproteins) of "good" cholesterol that keeps the arteries clear by scavenging fats from the artery wall. The LDL (low density lipoproteins) are the "bad" cholesterol that deposits the fats on the walls of our blood vessels.

How dangerous is cholesterol? Well, it is true that cholesterol is a component of the plaque that blocks our coronary arteries, but it is more complex than that. There are a handful of well-known risk factors that clearly contribute to heart disease. They include smoking, obesity, high blood pressure, sedentary habits, and poor diet.

Physicians are becoming more aware of nutrition lately, but it often seems that their only advice for preventing heart disease is to avoid cholesterol and saturated fat.

The public's awareness of cholesterol lacks an understanding of basic nutrition principles. Products like vegetable oils sit on supermarket shelves with bold "no cholesterol" labels. Consumers buy these products without considering that plants (vegetables) never contain cholesterol. Meanwhile that bottle of vegetable oil may contain a dangerously high amount of saturated fat or hydrogenated oil. This synthetic form of fat is hydrogenated into a solid fat for margarine. The link to heart disease may be incorporated into our cellular structures.

During the last few decades the cholesterol theory has spawned a huge economic bonanza for the food industry, the pharmaceutical companies, the medical complex that includes doctors, researchers, and academia. As Thomas Moore points out in his book, "Heart Failure," there's a vested interest in the cholesterol theory. "A whole medical-industrial-scientific complex feeds on it." The focus on cholesterol has obscured other more serious factors such as sugar, refined flour, margarine, hydrogenated vegetable oil, and food additives.

There are many studies which do not support the cholesterol hypothesis. They showed that people with low, high, and normal cholesterol levels were dying of heart disease. Recently, a Swedish researcher named Uffe Ravnskov did a longer trial (over five years) which showed a significant number of people dying or developing heart disease soon after cholesterol-lowering treatment was started, perhaps because of serious side effects of cholesterol-lowering drugs. In fact, in two cases, researchers who tested cholesterol-lowering as a preventive measure stopped their trials and didn't publish the full results because of side effects. What was the main side effect?- coronary heart disease. Other studies suggest long-term use of cholesterol-lowering may lead to cancer. The number of controlled cholesterol-lowering trials in which total mortality and coronary mortality were reduced equal the number in which they were increased this does not mean that there is no connection between cholesterol and heart disease. It does mean we should consider other factors just as seriously as we do cholesterol.

Does lowering cholesterol increase your life span? Not according to Dr. Taylor and his colleagues at Harvard who found that the net result of lowering cholesterol would be a few days to a few months of of life expectancy. Another respected medial professional, Dr. Eliot Corday, argues against mass cholesterol screening of the adult population. He comments, "we don't know what to do, but we spend billions of dollars... they had no right to go out frightening the hell out of the whole world about cholesterol without having the facts."

An even stranger twist to the cholesterol story is the fact that low cholesterol doesn't mean you're safe. Six percent of middle-aged adults with cholesterol counts below 160 mg/dl have a high risk of dying of lung cancer, liver cancer, respiratory disease, cerebral hemorrage, alcoholism, suicide, and accidents. Dr. William Castelli, a director of the Framingham heart Study has noted that just as many men and women who have a total cholesterol count under 200 have heart attacks as those with a total count over 200. He claims that HDL is the best predictor of a future heart attack. A total cholesterol to HDL ratio higher than 4.5 to 1 puts you in the high-risk category.

The cholesterol theory has scared people away from high cholesterol foods like eggs and butter, and created a market for margarine and egg substitutes. The surprising fact is that in most humans, dietary cholesterol actually has a minimal effect on the amount of cholesterol in the blood. The dangers of eating eggs and butter have been highly exaggerated. Look at your triglyceride level. If it is over 120 you should lower the amount of carbohydrates in your diet. A high carbohydrate diet can overload your body with glucose and increase your triglyceride level. Cholesterol is simply one of the several factors in a dynamic metabolic balance.

The American diet is a ticket to disaster. Although there is not one diet for everyone, there are some guidelines to follow in choosing what to eat. A basic principle in food selection is to choose foods that are rich in vitamins and minerals, fiber, and protein, and have a minimum of calories. Such a food is nutrient-rich salmon. It's loaded with protein, Vitamin A, selenium, and heart-healthy omega-3 oil. Another is broccoli, which has fiber, Vitamin C, the carotenoids, calcium, and cancer-preventive indoles. Think vegetables and fruits. They have fewer calories and animal studies show they sharply reduce the incidence of cancer and prolong life.

These days every major media is trumpeting the low-fat, low-cholesterol diet. Supermarkets boast that almost every product on their shelves is cholesterol-free. People believe that "fat is the calorie stuff that makes you fat and has something to do with heart disease, so eliminate fat and you'll stay slim forever and never die. Right? Wrong! The low-fat mania has resulted in excessive consumption of high-calorie foods like low-fat desserts, cookies, breakfast pastries, and pasta products made with refined flour.

I recommend the salmon and salad diet. The diet is extremely healthful and beneficial for weight loss, cholesterol, and blood pressure reduction, and control of diabetes. There are three key groups in the salmon and salad diet-the foods to emphasize, the foods to eat in moderation, and the foods to avoid. Fresh salmon, trout, tuna, and mackerel are good protein sources and contain beneficial omega-3 oils. You can also eat shellfish, shrimp, and lobster. Despite their cholesterol content eggs don't increase blood cholesterol levels. Skinless breast of turkey, chicken, and legumes and tofu are allowed. Eggs are exceptional (poached, hard-boiled, or scrambled). Drink herbal teas, fresh vegetable juice, and healthful green drinks which contain phytonutrients.

REVERSE HEART DISEASE NOW
STEPHEN T. SINATRA, M.D., JAMES C. ROBERTS, M.D., WITH MARTIN ZUCKER

Dr. Sinatra's Story

Dr. Jacob Rinse, 91 inspired Dr. Sinatra to learn that there was more to medicine than just drugs and surgery. That was the start of my career in integrative medicine. I recommended vitamin C and vitamin E, and talking about exercise. I went for a degree in nutrition. In the early 1980s I learned about CoQ10. It is critically important for the pumping of the heart. Plus it prevents the formation of plaque. I found major benefits using B vitamins, fish oils, green tea, etc. They unclogged arteries and my practice turned from crisis management to crisis prevention-from illness to health. My challenge became stabilizing and reversing plaque.

Dr. James C. Roberts

After years of treating patients with the same problems over and over, I began thinking seriously about prevention and alternatives after seeing several older patients with alarmingly high cholesterol levels, but totally normal coronary arteries. They were taking vitamins. I started putting patients on vitamins C, D, B-complex, magnesium, CoQ10, and selenium.

Prevention kept most of my patients out of the hospital. Today I regard a hospital admission as a failure on my part. My patients take their necessary medications. They also take supplements that minimize the damage to their arteries and heart cells. Over a 10-year period this approach has revolutionized my practice. Smart medicine doesn't choose sides.

Inflammation leads to blockages. If cholesterol was the cause of blocked arteries then everyone with heart disease would have high cholesterol. Yet half of all heart attacks occur in individuals with normal cholesterol.

The new paradigm in cardiology identifies inflammation as the most important factor in the formation of plaque and arterial disease. We predict that plaque reversal will become the new buzzword.

We may prescribe a cholesterol-lowering drug because it beats down arterial inflammation. We may start you on a regimen of fish oil, magnesium, CoQ10, niacin, Vitamin C, and nattokinase. They offer life-saving benefits without side effects.

We are more concerned with homocysteine. We check Lp(a), fibrinogen, ferritin, and C-reactive protein (CRP). We want to know the calcium score in your coronary arteries. It predicts heart attack risk better than traditional tests. "We can't change your present, but we can influence your future."

Inflammation is the body's first line of defense against injury or infection. It is what causes a burn to turn red or a bruise to swell. It's nature's design to help heal. But if it becomes chronic it can lead to disease.

The women's health study in 2000 revealed the role of inflammation in CVD. 28,000 healthy post-menopausal women put a new risk factor into the spotlight-C-reactive protein (CRP). People with the highest level of CRP had five times the risk of developing CVD and four times the risk of a heart attack or stroke compared to those with the lowest level. Paul Ridker led the study.

The CRP link explains why more than half of heart attack and stroke victims have normal cholesterol levels. We have moved so far in recent years that the model of diseased arteries clogged with cholesterol-laden plaque is as outmoded as the typewriter.

Life-threatening plaque is now regarded as an inflammatory injury- a lesion- that develops like a boil along the inner surface of arterial walls. The process unfolds slowly. In others, the deterioration occurs fast, leading to vessel closure, stoke, or sudden death.

The heart and its network of blood vessels deliver oxygen and metabolic fuel to the cells. The heart is a fist-sized cone-shaped muscular pump wrapped around four chambers. The chambers are connected by a series of one-way valves that let the blood flow in one side and out the other. Oxygen-poor "used" blood returning to the heart collects in the right atrium and is funnelled into the the right ventricle, which pumps it into the lungs to pick up oxygen. Oxygenated blood returns to the left atrium, passes through the mitral valve into the left ventricle, and is pumped out with great force into the main artery of the body, the aorta. From the aorta, other arteries branch off to feed the body including the two coronary arteries that supply the heart muscle.

Blood moves through the 60,000 miles of blood vessels known as the circulatory system. We are most concerned with the innermost layer of the artery wall known as the endothelium. A healthy endothelium allows for normal expansion and relaxation of blood vessels. Inflammation develops from a less than healthy lifestyle. Unhealthy habits include overeating refined packaged, and processed foods with lots of sugar, unnatural fats, and chemical preservatives, and not eating fresh fruits and vegetables and not drinking enough water, smoking, and not being physically active.

Circulation reported that 20 to 35 percent of people (14-35) autopsied after homicides, auto accidents, or suicide already had a major lesion in the coronary arteries. The major cardiac hotspots are the left main coronary   artery- the Left Main." The lesion grows and attracts CRP and fibrinogen. Plaque begets plaque. If you have it in your coronary arteries you most likely have it in your carotids and aorta. At some point, calcium becomes deposited in the arterial walls. Calcium makes up one-fifth of the plaque and contributes to the hardness. Hardened, constricted arteries cause the heart to work harder to pump blood through the narrower blood vessels. This can lead to angina-chest pains- associated with heart disease.

Many people with plaque-ridden arteries live well into their eighties and nineties- as long as the plaque is stable. Heart failure occurs if the heart cannot pump sufficient amounts of blood to the rest of the body. Fluid accumulates in the lungs, ankles, or legs creating general fatigue and shortness of breath.

Inflammation causes the plaque to rupture, and that is what kills most of the time. We used to call this stenosis. Now we call it plaque rupture. In emergency rooms we apply clot-busting medication. Then we do bypass surgery or dilate the narrowing and place a stent. This saves lives and limits heart muscle damage.

Years ago cardiologists couldn't understand how a cholesterol level over 300 did nothing to some patients. This was the cholesterol paradigm, a misconception dominating cardiology thinking for decades. Patients would say they had been taking vitamins and antioxidants. We were conventional cardiologists getting lessons from our patients. Cholesterol is not the culprit. Nature didn't equip you with a system designed to kill you. Contrary to cholesterol's negative reputation, you and your body cannot function without it. The liver produces about 800 mg a day.

Cholesterol is a fatty substance that is not soluble in water. If you eat cholesterol-rich foods your liver makes less. If you eat less cholesterol, your liver makes more. Cholesterol is wrapped in protein so it can travel through the circulatory system. HDL (high density lipoprotein) acts like a garbage truck, picking up oxidized LDL and bringing it back to the liver. LDL (low density lipoprotein) contributes to the many cholesterol needs of your body. It has gotten a bad wrap.

Lp(a) acts as a beneficial repair molecule, an artery patch. Too much Lp(a) is dangerous- it promotes the formation of blood clots on top of plaque. This narrows the vessel and worsens symptoms . In 1956, the American Heart Association used the conclusions of Ancel Keys (Seven countries Study) and the Framingham Study, and declared that, "the cause of heart disease was butter, lard, beef, and eggs." The medical world thus settled into a "cholesterol is the cause of heart disease" paradigm. Currently, the official target level for total cholesterol is 200 mg/dl or less and 40 mg/dl or higher for HDL. Though lower cholesterol may mean lower cardiovascular mortality, people with higher cholesterol have less cancer, respiratory failure, automobile accidents, and suicides.

Relevant studies point to the fact that high cholesterol is not the killer it has been made out to be. The tragedy is that the United States and the rest of the Western world has become obsessed with removing a substance from the body that nature intended us to have. In the new cardiology we think cholesterol is only a problem if is oxidized and contribute to the inflammatory cascade.

The Awesome Foursome

CoQ10, Magneium, D-ribose,and L-Carnitine. They energize heart muscle cells and the rest of you

Supplement Program

Multivitamin/mineral program
Fish oils   2-4 grams
Magnesium   400-800 mg
CoQ10   100 to 300 mg
L-Carnitine   1-3 grams
L-Arginine   6-8 grams
Detox   1 oz. twice a week
Nattokinase   400 units a day
Lumbrokinase   20 mg capsules
Vitamin C   at least 1,000 mg
B-complex vitamins
Vitamin E   200 IU
Garlic   1,000 mg
L-Lysine   2,000 twice a day
L-Proline   1,000 mg twice a day

The Future of Cardiology

The future of cardiology requires patients to do their share. We must integrate the principles of a holistic approach. There is still antagonism in medicine by orthodox physicians who don't tolerate alternative modalities.

However, the bitterness and badmouthing seem to be receding. The future must bring about a union in which there will be a separate alternative medicine and conventional medicine. Instead we must have smart medicine in which physicians consider combinations of nutrition, lifestyle, pharmacology, and surgery to prevent or treat CVD. Hopefully, the union will occur in time to help you and your family, and before our expensive disease management approach bankrupts the Medicare and Medicaid programs.

THE PH MIRACLE DIET
ROBERT O. YOUNG AND SHELLEY REDFORD YOUNG

The pH Miracle Diet is a medical breakthrough in the understanding of the basic cause of disease. Dr. Young's concept is a major contribution to natural healing. It is a continuation of the brilliant work of Antoine Beauchamp and Claude Bernard who taught that a person's (psychic, physical, and biochemical) was the most important factor in whether a person remained healthy.

Florence Nightingale in the 1850s said, "The swamp breeds mosquitos, the mosquitos do not create the swamp." Even Pasteur, on his deathbed stated that the terrain is everything-Claude Bernard was right.

When you create a healthy pH, you create a disease resistant body. The healthiest pH level is 7.46. Dr. Young teaches us to minimize especially sweet fruits in our diet. The other components of the healthy alkalizing diet are good hydration, high oxygen intake, and a highly mineralized food intake. This book is a classic in natural healing literature.

Synopsis

The work of some great pioneers has been overlooked by the medical mainstream. Medicine is so deeply mired in their own myths that it is blind to larger truths, until now.

It's all about balance- pH balance. When imbalance occurs, we get the signs of disease. Imbalance causes low energy, fatigue, poor digestion, excess weight, foggy thinking, aches and pains, as well as major disorders. This book is about reclaiming balance, energy, mental clarity, smooth operation of all body systems. Clear bright eyes and skin, and a lean, trim body. This book will show you how all that can be yours in a few weeks.

Most people you see today are obese. Chances are that one person you love is suffering from the top three killers- heart disease, cancer, and diabetes. We've forgotten that it is natural to die- and to live- healthy. In fact it is your birthright to live healthy, right up until the day you die. The good news is simple, and available right here and now. Today all three top killers are directly linked to diet. Eating the proper foods will help you avoid all that.

America's agribusiness industry and the advertising world have misled us about the food sold in our grocery stores and served in our fast-food restaurants. The result? We are a country that is fatter than ever and we're certainly no healthier.

Forget cholesterol, forget calories, forget blood pressure, blood sugar, hormone levels. It turns out that the single most important measurement to your health is the pH level of your blood and tissues. How acidic or alkaline it is.

The goal is to create the proper balance within your body. The way to do that is by eating the proper balance of alkaline and acidic foods. That means that 80% of your diet must be alkalizing-foods such as green vegetables.

That's it. That's all there is to it. I guarantee you'll see immediate improvement. Your energy will increase. You'll look better. With the healing you'll experience vibrant, energetic, personal health. Shelley and I have been on the pH miracle diet for more than ten years. We'll never go back. Even as we get older, we keep feeling better. We invite you to begin this journey and experience the results for yourself.

It's all About Alkalinity

The pH balance of the human bloodstream is one of the most important biochemical balances in all of the human body chemistry. The human body is meant to be alkaline, but all body functions produce acidic effects. Overacidification of body fluids and tissues underlies all disease. Good health requires a body in proper acid-base balance. Proper diet and lifestyle choices (like the ones laid out in this book) are the only way to ensure that.

pH stands for "Potential Hydrogen." The scale is 0-14. On that scale

7 is neutral. Below 7 is acid and above it is basic or alkaline. A pH of 5-acid is ten times as alkaline as a pH of 6; a pH of 8 is ten times as alkaline as a pH of 7 Acidity reveals itself in seven stages:

- Loss of energy.
- Sensitivity and irritation (as in IBS).
- Mucus and congestion.
- Inflammation.
- Hardening of soft tissue.
- Ulceration.
- Degeneration (cancer, heart disease, stroke, AIDS, ALS, MS, and diabetes).

Microforms

Bacteria, yeast, fungus, and mold are biological transformations of you and live and thrive in acidity. They have to swim in their own waste products. They also love the low oxygen levels that come with acidity. All that is required in alkalizing your blood and tissue pH are appropriate nutritional supplements and an alkaline lifestyle. Then your body goes from acid back to base. Bacteria, yeast, fungus, and mould stop developing. Then you once again become benign. Their left-over toxins can be bound up by certain fats and alkaline minerals and eliminated from the body.

Acid imbalance is perfectly natural--when we're dead. When our body stops breathing, oxygen levels decrease, creating the anaerobic (without oxygen) environment in which microforms thrive. Biologists call it the carbon cycle. It is the literal meaning behind "ashes to ashes, and dust to dust." Acid is what makes our corpses rot. (the scary part is that it does the same thing to us while we are living). "When we are acidic we are basically rotting inside."

You can check your pH levels at home with pH paper strips, available at many pharmacies. The strips are inexpensive and should be easy to test in saliva or urine. You are better off testing our urine. Ideally, it will be mildly alkaline: pH at 7.2 or higher. If you find that your results are below 7.0 you can correct it immediately by eating alkaline food like cucumber, broccoli, asparagus, or avocado, or taking 3 tablespoons of mineral salts in 6 ounces of water. It is best to rest your urine and do it first thing in the morning. The ideal blood pH is 7.365

The blood never lies. It is a direct reflection of your health and what you are eating and drinking, etc. There are only two types of blood: healthy and unhealthy! The pH Miracle diet and lifestyle program restores health, harmony, and balance to your body through a diet of alkalizing vegetables, sprouted and soaked nuts and seeds, essential oils, unprocessed salts, low-sugar fruits, and alkaline water.

Symptoms and Disease

Symptoms are just indications that you are overly acidic. Symptoms are caused by acidic food and lifestyle choices. The so-called disease is a general, underlying condition of acidity. Germs are just the expression of the underlying so-called disease. It is the acid that kills, not the associated germs.

There is almost no research where the problem is and where the solution lies... at the intersection of nutrition and blood. There is only "one" disease and that disease is acidosis. As you restore a healthy balance in your body's environment on a basic (alkaline) diet, you will stabilize at your ideal weight. If you are excessively thin, it is no healthier than being overweight. Healthy bodies are not overweight or underweight.

Allergies

Allergies are 100% reversible with an alkaline diet and lifestyle. Ten foods that cause allergic and acidic reactions:

- Dairy products
- Meat and shellfish
- All forms of sugar
- Vinegar
- Mushrooms and algae
- Peanuts and peanut oil
- Corn
- Fermented foods (soy sauce and miso

- Eggs
- Alcohol

Fatigue

Fatigue is the first stage of overacidity and microforms are the major players in chronic fatigue.

Diabetes

Low blood sugar (hypoglycaemia) and high blood sugar (diabetes) are really just low energy and high acidity- they are rampant today and devastate a lot of lives. They both stem from dietary and metabolic acids. Sugar is not a source of energy. The more sugar we eat, the more we risk an increase in bacteria, yeast and moulds. The solution is straightforward, cut out all forms of sugar, eliminate animal proteins, and get regular exercise.

High Cholesterol

If your body is acidic, the liver increases cholesterol production to buffer those acids. Cholesterol is there to help us. It isn't cholesterol that causes heart attacks and strokes-dietary acids do. We have been trained to avoid high cholesterol at all costs, but lowering cholesterol with drugs, without lowering our exposure to acids, is a recipe for disaster.

Foods to Avoid

Meat, eggs, and dairy
Processed and refined foods
Yeast products and grains
Fermented foods
Artificial sweeteners
Sweet fruit
Natural and artificial sugars
Alcohol, coffee, and chocolate
Black tea and sodas

Alkalizing Foods

Vegetables
Avocado
Tomato
Cucumber
Bell pepper
Grapefruit
Lemon
Lime
Sprouted seeds, nuts, and grains
Grains are acidifying-raw foods are alkalizing
Cooked food is more acidifying
COWS - stands for "chlorophyll, oil, water, and salt
Chlorophyll comes from green vegetables
O is for oils (essential fats)
EFAs are essential fatty acids
Polyunsaturated fats such as flaxseed and hemp oils eliminate acids
W is for water (alkaline water)
The body is 70% alkaline water
Eyes are 98% alkaline water
Blood is 94%

Getting the right water is the most important part of the pH miracle plan for health. You should drink two and one half to three litres of fluid a day, the amount we lose each day through breathing, sweating, moving, even sleeping. If you don't get enough water, you'll get fat. An acidic body pulls water into the tissues to try to neutralize the acids there. Lack of water can kill you. Avoid dehydration. Most people exist in a chronic state of low-level dehydration for most of their lives. No wonder so many of us are fat and sick and tired!

S- for Salt

We cannot live without healthy alkalizing salt. It is as important to our bodies and our health as water or air. We need all three to survive. Our bodies contain about a pound of salt. Our blood, sweat, and tears all contain salt. So does our saliva. In fact, all our body fluids are salty. Without enough salt we get muscle cramps, dizziness, and exhaustion. We need to replenish the salt the body uses up in maintaining our normal health, vigor, and alkalinity.

We are right when we think that salt is bad for us. Standard, overprocessed, demineralised salt is bad for us. The average person eats four to six thousand milligrams of salt each day. Table salt is absolutely useless and potentially destructive.

You cannot consume too much natural, unrefined salt. Salt that hasn't been processed is full of minerals, is healthy, and alkaline. The salt will provide potassium, calcium, magnesium, and every known trace mineral. Sea salt, Celtic salt, Himalayan salt, and real salt from Redmond, Utah are recommended. One teaspoon in 3 ounces of alkaline water, three times a day will keep your pH at 7.2 or above. Sodium bicarbonate or baking soda can be used with mineral salts. It has a pH in the 8s. Raw foods are the best because they contain electrical energy or life force. Fresh organic foods (think salads, great big salads are preferable. They are more nutritious as well.

What to eat and What to Avoid

There are thousands of alkaline vegetables. We need them for overall energy reserves and good health. Government guidelines recommend 5 to 6 servings of fruits and vegetables a day. We really should be easting 3 to 4 times that!

Some of the vegetables on the list are:

Asparagus	Onions
Broccoli	Peas
Cabbage	Radishes
Carrots	Red, yellow, and green
Celery	peppers
Scallions	Turnips
Eggplant	Water chestnuts

In addition- avocados, tomatoes, sprouts, lemons, non-sweet grapefruit, pomegranates, herbs and spices, vegetable juices

High-carbohydrate vegetables like potatoes, winter squash (acorn, butternut, and pumpkin), yams, and sweet potatoes can be eaten in moderation. Make sure they are fresh.

Protein

The average American who eats meat, eggs, and dairy gets 75 to 125 grams of protein a day. That is -3 to 5 times more than we actually need. I believe protein should comprise 5 to 7 percent of our total healthy diet. Our bodies are just 7 percent protein. Some of the strongest animals in the world, the gorilla, the horse, and the elephant eat no meat. They eat grass and leaves.

"We eat fish once every month. We eat tofu a couple of times a month. All the protein we need we get from greens. Eating more protein than you need can make you tired, weak, and sick. Animal proteins contribute sulphuric, phosphoric, and uric acid to the body.

This revised edition has made a significant and healthy step away from recommending all forms of soy as part of the diet. The decrease in emphasis on soy shows how the evolution of thinking as new information emerged since the first edition.*

* Gabriel Cousens, M.D. (from the preface)

What to Avoid

Sugar (all forms of sugar). Avoid white sugar, brown sugar, beet sugar, cane and corn syrups, maple syrup, honey, molasses, sucrose, fructose, maltose, lactose, glucose, mannitol, sorbitol, galactose, monosaccharides, date sugar, turbinado sugar, candy, soft drinks, pastries, ice cream, chocolate, carob, and even sugars from fruit.

Simple carbohydrates are acidic. Skip junk food. That means chips, cookies, doughnuts. Stay away from fast-food restaurants.

Sugar is sugar and acid is acid. It doesn't matter if it is honey or maple syrup. Fruit juice is even worse-acid sugars are more concentrated.

Dairy Products

All dairy products produce lactic acid. Cheese and yogurt are made by fermentation. Dairy products form sticky mucus. It is highly acid forming.

Pasteurized milk left out will rot and stink, whereas raw milk curdles naturally and is edible. Eliminate dairy products and try soy, almond, or hemp milk. If you must have milk, use unprocessed goat's milk. Milk is simply not a human food. It takes 240 cups or 15 gallons of something alkaline to neutralize one cup of ice dream.

Fats

The wrong fats are villains. Hydrogenated or partially hydrogenated vegetable oil, margarine, butter, saturated fats, and most all fats from meat, poultry, eggs, and dairy should be eliminated from your diet because all of these are dangerous. The good fats are olive oil, flaxseed, and grape seed.

Meat and Eggs

All animal products –meat, pork, beef, lamb, chicken, and turkey and eggs are filled with acidic hormones, pesticides, steroids, antibiotics, etc. And the saturated fats contribute to heart disease, strokes, and cancer. Don't have anything to do with them. Humans are designed to be vegetarian.

Alcohol

Alcohol is an acid. This includes wine, beer, whiskey, gin, rum, and vodka.

Caffeine

Chocolate, cocoa, tea, sodas, and all forms of coffee are acidic.

Artificial Sweeteners

Aspartame (Nutrasweet), saccharine (Sweet and low), sucrose (Splenda) etc. Are acidifying. Safe sweeteners are natural plant sources such as Stevia and chicory

THE SECRETS OF PEOPLE
WHO NEVER GET SICK
GENE STONE

The search for "The Fountain of Youth" continues. This work adds 25 ways to extend the quality of life and live until 100 years of age. It is important where you live, what you eat, your supplement regimen, and your exercise level. The lessons in this book will help to improve your chances to achieve Ponce De Leon's dream of living a long and healthy life.

Synopsis

Blue Zones

The geographic areas which have the highest concentrations of the world's longest-lived people: So far five blue zones have been confirmed.

- Barbagia, Sardinia, Italy- shepherds frequently live over 100 years.
- Okinawa, Japan- has the most centenarians in the world.
- Loma Linda, California- 9,000 Seventh Day Adventists are the longest-lived people in America.
- Icaria, Greece- the highest percentage of ninety-year olds on the planet.
- Nicoya, Costa Rica- strong family and social networks, a commitment to the environment. This prolongs lives. They enjoy a healthy diet in nutrients and calories, don't overeat, many centenarians.

Brewer's Yeast

Barbara Davis is an 83-year old who uses Brewer's Yeast as the core of her program. B-vitamins, minerals, etc. Are essential for growth. They are good for healthy hair, skin, nerves, blood cells, hormone producing glands, and the immune system. Brewer's Yeast is a good source of selenium, copper, iron, zinc, potassium, magnesium, and chromium.

Caloric Restriction

George Burns, the legendary comedian died in 1996, just after his one hundredth birthday. His secret was eating half as much as most people. Many studies show the benefits for longevity by restricting calories. Unfortunately, most people are unwilling to eat only half the food on their plates.

Chicken Soup

I learned from my sixth grade teacher that consuming several bowls of chicken soup a week prevents colds. She learned this from her mother, who learned it from her mother. Chicken soup is called the "Jewish Penicillin." Irwin Ziment, M.D. at the UCLA School of Medicine found that chicken soup contains an amino acid called Acetyl cysteine-which is prescribed for bronchitis and other respiratory ailments.

Cold Showers

Cold showers have been around for a long time. The Greeks, the Egyptians, and the Romans believed in hydrotherapy as a way to treat disease. Paul Newman dipped his face in a bucket of ice-cold water to keep his skin taut and healthy. Cold showers are making a comeback. Proponents claim that they:

- Improve circulation
- Strengthen the skin
- Bolster the immune system

- Better you mood
- Invigorate your body

Detoxification

Toxic substances must be eliminated from the body. Some of the culprits are synthetic chemicals, metals, and unhealthy foods. If you detox, your health will improve.

Eating raw foods, organic foods, and fasting will help you clear your body of unwanted chemicals and other toxic products.

Garlic

Early civilizations used garlic to treat fevers, inflammation, and injuries. Sumerians, Egyptians, Israelites, Romans, and Greeks were aware of the benefits of garlic.

Herbal Remedies

Chinese medicine has used herbs for thousands of years. 5,000 herbs have been studied for their medicinal benefits.

Hydrogen Peroxide

The applications of hydrogen peroxide are myriad: making rocket fuel, removing ear wax, whitening teeth, bleaching hair, cleaning clothes, vegetables and fruits.

Lifting Weights

Weightlifting is good for health. Barbells have made weightlifting more practical and efficient. Strength training can help to build and maintain healthy muscles, bones, and joints. It can lower your biological age. It is good for seniors. It rejuvenates the body, provides energy, and fortifies the immune system.

pH Balance

Your health is entirely dependent on your acid/alkaline balance. The term pH means "potential hydrogen." pH is measured on a scale of 0-14. 7 is neutral.

Most vegetables are alkalizing, especially leafy greens, but raw and cooked green beans, asparagus, carrots, and collards are safe bets. Some fruits are alkalizing, including cucumbers, coconuts, and avocados.

Probiotics

The term probiotics was coined in 2001 by the food and agriculture organization of the United Nations which defines them as "live microbes which when administered in adequate amounts confer a health benefit on the host." Probiotics increases the population of friendly bacteria.

Vitamin C

"Vitamin C and the Common Cold" was written by Double-Nobel Laureate Linus Pauling in 1970. He recommended megadoses of vitamin C for optimal health. It is one of the best antioxidants. Pauling and Dr. Robert Cathcart believe that megadoses of vitamin c are effective in treating diseases ranging from cardiovascular disease to cancer. It is ironic that the medical establishment's attacks on Pauling and Vitamin c provided the catalyst for its widespread popularity.

Although the powerful pharmaceutical industry still manages to downplay the benefits of vitamin C many people still find it prevents colds and viruses when taken in the proper dosage.

THE IMMORTALITY EDGE
MICHAEL FOSSEL, M.D., PH.D. GRETA BLACKBURN AND
DAVE WOYNAROWSKI, M.D.

Telomere biology represents a paradigm shift in medical research. It is now possible to dream of the day when we can delay our mortality and promise us a long and healthy life. Telomeres determine the life span of a cell. They don't cause aging, but they do play an important role in controlling the aging process. Carol Greider, Elizabeth Blackburn, and Jack Szostak were awarded the Nobel Prize in 2009 for their research on the role of telomeres and chromosomes, and for the discovery of in 1984 of telomerase by Greider and Blackburn. Telomerase is an enzyme that causes the ends of chromosomes to grow. What these scientists discovered will inevitably lead to a universal cure for all forms of cancer. They have indeed discovered the secret of immortality.

Synopsis

Breakthroughs in DNA research have made it possible to extend your life expectancy beyond 100 to 120 years while maximizing your strength and vitality. Imagine a centenarian playing with his great-grandchildren and still having a great sex life. All this and more is possible, without worrying about the degenerative diseases that plague older people. It sounds too good to be true, but it isn't.

The double helix, twisted strands of DNA, on which genes are found contain our chromosomes. They are organized in pairs, like two sausages, every single cell has 46 chromosomes-one from the mother and one from the father. The DNA in our chromosomes defines everything about us- every genetic trait that we inherit. Chromosomes are important to all forms of life. They are found in every living thing.

Telomeres can be compared to aglets, the plastic caps at the ends of shoelaces. Aglets keep shoelaces from falling apart at the ends, telomeres keep the ends of DNA from fraying. Infants have long telomeres-adults have shorter telomeres. Adults who have longer telomeres are destined to live a long life.

High levels of stress hormones, inflammation, insulin, and blood sugar etc. Are all linked to shorter telomeres and lower telomerase levels. The trillions of cells that make up a person continue to divide, grow, and replicate. With each cell division a few base pairs at the tips of the chromosomes (telomeres) are lost, until the critical limit is reached. Telomeres die when they become too short. Leonard Hayflick must have been correct after all. He is known for the "Hayflick Limit." However, scientists have found that telomeres in some cells become shorter, but a few telomeres become longer. The reason is the biochemical catalyst or enzyme telomerase.

After many months of failed experiments, Blackburn and Greider discovered the enzyme telomerase. It is present in germ cells and cancer cells. These cells never reach senescence. The telomerase gene is found in all other cells, but normal cells don't express telomerase because that gene is repressed in them. The key to immortality is turning the telomerase gene from off to on.

We have a goal in creating "The Immortality Edge" program. We want you to be forever young and disease-free. If you keep your telomeres long enough and grow them even longer, you will never have to face the deterioration of getting old. You will remain forever young.

How Will the Earth Hold us All?

It stands to reason that life extension will increase the world's population. In just over a century, the average life expectancy of a person living in the United States has increased from 47.3 years in 1900 to 78 years in 2008. Technologies such as vaccines, antibiotics, chemotherapy, and antioxidants have contributed to this, but something interesting has also happened. The birth rate fell rapidly, and the average number of children in the U.S. was more than cut in half from 6 to 2.4.

Today, population researchers think the world is headed quickly to a stable population as resources become scarce, prices rise, and as prices rise, family sizes shrink. Let's be realistic. Unless this book outsells the bible, we don't have much to worry about.

How many people even want to have an indefinite life span? We think it is sad that most people accept death as inevitable, and it will be a very long time before the majority realizes that this is no longer the only option.

Death is not Inevitable

A famous neuroscientist, Anders Sandberg points out that "every time a human being dies, a library burns." It is a horrible tragedy that all our life experiences get lost, "both the good and the bad." It is worth stating again and again, "Death is not inevitable." Aubrey de Grey, the Oxford biogerontologist is quoted as saying, "once we are able to implement comprehensive repair and maintenance technologies, we'll be able to do the same for the human body. The first human being to live one thousand years is already among us." He is referring to the "one-hundred-year old cars that are working just as well as they did when they rolled off the production line."

If you believe that you have no purpose in life and nothing to contribute to other people, then this book is not for you. However, if you are living as long as possible, then you can achieve more and become a more valuable person.

There are many ways to keep your telomeres long and healthy. You can start today by eating telomere friendly foods, exercising the right way, meditating, taking supplements, and making other lifestyle changes. By reading this book you will be part of the first group of human beings to blast through the "Hayflick Limit."

The Aging Cure

Unlike germ cells, some cells contain a gene that controls the production of telomerase, and this gene is turned off. Without the ability to produce telomerase, the telomeres of somatic cells grow shorter with each replication, until the cells die.

As you mature into an adult your body is no longer able to build new proteins. Protein synthesis declines by more than half. As the balance shifts toward the forces of decay, we age faster. The pace of telomere shortening picks up. Old age underlies most diseases, but we do not have the "magic bullet" to indefinitely extend human life. We believe that it will be available in the next twenty years. It will be a drug therapy that turns on the telomerase gene in healthy somatic cells. All of the current theories of aging are related to accelerated telomere loss and damage. We are quite positive that the solution to aging lies in telomere biology.

The Major Aging Factors

The three major aging factors are oxidation, inflammation, and glycation. They wreak havoc in our bodies. How to minimize the impact of these aging factors is the purpose of this book.

Oxidation- free radicals are unstable molecules that have a single unpaired electron. They are infectious. As you age free radicals damage to your DNA increases. Supplement and nutrition which will be discussed later can minimize the damage to your telomeres.

Inflammation- Arthritis and Asthma are inflammatory diseases. Cardiologists thought heart disease was caused by cholesterol. Now we know that inflammation is the culprit. Chronic inflammation causes Alzheimer's disease. Inflammation plays a role in all non-genetic disease. It causes telomeres to shorten at a faster rate.

Glycation- Sugar is sabotaging your health and making you age faster. Carbohydrates convert to sugar and the glycation process begins. The sugar molecules attach themselves to proteins and fats. The result is called cross-linkages. The molecules involved become damaged, the cell membranes become less elastic, and some cells die.

The Lucrative Side of Longevity

Instead of longevity, national companies will flourish. If you make lifestyle changes, follow the fitness and nutritional guides, you should be able to extend your life span and activate the telomere gene. Your telomeres will grow, and as you become chronologically older, you will become biologically younger.

Supplements
Stage one

Omega 3 fish oil   6 grams (6,000 mg)
(DHA and EPA)   3,000 twice a day
Acetyl-L-Carnitine   2,000 mg. 1,000 in the morning and 1,000 in the evening
Extracts containing Anthocyanins 700 to 2,100   700 with each meal
N-Acetyl Cysteine   1,200 mg   600 in the morning and 600 in the evening
A super multivitamin

Stage two

CoQ10   200 to 600 mg
L-Carnosine   1,000 to 5,000 mg.
Phosphitidylserine   100-800 mg.
Alpha-Lipoic acid   50-300 mg.
Vitamin D   2,000- 10,000 mg.

TA-65 costs $8,000 a year. A lower dose half as much and a quarter dose costs $2,200 a year (geared to younger people)

The Fitness Plan

Study after study reinforces the fact that exercise is important. Lack of exercise may speed up the time of your death. Exercise is linked to lower rates of cancer. Before you start any exercise program, check with your primary care physician. Shorter and faster exercise is better than long and repetitive exercise

Each time you exercise your muscles get stronger, blood flows to your brain, and the immune system is invigorated. The programs in the immortality edge are skewed toward high-intensity, non-cardio kinds of training. A recent Harvard Study of Boston marathon runners found that nearly all of them suffer some heart damage. It is common knowledge that football players and boxers develop long-term brain damage (Mohammed Ali) and severe arthritis.

YOUNGER BRAIN, SHARPER MIND
ERIC R. BRAVERMAN, M.D.

Overall good health cannot occur without a healthy brain. When I was in medical school science was absolutely certain that brain cells cannot be replaced. That assumption has been proven to be entirely false. Today, we know that the brain can repair itself and adapt to change.

Synopsis

We do this by a process of neurogenesis- the growth of new brain cells. The brain controls all aspects of your health. We are born with 100 billion brain neurons. Every neuron has a nucleus (head) arms (called dendrites), and legs (called axons). Each neuron has 10,000 axons and dendrites which connect to each other to create your body's electrical network. The space between neurons is called the synapse. Each of us has 100 trillion synapses.

Brain Chemistry

- Dopamine determines voltage.
- Acetylcholine determines your brain's processing speed.
- GABA (Gamma-aminobutyric acid) determines your electrical balance. It affects your stability. It is the brain's natural valium.
- Serotonin provides healing, nourishing, satisfied feeling to the brain and the body.

The Anatomy of the Brain

The brain is divided into three parts: The cerebrum, the brain stem, and the cerebellum. The cerebrum is divided into two hemispheres. These hemispheres have identical areas that are called lobes. Each hemisphere is divided into four lobes, and the cerebrum houses three. All of these lobes in conjunction with the brain stem control the automatic processes, such as breathing, digesting, and manage all our other internal systems. Each lobe also directs mental functions, how we think, reason, create, and remember.

The Cerebrum

The largest part of the brain, the cerebrum, comprises both the right and the left hemispheres of the brain, each of which contains four pairs of lobes. Each pair is dominated by one of the four primary chemical families. They ultimately control your thinking, personality, and health..

Frontal lobes- controls you brain's voltage

Parietal lobes- located just above the ears. Directs the brain's ability to store memory and language

Occipital lobes- are found at the rear of the brain- they control vision

The Corpus Callosum- is the internet of the brain. It's the place where every brain cell has to connect so that the brain and the body work as a whole. It is the electrical network that allows the two sides of the brain to consolidate their tasks.

The Brain Stem

The brain stem is the point where electricity is transferred between the brain and the body.

The Cerebellum

It is located just below and behind the brain. The cerebellum controls balance and arm and leg coordination.

Cerebrospinal Fluid

I call cerebrospinal fluid the ocean of life. New neurons are created and travel in the fluid and eventually settle in their particular locations. Hydration is essential. Without water the brain would shrink, harden, and eventually die.

The Braverman Protocol

Step one--Early Testing:

A full health checkup is the only way to start an effective early prevention program. There are complex and accurate imaging techniques as well as my own tests and quizzes that can help determine whether you have a brain chemical imbalance

Step two--Smart Lifestyle Changes:

• Treat yourself to a massage- it relieves stress, controls blood pressure, and manages depression and pain
• Practice quiet meditation- meditation allows the brain to slow down and rebalance.

Diet and Nutrition

The following foods should be in your diet. They stimulate leptin production which helps you maintain your ideal weight. Apples, berries, broccoli, carrots, coconut oil, cruciferous vegetables, eggs, flaxseed oil, leafy greens, lean meats, low fat yogurt, olive oil, pears, plums, poultry, salmon and other fatty fish, spinach, and unsalted almonds.

10 Rules for a Younger, Smarter You

• Add spice to every meal
• The right caffeine improves cognition
• Eat yogurt every day
• Lean protein creates the most brain power

- Kick the sugar habit
- Choose fiber to cleanse your body
- Drink water
- Eat fruits and vegetables
- Eat high quality produce
- Include three food groups-carbs, protein, and fats

Nutrients That Make you Smarter

Amino acids, choline, chromium, essential fatty acids, folic acids, iron, magnesium, riboflavin (B-2), selenium, sodium, thiamine (B-1), vitamin E, and zinc

Step three--Exercises That Boost Your Brain

Phase 1.   Stretching, walking for about 15 minutes a   day
Phase 2.   Yoga, pilates, and low-intensive aerobics
Phase 3.   Running, speed walking, swimming, tennis, and basketball
Phase 4.   Weightlifting to strengthen muscles and bones
Phase5.   Cross-training- the highest level of exercise for peak performance

Step Four--Natural hormones Jump-Start Quick Training

When hormone output is high, you feel healthy, smart, and young. As you get older, your organs slow down their particular hormone production. As each organ begins to fail, it affects every part of your health, including your cognition

I have been using more than 20 bio-identical hormones supplements for more than two decades. My program makes it possible for you to get sharper as you grow older. Hormone replacement won't bulk you up or cause cancer, or any other misguided rumors you might have heard. In fact, many of the supplements I prescribe are so gentle that they are sold over-the-counter.

Bio-identical hormones are created at compounding pharmacies, not by the big pharmaceutical companies. They are often made from plant sources as opposed to compounds made from human cadavers or horse urine that have been directly implicated in cancers and disease.

18 Hormones you Need to Know

- Aldosterone
- DHEA
- DHEA-sulfate
- Erythroprotein (EPO)
- Estrogen
- Estradiol
- Estriol
- Estrone
- Human Growth Hormone (HGH)
- Increlex (insulin-like growth factor (IGF)
- Melatonin
- Parathyroid hormone (PTH)
- Pregnenolone
- Progesterone
- Testosterone
- Thyroid- T3 and T4
- Vasopressin
- Vitamin D

Step Five--Brain-Balancing Medications

Medications that enhance acetylcholine production will improve your memory

The GABA medications will relieve anxiety

Dopamine medications will enhance your attention

And lastly, serotonin medications treat depression and sleep issues

"It has been said that we only use 10 percent of our brain's power. Now let's see what we can do with the other 90 percent of our brain. The ability to learn from the past to shape a better future will lead to greater character in the same way that literacy over the past 2,000 years has led to greater intelligence.

By biggest hope is that you can imagine a world of peace, tolerance, and intelligence, and harness your better brain to help create it.

CANCER'S CAUSE, CANCER'S CURE
MORTON WALKER, D.P.M.

Cancer is a dread disease that has haunted us and killed our loved ones. In the 1960s, Richard Nixon declared war on cancer. It is a war we have lost. The large pharmaceutical companies which make billions from the cancer business have been accused of not really searching for a cure. We are faced with the dilemma of record deaths which have recently exceeded the numbers of cardiovascular deaths. Cancer is number one.

Ten years ago I retired from active participation in medical journalism. But cancer took my wife, my mother, my sister, and my fiancée. I had to uncover which alternatives really worked and let the world know about it.

I found a humble scientist who worked at the Pasteur Institute in Paris, who was a genius in discovering how cancer works in the DNA of our cells. This book presents the work of a French biochemist, Mirko Beljanski, Ph.D. He died in October, 1998. He was a Yugoslavian born French citizen. He was forced out of the Pasteur Institute, but his work didn't stop. For two more decades of independent research Beljanski struggled to find the answer to cancer. He didn't want to see people die and he knew he could do something about it. His findings deserve the highest accolades anyone can give another human.

Beljanski had a holistic orientation. He believed in alternative forms of healing. His career spanned forty-five years. He discovered what happens to a cell at the molecular level, thereby discovering the DNA of cancer. Once he understood how a cell becomes cancerous, he was able to find and perfect the application of anticancer botanical approaches which can handle most cancers.

As a medical journalist, I have dedicated my life to bringing important discoveries in holistic medicine to the public. This is my 92nd book and I believe it is my most momentous. I came out of retirement because I believe that Beljanski's discoveries could save millions of lives.

In the spring of 2003, I learned about Mirko Beljanski at an ACAM (American College of Advancement in Medicine) conference. ACAM has 2,500 holistic medical practitioners. Dr. Michael Schacter kept my beautiful wife Joan healthy and thriving for thirteen years. He invited me to the ACAM conference. My respect for Dr. Schacter is immense. His talk on cancer and Beljanski's concepts were worthwhile to hear. I was introduced to Beljanski's wife and daughter, and they invited me to attend a picnic in Charente, France in September, 2007 conducted by CIRIS (Centre D'enformation de Recherchement D'enformation Scientifiques). CIRIS is an organization whose membership is between 3,400 and 5,000 French men and women, all of whom had been saved from cancer or AIDS by application of Beljanski's discoveries.

I was astonished by what I found and I believed that I had come across knowledge about the most viable weapons to date to fight cancer. I bought Beljanski's products for my sister. She was suffering from lung cancer and was dealing with radiation and chemotherapy. She longed for death and she entered a hospice to anticipate the end of her life.

My sister Phyllis benefitted from Beljanski's formulas. Her oncologist took credit for her improvement. I didn't tell him about the herbals Phyllis was taking. When the nurses and aides noticed the improvement from the herbals they took them away. I was outraged when I discovered that the hospice requires that nothing be done for the dying patient but to allow him or her to ease their way into the next life. My sister quickly succumbed to the lung cancer. I believe she would still be alive if she continued to take Beljanski's botanicals. I vowed at her death that I would make sure the world knew about this amazing man and his anti-cancer botanicals.

Before my sister died I met an attractive woman. I had been a widower for three years. We toured nine cities in Spain. We planned to be married in early 2005. My fiancée was admitted to Massachusetts General Hospital with pancreatic cancer. Her doctors were recommending radiation, chemotherapy, and surgery. They appeared "like used-car salesmen and I was astonished at how they discussed the side effects of their treatments.

"No side effects."

I knew they were lying. I tried to convince her to check into a program of a friend, a holistic oncologist named Nicholas J. Gonzalez, M.D. of New York City. He was ready to take her into his program. The Gonzalez patient investigation was funded by the U.S. Government as a research program using enzymes from New Zealand lambs. My fiancée refused Dr. Gonzalez's offer.

I encouraged her to take Dr Beljanski's botanicals. He two sons did not understand how and why they worked. They flushed Beljanski's herbals down the toilet. They thought holistic theories were outright quackery. They insisted that I leave Massachusetts altogether. They said, "get out of my mother's life! Go home to Connecticut." She died two months after her sons sent me away.

The traditional treatment for cancer is well known. Radiation and chemotherapy are designed to kill cancer cells. The problem is that the treatment often kills the patient. The treatment kills all cells. In the medical journal Oncology three eminent cardiologists stated that the benefit of cytotoxic chemotherapy has been overestimated for cancers of the esophagus, stomach, rectum, and brain.

Beljanski's botanicals target the cancer cells and destroy them. They also leave the healthy cells undamaged. This is a highly important subject- vital for saving lives. Beljanski's approach is scientifically based, tested, and proven both in the laboratory and in human clinical trials. We must unite and work together to win this war on cancer if we use the discoveries of Dr. Mirko Beljanski.

Before exploring the life of Mirko Beljanski it is important to hear the amazing story of a journalist, M. De Perlier, who was asked to write an expose of a maverick microbiologist who was affecting the sale of drugs with his botanicals. He is a quack and must be stopped. M. De Perlier interviewed many people who were taking Beljanski's herbal preparations, but they all had good things to say about them. It was also soon discovered that Francois Mitterand was using Beljanski's supplements to cure his prostate cancer. Mitterand was France's president. Not only was M. De perlier not able to write an expose of Beljanski, but his editor wanted him to write an article praising the microbiologist who was extending the life of France's president.

Suddenly, in an ironic twist of fate, de Perlier was diagnosed with colorectal cancer, and his oncologist told him that he had only three months to live. De Perlier was settling his affairs in preparations for dying when he received a package of botanicals from a friend who was cured of cancer by Beljanski after taking the supplements. De Perlier was miraculously cured and was alive and well and able to tell me his fantastic story of how he was saved by Mirko Beljanski's preparations.

Mirko Beljanski was born in 1923, in rural Serbia, which was part of Yugoslavia, As a youth he had a positive attitude and wanted to do things with his life. Mirko was not interested in politics, but he did enlist with the partisans during the war. But by a stroke of good luck he received a fellowship to study in Paris. He attended the Sorbonne and intended to obtain a doctorate in science. He joined the Pasteur Institute and worked in a laboratory in the department of cellular biology. He acquired his doctorate in 1951 in molecular biology. He was drawn to the science of microbiology. He married Monique Lucas, a beautiful French girl.

Initially Beljanski worked under professor Macheboeuf. In 1952, Mirko's beloved mentor died suddenly. Pasteur's board named Jacques Monod, Ph.D. as a successor. That created a problem. Mirko and Monod did not like each other at all. Jacques Monod craved praise. He was ego driven. Mirko Beljanski did not feed Monod's ego. They were two strong egos that were not made for cooperation.

Beljanski was able to spend two years at N.Y.U. in New York, but Monique presented Mirko with two children, a boy and a girl, and Beljanski wanted to have their children grow up in France. Monod was a brilliant man and in 1965 he shared the Nobel Prize with two other researchers for their work concerning the control of the genetic expression in DNA (the part of the DNA that has to do with the pattern of physical characteristics of the human body). In spite of the clash of personalities, Beljanski continued to work at the Pasteur Institute for almost twenty-five years under Monod.

There are two acids in the nucleus of a cell-DNA (Deoxynucleic acid and RNA (Ribonucleic acid). Cancer is a disease where the body's cells become abnormal and continue to divide indefinitely. Healthy cells are pre-programmed to die. This is called apoptosis. The rogue cells multiply forming a tumor. Eventually, the cancerous cells metastasize and spread to other parts of the body. There are over one hundred types of cancer and not all cancer cells behave the same.

In 1962, Watson and Crick and Wilkins were awarded the Nobel Prize for discovering that the long strands of DNA (genetic material) were contained in a double helix (two spirals that are twisted together). The DNA contains all the information needed to make and control every cell. DNA has two main functions: genetic and self-replicating the pairing of the genes. They govern all of your physical appearance –eye color, hair color, height, weight, and sex. Self-replication is crucial for the durability of the species. Because that is how cells produce more cells which allow life to continue, the structure of the DNA molecule fascinated Beljanski. He concluded in the late 1980s that cancerous behaviour is cause by structural corruption of the DNA. The idea was revolutionary because since the 1950s the scientific world was wedded to the idea that the cause of cancer was gene mutation.

Oncologists have yet to accept Beljanski's cancer-causation finding (DNA destabilization). Therefore the cause of cancer continues to elude them. Dr. Mirko Beljanski deserves but has never been awarded the Nobel Prize for tracing the cause of environmental cancer at its core, in the DNA of the cell. Perhaps history will somehow rectify this mistake.

Cancer is a battlefield whose opposing forces have fought to use their protocols to make many billions of dollars. About fifteen hundred people die of cancer every day. The orthodoxy uses chemotherapy, radiation, and surgery. Billions are spent in research. Cancer rates keep growing which proves that the war on cancer has been lost. Massive amounts of money are involved in the sale of both "natural cures" And pharmaceutical drugs.

One of Beljanski's botanicals is a plant named Pao Perera that is derived from the powdered bark of a Brazilian rainforest tree. His team found that the bark of the Pao Perera induced apoptosis. This gets the cancer cell to kill itself. For over thirty years two botanicals- Pao Perera and Raowolfia Vomitoria have been used successfully to manage cancer and viral pathologies throughout Europe. They remain almost unknown in the United States because of the monopolistic practices of America's Big Pharma.

These two alkaloid extracts have saved so many people in Europe from dying of malignant tumors. I have made it my mission to help the American medical consumer become aware of the possibilities they offer. I receive no pay from the Beljanski foundation. I use these herbs myself and pay for them as does any consumer or health professional.

From colon cancer to liver, skin, ovary, pancreatic, prostate, and thyroid cancers, Pao Perera showed remarkably high in vitro kill rates for all these cancer cells- all in the 80 to 90 percent range. Dr. Mirko Beljanski passed away in October, 1998.

Dr. Aaron Katz learned about Beljanski's botanicals through Dr. Michael Schacter. He met Monique and Sylvie and they gave him some peer-reviewed scientific articles about Mirko's projects. Dr. Katz is the director of Columbia University's Center for Holistic Urology. (He is now at Winthrop Hospital in Long Island). Columbia's research team tested both botanicals in vitro again and again. The results were published in 2009 and written up in "Integrative Medicine." We now know that the two extracts lowered PSAs. The Columbia studies lend a great deal of scientific credence to the work of Beljanski's team in France.

Dr. Samuel Epstein, M.D. in his 1998 book, "The Politics of Cancer Revealed," states, "The National Cancer Institute and the American Cancer Society have misled and confused the public and congress by repeated false claims and these are claims made to create public and congressional support for massive increases in budgetary appropriations. Cancer is a major cause of misery and death. To say that cancer is incurable is a myth perpetrated by the greedy people who want to keep the cancer machine alive. Dr. Mirko Beljanski and his dedicated team of researchers have given us a way to treat and prevent cancer from occurring in the first place. We need to fight to bring to the forefront cancer therapies that are proving themselves scientifically to be more effective than the current conventional treatments. We in the United States need to work together if we want to win the battle against cancer.

A Lasting Legacy

Dr. Mirko Beljanski died on October 28, 1998. He succumbed to acute myeloid leukemia, a cancer that he may have treated with his botanicals, if he had access to them. The French government and pharmaceutical industry combined to make life miserable for this hero researcher who, worked against all odds for a cure for the most dreaded disease in modern history.

French Special Forces raided Beljanski's lab. Helicopters were overhead, German shepherd dogs lunging at the end of their leashes, and a swat-like team with guns drawn invaded Beljanski's lab, forced open locked closets, confiscated computers and notebooks, removed all nutrients and medicines, and herded together rabbits, guinea pigs, and mice.

A man's life's work was destroyed without due process of law. Shortly after, Beljanski was roused from his bed and arrested and held in jail for 24 hours.

In a cruel irony, Dr. Mirko Beljanski died of the same illness he had fought against for 45 years. At 74, he might have saved himself from dying if he had access to his own supplements. This Greek tragedy was played out and Dr. Beljanski was hounded by jealous associates, competitive drug executives, and zealous bureaucrats who prevented him from his life-saving discoveries to the world.

THE HEALING CELL
ROBIN SMITH, M.D., MSGR. TOMASZ,
AND MAX GOMEZ, PH.D.

This is a book about improvements and cures using of stem cell treatments. It is also about the ethical science behind these successes. People have received significant benefits from medical investigation into stem cell therapies.

You'll meet the people who are waiting desperately for cures, and who've lost precious time during their wait. This science has been decades in the making, that is now paying off with treatments that repair damaged hearts, restoring sight, killing cancer, curing diabetes, and stopping the degenerative diseases such as Alzheimer's, multiple sclerosis, and Lou Gehrig's Disease (ALS).

These treatments aren't science fiction. They are rather the authors' vision of the future. These therapies are used in hospitals and are moving through promising clinical trials.

The stem cell landscape is populated by smart, motivated, and ethical scientists, but also by hucksters, peddlers, and snake oil salesmen.

This book will present the facts, and you can draw your own conclusions. Stem cells promise to revolutionize the world of tomorrow. Doctors have already used stem cells to grow new vessels, build liver tissue, insulin secreting cells of the pancreas, and cells that support a beating heart.

It is premature to claim that stem cells cure any disease, but soon they actually might—and in some cases they already have.

The use of adult stem cells allows researchers to use a patient's own cells . They are called "autologous cells." They sidestep the difficulty of rejection. This book is about life and death. It details the science and the successes of adult stem cell therapies. These successes are many and they are powerful. They can extend the lives of billions of people around the world. These stem cell therapies may change your life.

Stem cells are here. They are no longer a vague dream about future therapies. Autologous stem cells (adult) are showing great promise in a variety of areas. There are 4,700 studies underway at this moment. We will be hearing exciting results in the coming months and years.

The stem cell industry has been held back by the controversy surrounding the ethics of using embryonic stem cells. Adult stem cells have shown their efficacy in the treatment of many diseases, and they are approved for use in many countries around the world where there are less regulations than in the United States.

This book by Robin Smith, Max Gomez, and Msgr Tomasz spotlights the progress made in organ creation, cardiovascular, cancer, arthritis, and psychiatric diseases.

I predict that within a decade, stem cells will be a flourishing industry saving millions of lives.

Synopsis

Organ Regeneration

Katherine Manner's spinal cord had a hole, and the sheath that holds the spinal cord failed to close. When she was born she had spina bifida. It affects 1,500 babies every year. Katherine's cerebrospinal fluid wasn't circulating properly. This condition produced hydrocephaly or water on the brain. In 1900, life expectancy for her would be 21.

Surgeons insert a shunt to drain excess fluid. As she learned to walk, she was fitted with arm-brace crutches that she would use for the rest of her life.

Katherine's bladder lost the ability to hold liquid. Her family worried about renal failure. Her best option was a kidney transplant, but more than 100,000 people are waiting for a kidney. Her damaged bladder would eventually destroy it as well.

Katherine's family enrolled her in a clinical trial at Boston Children's Hospital in partnership with Dr. Anthony Atala at Wake Forest's Institute for Regenerative Medicine.

Instead of waiting for a donated bladder, Katherine would grow a replacement. Dr. Atala used 10,000 stem cells from her bladder and grew them to 1.5 billion cells in a couple of weeks. He had a perfect replacement in a dish in his lab at WakeFforest. It was Katherine's own body because it was built from her own cells. Surgeons removed her dying organ and replaced it with the new one. She didn't have to wear a diaper. Dialysis—gone! A lifetime of incontinence—gone!. The Junior Prom? Six other cases of spina bifida benefitted from the same clinical trial.

Body parts being explored for stem cell regeneration at Wake Forest include blood vessels, bone, cartilage, cornea, ear, heart, heart valves, nerves, ovaries, pancreas, prostate, muscle, and uterus.

Some are ready for installation, others will be soon. Today medical science is reaching levels of knowledge that only science fiction writers could dream up. Tomorrow it will be common to replace a malfunctioning organ.

Heart and Vascular Disease

Karen Parcher had 4 heart attacks. Her family had a history of early death from heart attacks. All the males for three generations died before 50. She enrolled in a clinical study- 20 would have stem cells injected into their hearts and 10 would receive a placebo.

Bone marrow had worked with mice, and now it was being tried with humans. Karen would learn on her six month's visit if she had been injected with stem cells or a placebo. She received stem cells. Stem cells can encourage donated tissue to grow, repairing hearts.

The injection of stem cells into Karen's heart made a dramatic difference in her life and allowed her to resume her regular activity in her catering business.

"Now I can walk three blocks without getting winded. It's a miracle. I feel blessed."

Today Attorcyte, a subsidiary of Neostem, is developing a therapy that can harvest CD 34+ cells without the use of Neupogen, which dumbs down the ability of stem cells to naturally migrate to damaged areas. Therefore, stem cells can be injected into the artery that was blocked, where they can navigate to the areas in need of repair.

The 31 person Amorcyte (AMR 001) trial showed that patients who were being treated with 10 million of their own stem cells had an increase of oxygenated blood through blood vessel formation feeding the damaged and surrounding heart muscle than did patients with fewer or no stem cells. The FDA has approved a 160 person study –Phase II clinical trial using AMR 001.

With clinical trials run by Harvard, Emory, the Mayo Clinic, the University of Pittsburgh, and the Texas Heart Institute, and reports published in such top scientific journals as Nature, NEJM, and Circulation, the clinical journal of the AHA. The application of adult stem cells harvested from a patient's blood, and restored to their heart is one case in which stem cell treatments are more than a futurist's pipe dream-they're a pragmatist's go to treatment.

In 2004, the Lancet said, "intracoronary transfer of autologous bone-marrow cells promotes improvement of left-ventricular systolic function in patients after acute myocardial infarction."

Burns

There now exists a spray gun that can coat ulcers and burns with a fine layer of stem cells. It heals severe burns and other skin defects in days. The skin is the body's biggest organ. Dr. Vincent Falanga, at the Boston University School of Medicine is working on a fibrin and stem cell mixture that can be applied in three treatments to a burn to get closure. The U.S. Department of Defense has funded Neostem research to accelerate this approach to rapid wound healing.

This will make a great difference for the over one million fire fighters in the United States. In 2010, more than 3,000 fire fighters suffered burns. Imagine how valuable this treatment can be for fire fighters or soldiers injured in combat..

In 2002, a suicide bomber in Bali exploded a 2,250 pound van-bomb. More than 500 people were burned. Twenty-eight victims were flown to Perth. There wasn't enough skin to perform grafts from their bodies. Instead, Dr. Fiona Wood, head of the Royal Perth Hospital burn unit reached for her device, a spray-skin gun she had spent years in developing. She mobilized the stem cells with nutrients and growth factors, and sprayed the cell-rich cocktail onto the red and blistered burn areas.

The stem cells quickly got to work generating new tissue. In less than a week, with this spray-gun, the skin had healed. Many of these horribly burned patients walked out of the hospital, with practically reduced scarring.

Gregori Venadich, one of the patients, was quoted as saying, "It feels fantastic; words can't describe it." It was what he called, "divine intervention," escaping from the burning rubble and Dr. Wood's stem cell treatments.

In 2009, Wood's Recell technology, which had previously been approved for use in Canada, Mexico, Europe, and many other countries is now in clinical trials in the United States.

Brain Trauma and Stroke

The Memorial Hermann Hospital (where Gabrielle Gifford recovered after being shot in the head) was enrolling patients in an early clinical trial that involved using patients' mesenchymal stem cells, and injecting them into damaged areas of the brain. Jackson Dwyer was in a car crash in Texas and he was rushed to the hospital. He had a massive concussion and a stroke.

Jackson's parents signed the forms and the results were dramatic. Eight days later, he walked out of the hospital with no apparent brain damage. He played baseball and made the honor roll that year. His father said, "We did feel incredibly lucky that not only can we hug him, but he can hug us back." Almost all the kids in the University of Texas study performed at Memorial Hermann benefitted from the procedure.

Gary Steinberg at the California Institute for Regenerative Medicine (CIRM) recently opened enrollment in a Phase 1 "safety" trial using MSCs (bone-marrow derived) mesenchymal stem cells, which surgeons will implant in patients who have had a stroke 6 months and a year ago.

Steinberg said, "I believe that stem cell transplantation for stroke holds great promise. Over the next two decades we will see remarkable advances."

In the clinical trials with stem cells for brain conditions, stroke, and cerebral palsy, there are signs of initial promise. There are legitimate success stories. There is hope. But there is a long road ahead. Even when Jackson Dwyer's stroke could be considered a cure, we are tipping from theory to practice. The future is looking better all the time.

Alzheimer's, Parkinson's,
and Other Neurodegenerative Diseases

Alois Alzheimer described the disease in 1906 (after more than 100 years and 750 clinical trials) we still aren't exactly sure what causes it. One feature of the disease is the loss of connections between the neurons called synapses. There are drugs that help, but they don't cure the condition. Plaque in an Alzheimer's brain is a protein fragment called beta amyloid. These fragments accumulate and form hard and insoluble plaques.

No matter what the cause. the disease marches on. Short-term memory loss is followed by a steeper cognitive decline, and eventually by the shutdown of bodily functions and death. Five percent of the U.S. population is affected by age 65, and 25 percent by age 85 or older. 100 million people worldwide, one in every 85 people will show symptoms of Alzheimer's by 2050 according to the United Nations Department of Economic and Social Affairs.

Frank La Ferla, Ph.D. was a skeptic. He had little hope that stem cells could reverse the course of Alzheimer's. He is the director of the Institute for Memory Impairments and Neurological Disorders at the University of California, Irvine (UCI MIND).

The hippocampus is the area in the human brain for coding new memories. It is one of the areas in the adult brain that continues to make use of its stem cells throughout your life. The hippocampus is always growing new neurons, but in Alzheimer's the growth doesn't match the rate of neuron death.

La Ferla injected rats hippocampus neuron stem cells. It had no effect on the tangles or plaque, but the number of synapses bloomed. La Ferla said, "That was very interesting, because the best correlation of cognitive decline (due to Alzheimer's disease) is not plaques but the decrease of synapses. Essentially the cells were producing fertilizer for the brain," La Ferla said.

Now we know stem cells don't need to replace neurons by implanting stem cells into brains, there is almost a doubling of synaptic density."

This is stem cell treatment at its most promising. For sufferers of Alzheimer's , Huntington's, Batten, and Parkinson's diseases, stem cell treatments offer more than hope in a few preliminary trials, they offer good years of life, perhaps soon they'll offer a cure.

Cancer

Leukemia is a story about blood. Patients with reduced platelets bleed uncontrollably. Patients without white blood cells are prone to infections. Patients whose red blood cells have been squeezed become anemic. Leukemia cells become the blood system's dominant life-form, and without treatment it is universally fatal.

Every four minutes one person in the U.S. is diagnosed with blood cancer, and every ten minutes someone in the U.S. dies from blood cancer. This represents nearly 145 people each day or more than six people every hour. The Leukemia and Lymphoma Society estimates that there are 275,000 with leukemia in the U.S., and more than 44,000 new cases will be diagnosed in 2011. According to the American Cancer Society global cancer cases could increase to 21.4 million by 2010.

The problem with leukemia is that you can't remove a tumor, you are limited to chemotherapy and radiation. The hope is that the treatment would kill the leukemia before it kills the patient. In 1968, doctors at the University of Minnesota performed the first successful bone-marrow transplant. They didn't know it, but they were using stem cells therapy.

The bone-marrow produces the components of your blood system including the red blood cells that carry oxygen and the white blood cells that keep your body clear of disease and infection. The factories within the bone-marrow that create blood are stem cells. Since 1968, doctors around the world have refined the technique of bone-marrow transplantation to point the way to health for 20 to 75 percent of patients with leukemia.

For Ellie Kranzyk it was too late. She had Glioblastoma, a brain cancer. Her doctors told her that there was nothing that they could do. She died on Christmas Eve 2010.

Stem cells are today's engine of repair, and they know where repair is needed. That's where they go. Doctors at the city of Hope Hospital in Duarte, California injected Ellie's brain with 10 million of her own neural cells, which migrated to the tumor site and attached themselves to cancerous cells.

Before injecting these neural stem cells, doctors had genetically engineered them to carry a special package, the ability to make a benign protein. Then the patient takes a pill which is also a benign little chemical that easily crosses the blood-brain barrier. Now, crossing independently, the neural stem cells and the pill have smuggled two pieces of a powerful weapon into the brain. When the pill has the protein made by the neural stem cells, the two combine to form a powerful poison. This powerful poison kills only the cancer cells.

Ellie had taken the first step on the moon. After her treatment the therapy went into a clinical trial with 16 patients newly diagnosed with Glioblastoma. The results were miraculous. At the time of this writing 3 of the 16 were free of the disease. 80 percent of the patients were still alive.

It is too soon to tell whether this treatment is a cure or a temporary fix. But all 16 of these early patients were given years of life.

On January 19, 2011, the biotechnology companies Neostem and ImmunoCellular teamed up to launch a Phase II study of this therapy in nine clinics around the country. They hope to expand this trial to twenty or more clinics and to treat 200 patients.

Arthritis

CNN estimates that more than 500,000 Americans have knee replacement surgery. The NIH estimates that in 2003 300,000 knee replacement operations were performed.

Sylvia Bell was 72 years old, and she was told she needed a double-knee replacement. Sylvia decided to try an experimental stem cell therapy. Dr. Christopher J. Centeno had performed the procedure on more than 200 patients since 2009. He harvests mesenchymal stem cells from a patient's hip, expands the cells in the lab, and then injects them into the patient's arthritic joints. It is an outpatient therapyafter which patients walk out of the clinic with a knee brace.

Dr. Centeno states, Because the stem cells come from your own body there is little chance of infection or rejection." Two-thirds of Centeno's patients received greater than 50% relief, and 40% reported more than 75% relief one to two years afterward. The treatment is less expensive than knee surgery. Because the procedure isn't FDA approved and insurance doesn't cover it, some patients travel to the Cayman Islands for treatment.

Sylvia Bell claims, "Almost from the moment I got up from the table, I was able to throw away my cane." Now I am biking and hiking like a thirty –year old.

Summary

The Information in Cellular M Society (ICMS) represents 1,000 physicians, researchers, and patients from over 35 countries on 5 continents. It offers links to the largest research on stem cells . the research section of the ICMS points to the latest published articles for many of the conditions described in this book

But despite the regulation of clinical best practices and the attempt to reign in unfounded claims of miracle cures , it's also a bit unclear where the ICMS draws the line between (nearly proven) effective treatments such as the Centeno & Schultz Clinic offering and extremely unproven stem cell treatments for conditions like cerebral palsy, epilepsy, autism, spinal cord injury, and Lou Gehrig's disease.

Certification of stem cell clinics can help ensure conformity to safety. This doesn't imply that the treatments of every certified clinic are effective. It's an industry in which it is almost impossible to pin down what works and what doesn't yet work- and there is an ever moving force that divides real treatments from shams.

Here is this book's best attempt at a hard and fast rule; improvement in musculoskeletal injuries and other conditions can come from clinics, but "miracle" cures almost exclusively come from U.S. FDA-approved treatments and clinical trials described previously.

There are exceptions to this rule, but your best chance for success lies along the same path as the people in this book who pursued FDA-approved trials and treatments.

When scientific inquiry is compiled with high ethical values, it serves society best of all. This applies especially for adult stem cell research, which holds such tremendous promise to treat illness and alleviate suffering around the world.

For reliable investigation on current developments in adult stem cell research, as well as our unique partnership with the Vatican, to explore the cultural, ethical, and human implications of adult stem cell use, please visit our website at the stem for life foundation.

SUPERNUTRITION
RICHARD A. PASSWATER, P.HD.

Supernutrition is a program for good health based on a diet of good foods supplemented by vitamins and minerals. It is an idea that has come just in time for millions of Americans who suffer diseases each year that supernutrition can prevent. Extensive research has proven that fact. The author believes that his program can prevent 500,000 to 1,000,000 premature deaths each year. In addition to explaining the benefits of supernutrition, Passwater makes a point of criticizing the myths fostered by the FDA, the AMA, the USDA, and the food industry.

Synopsis

A shocking confirmation of our nutritional status was articulated by Jean M. President of Tufts University. As chairman of the White house Conference on food, Nutrition, and health, he reported, "In almost thirty nations, life expectancies for adult males since 1950 have been greater than they were in the United States." Moreover, 10% of us are anemic, 25% are overweight, and more than half the population doesn't eat well enough to be half-alive. The same is true in England.

Food rapidly loses its nutrients in cooking, freezing, and canning. The loss in nutrition through processing foods is as follows: fresh foods lose 56% of their nutrients during cooking, frozen foods lose 25% in scalding, 19% in freezing, 15% in thawing, and 24% in recooking, for a total of 83% loss; canned foods lose 30% in scalding, 25% in sterilization, 27% in liquor diffusion, and 12% in reheating, for a total of 94%.

A balanced diet should consist of something every day from each of the following 7 groups:

- Green and yellow vegetables
- Citrus fruit and tomatoes
- Potatoes, rice, and fruits
- Milk and milk products
- Meat, poultry, fish, and eggs
- Bread, flour, and cereals
- Butter

Many people think that physicians are experts in nutrition. The truth is that very few are tasught to prevent illness; they instead devote most of their time in medical school in learning about drugs, and their complications. They are trained to diagnose illness, administer drugs, and perform surgical procedures. Most physicians are not experts on dietary cholesterol, sub-clinical scurvy, and long-term dietary studies. Medical schools with nutrition departments are rare. Most don't even offer separate courses in the subject. In fact, "not one medical school can honestly say it teaches nutrition seriously. "However, physicians often downgrade the importance of vitamins by making statements such as, "Forget the baloney about vitamins and worry about being fat."

The value of supernutrition is easily demonstrated by vitamin C. Humans and a few other animals cannot manufacture it. We therefore have to get it from the foods we eat or through supplements. The original research on this vitamin was done by Dr. Irwin stone, who spent 10 years writing "The Healing Factor: Vitamin C Against Disease" Dr. Fred Klenner, a North Carolina physician, has been a pioneer in using massive doses of vitamin C to detoxify poisons and cure bacterial infections. Of course, the impact of Linus pauling's book, "Vitamin C and the Common cold" brought the vitamin C story to the attention of the public. Dr. Pauling recommends 1 to 5 grams immediately and every hour until the cold is thwarted. Many studies confirmed Pauling's findings. In Glasgow, Scotland, a test with 90 volunteers gave evidence that those who took vitamin C had 50% fewer colds. Drs. Mary Clegg and Sheila Charleston concluded that no further testing was needed. As far as they were concerned, large doses of vitamin c help prevent the common cold.

Megavitamin therapy is very effective in curing the mentally ill. Dr. Abram Hoffer started in 1952 to use massive doses of niacin (B-3) to treat schizophrenia. Schizophrenia and depression affect 10 million Americans each year. After more than 20 years of success with this megavitamin therapy there are still those who denounce the concept. Psychiatrists refuse to consider seriously the possibility that this method will work. Yet someone in need of psychiatric care should be treated by a scientific psychiatrist. Dual treatment is required. The vitamins used in megavitamin therapy are inexpensive and reduce the need for expensive drugs. Generally speaking, when megavitamin therapy is combined with conventional drug treatment, it is twice as effective as drug treatment alone. Dr. Hoffer has reported a 93% cure rate for patients in combined therapy who are ill for less than 2 years.

Cholesterolphobia has changed the eating habits of the country. Physicans are almost unanimous in their recommendation of diets that restrict foods containing fats and cholesterol. Our intake of polyunsaturated fats are at an all-time high. In spite of that the heart disease rate is reaching epidemic proportions. It Appears that low-cholesterol diets have not done the job. In fact, there is evidence that the unbalanced diet and lack of many nutritious foods such as milk, butter, and eggs have actually contributed to or caused the disease they were designed to prevent.

There are very few foods in our diet that are as complete as eggs and milk. Most doctors fail to realize that egg protein contains trace nutrients such as minerals, B complex vitamins and sulphur and selenium compounds. They also appear not to know that the fat and cholesterol in whole milk is essential for the myelin sheaths of nerve fibers It is true that a certain level of polyunsaturated fats is required for proper nutrition, but there are now good reasons to question the necessity for a low-cholesterol diet. The American diet is now much higher in polyunsaturates and the heart disease rate is still increasing. Another very important fact is that the body produces cholesterol in the liver and other areas; if dietary is reduced, more will be made in the body. Cholesterol has important functions in the body. It is involved with hormones, bile, and important function in the brain. The Madison Avenue advertising blitz, with a strong assist from the medical profession, has obscured the fact that there never has been a proven, scientific relationship between lowering blood cholesterol and preventing heart disease.

If cholesterol doesn't cause heart attacks, then what does? Personality type and smoking have an effect since stress and nicotine consume nutrients. Heart disease is caused by undernutrition coupled with insufficient activity. Supernutrition will improve your chances for good health.

Here is a brief look at the benefits of certain nutrients, in order of importance. Vitamin E is more than just a vitamin. It does the following: prevents the formation of active sites for cholesterol plaques in the arteries; prevents blood clots; influences seum cholesterol levels; improves blood circulation and blood-oxygen efficiency; reduces scar formation in the heart due to infarcts; prohibits the forming of free-radicals and dienes(small unmetabolized particles of food that travel through the bloodstream and can cause damage to cells); offsets the carcinogens produced by chlorine in our water; strengthens heart contractions by increasing energy production and utilization; and helps in lowering triglyceride levels. Selenium is an antioxidant that complements the action of vitamin E. Natural sources are brewer's yeast, eggs, onions, and garlic. Vitamin C is found in low levels in heart attack victims. Smokers and other people under stress have lower levels of vitamin C. Ascorbic acid detoxifies the poisons in the blood and clears cholesterol from artery walls. B complex vitamins are critical in avoiding heart disease. Vitamin B-6 is particularly important because it is used to make lecithin, which dissolves cholesterol.

Supernutrition plays an important role in the prevention of hypoglycaemia, cancer, and aging. It is a startling fact that the life span for people 20 years of age or older has not increased since 1800. For individuals reaching 55 there is only a difference of 2 years between the figures for 1900 and 1968. For 60-year olds there is only a one year difference in life expectancy between the eighteenth century and today. Cellular aging is the real cause of aging. The body consists of 60 trillion cells of various types. These cells age at different rates and there are several underlying causes for their aging. Some of the theories advanced by researchers stress the following contributing reasons for the aging process. (1) free radicals. (2) Damaged DNA. (3) Missynthesized protein. and (4) Cross-linking. To help retard the aging process and promote longevity you should eat a balanced diet , take extra vitamins, especially vitamins E and C , keep trim, be active, avoid smoking, learn to cope with stress , enjoy life.

Extensive research reveals that supernutrition can save 500,000 to 1,000,000 lives each year. Other benefits are as follows:

- Heart disease will be reduced by 60% to 80%
- Cancer will be reduced by 30% to 40%
- Air pollution damage will be reduced by 95%
- The cure rate for schizophrenia will increase by 500%
- Individuals will live better and stay young longer

The facts argue strongly for the adoption of a supernutrition plan to augment a varied diet from the seven food groups. Remember, just because you are taking vitamins, minerals, and food supplements, you cannot neglect your basic diet. Supernutrition can lead each individual to optimum health and happier, disease-resistant life. Orthomolecular nutrition is a therapeutic approach toward disease for those who have succumbed to the country's poor diet and lack of proper nutrition. Passwater's method is a roadmap for preventing illness and prolonging a youthful and vigorous life.

ABOUT THE AUTHOR

Sheldon Zerden has had a successful career in Wall Street as an investment advisor. He is the award-winning author of several books on finance including "Best Books on the Stock Market," the Outstanding Book of the Year Award in Finance by the American Library Association. Margin Power in 1981, The Best of Health: the 100 Best Health Books in 2004. This 3rd edition of The Best of Health: the Best Health Books in the World combines the thoroughness of a stock market strategist and a serious interest in health issues to create a work of lasting importance.

Sheldon Zerden is currently the author of a weekly column called, "Health Beat" that has a large readership in the New York Metropolitan area.

He also writes for the Epoch times, which is the most widely distributed newspaper in the world. It is online and is translated into 18 languages in 35 countries. There are print editions in Australia, New Zealand, and all over the United States and Canada.